Palgrave Studies in Fashion and the Body

Series Editors

Jane Tynan
Department of Art and Culture, History and Antiquity
Faculty of Humanities
Vrije Universiteit Amsterdam
Amsterdam, The Netherlands

Suzannah Biernoff
Department of History of Art
Birkbeck, University of London
London, UK

Palgrave Studies in Fashion and the Body publishes research that offers a fresh perspective on the contemporary and historical significance of fashion as a bodily practice and cultural industry. A vibrant and growing field, fashion studies touches on disciplines such as art, film, history, design, sociology, literature, politics, geography and anthropology. The series explores modes of representation that fashion has taken historically, but also considers the cultural contexts for new directions, at a time when the fashioned body is increasingly implicated in the negotiation of individual and collective identities. By following new circuits of production and consumption the series highlights the range of social and political forces shaping fashion practices today. Looking to recent developments in new materialisms, medical humanities, disability studies, the posthuman, intermediality, decolonial and pluriversal perspectives, books in the series consider fashion's role in anticipating new cultural transformations.

Dawn Woolley • Fiona Johnstone
Ellen Sampson • Paula Chambers
Editors

Wearable Objects and Curative Things

Materialist Approaches to the Intersections of Fashion, Art, Health and Medicine

palgrave
macmillan

Editors
Dawn Woolley
Leeds Arts University
Leeds, UK

Ellen Sampson
School of Design
Northumbria University
Newcastle upon Tyne, UK

Fiona Johnstone
Institute for Medical Humanities
Durham University
Durham, UK

Paula Chambers
Leeds Arts University
Leeds, UK

Palgrave Studies in Fashion and the Body
ISBN 978-3-031-40016-2 ISBN 978-3-031-40017-9 (eBook)
https://doi.org/10.1007/978-3-031-40017-9

This Palgrave Macmillan imprint is published by the registered company Springer Nature Switzerland AG.
The registered company address is: Gewerbestrasse 11, 6330 Cham, Switzerland

Paper in this product is recyclable.

Contents

Notes on Contributors

Lucie Armstrong is a photographer and senior lecturer in BA (Hons) Fashion Photography at Leeds Arts University. Lucie's photographic practice revolves around communicating aspects of life experience and the everyday, working with performative and auto-ethnographic collaborative research methods to create photographic narrative. Approaches utilised to create narrative include experimentation with still and moving image, constructing the photograph and the use of cultural signifiers and exploration of direction, choreography and improvisation. Lucie produces personal projects alongside editorial and client-based commissions, building upon their research into photographic visual language and aesthetics that cross between fashion and art-based contexts. Lucie has exhibited at international photographic festivals and edited the work of other photographic artists as part of a self-published print publication titled *Forme Journal.*

Garry Barker is an artist and lecturer. He has delivered conference papers on various aspects of drawing, has published and exhibited widely, winning the 2017 Rabley Drawing Centre 'SKETCH' first prize, and has been selected for the Trinity Buoy Wharf drawing prize, and the Pinault Foundation's 2020 exhibition 'Untitled, 2020: Three perspectives on the art of the present'. Recently commissioned for the Leeds Arts Wellbeing and Health network, he uses a variety of methodologies to develop responses to individual and community concerns, using drawing, ceramics, printmaking, jewellery, sculpture and writing as tools to communicate ideas, drive narratives and create visual allegories.

Emily Beaney is an artist, filmmaker and AHRC PhD researcher at Edinburgh College of Art, University of Edinburgh. Her practice-based research centres on themes of care, control and health inequalities. Working collaboratively with family, friends and community groups to explore lived experiences of embodied difference, illness and disability, her projects seek to communicate with, through and between bodies to reveal that which remains hidden/unheard. Emily has shared projects across the UK and internationally in festivals, conferences and with organisations including the Southbank Centre, Alchemy Film and Arts, the Royal Scottish Academy, Creative Scotland, British Council and Unlimited.

Sonia Bernac is an artist and a PhD candidate at the Royal College of Art. She is also a researcher at the Artificial and Distributed Intelligence Lab based at the RCA and a recipient of London Arts and Humanities Partnership Scholarship. She was a co-founder of the Idle Institute (2016–2020)—a storytelling lab and a collective of writers, musicians and engineers, researching the role of fiction in anti-fascist resistance. She exhibited and published internationally, her selected projects, publications and papers include: *Cartographic bestiaries of the fascistic* at *Posthuman Mimesis: Embodiment, Affect, Contagion* conference, KU Leuven, *Curative Things: Medicine/Fashion/Art* conference, Northern Network for Medical Humanities Research, Wellcome Trust, *The New Solarists*, Summa Technologiae conference by e-flux, *Fictioning as resistance*, RCA conference London, *Enigma*, Folium, Lily Brooke Gallery, London, *Miracle Measure. The SSN conference's answer to the imprecision of doits and tinkers*, Science Museum, London, *Cybernetic Fairytales*, Xero, Kline & Coma, London, *The trials of mosquitoes*, Red Gate Gallery, Bejing, *The itches. A gym for public embarrassments*, Xero, Kline & Coma, London.

Rosie Broadhead is a designer and researcher specialising in biomaterials in the fashion industry, Founder of therapeutic clothing brand Skin Series, Textile Scientist at Ghent University, and Co-founder of Surface Tension, a platform centred around realising the positive potential of materials. Her research focuses on the skin microbiome and probiotic therapy as a solution for antibacterial finishes in textiles using technology naturally found on the skin. Rosie is a graduate of Central Saint Martins' MA 'Material Futures' course and has a background as a designer and Head of Sustainability at sportswear brand Perfect Moment and R&D at Rapha. Rosie's work has been showcased during Milan Design Week, Dutch Design Week, London Design Festival, and exhibited at museums internationally such as The Design Museum, London and Design Museum Gent. Her work has been featured by the BBC and in publications including *Forbes*, British *Vogue*, *i-D* and *The New York Times*, as well as academic journals and book chapters. Through her interest in skin and clothing interaction, her research focuses on how science and technology will influence the future of fashion.

Paula Chambers is an artist, academic and arts educator. She has exhibited widely including most recently the solo exhibitions *Working Girls* at The Whitaker, and *Not at Home* at the Art House, Wakefield. Paula is Subject Leader for Sculpture on BA(Hons) Fine Art at Leeds Arts University. She has presented at national and international conferences on feminism, contemporary art and the domestic and has chapters included in *Feminist Art Activisms and Artivisms, Feminist Visual Activism and the Body* and *An Artist and a Mother*. Also, journal articles published in the journal of *Psychoanalysis, Culture and Society*, and in *Performance/Research Journal* (special issue *On the Maternal*).

Alison L. Goodrum is an interdisciplinary researcher, traversing dress history, cultural geography and the creative arts. With over 20 years of experience as a career academic, she has worked in universities in New Zealand, the USA and the UK. Currently, she is Director of Research Development at Norwich University of the Arts, England. Alison employs a mix of ethnographic, creative and archive approaches, pursuing projects relating to the Interwar years, sportswear, millinery, weather/ing and the American designer-activist, Elizabeth Hawes (1903–1971).

Andrew Groves is Professor of Fashion Design at the University of Westminster, and the director of the Westminster Menswear Archive, which he founded in 2016. It is the world's only public menswear archive, establishing a space where students, academics, and designers in industry are co-located to conduct object-based research. It houses over 2000 examples of some of the most significant menswear garments from the last 250 years, including designer fashion, streetwear, everyday dress, sportswear, workwear, and uniforms. In 2019, Groves co-curated *Invisible Men: An Anthology from the Westminster Menswear Archive*, to date, the United Kingdom's largest menswear exhibition.

Anna Jamieson is an interdisciplinary art historian and a British Academy Postdoctoral Fellow at the University of Birmingham. She specialises in visual and material cultures of the late eighteenth and early nineteenth century, with a particular interest in the history of psychiatry, women, patient agency and dark tourism. She is an associate editor at *The Polyphony* and has held research fellowships at the Lewis Walpole Library (Yale University), the John Rylands Research Institute (University of Manchester) and the Northern Network for Medical Humanities Research. She is currently writing a monograph exploring asylum tourism in England between 1770 and 1845 and has had her research published in *Eighteenth-Century Studies* and *Journal of Eighteenth-Century Studies.*

Fiona Johnstone is an art historian, specialising in the intersections between art, health and medicine. She is the author of *AIDS and Representation* (Bloomsbury 2023) and *Anti-Portraiture* (Bloomsbury 2020), as well as numerous journal articles, book chapters and other writings. For 2021–2023 she is co-director of the international seminar series *Confabulations: art practice, art history, critical medical humanities.* She is currently Assistant Professor in Visual Medical Humanities at the Institute for Medical Humanities, Durham University, where she is working on a new monograph, provisionally entitled *Critical interlopers: contemporary artists as researchers and collaborators in healthcare and medicine.*

Katharina Ludwig is a researcher, artist and writer working with text, installation and objects. Her research is concerned with narrative holes in women*'s writing and the insurrectionary poetics of the 'wounded text'. Katharina tries to activate textual holes as a feminist practice of resistance with subversive potential that treats the textual wound as a political and writerly strategy in opposition to authoritarian systems. Her work has been shown, performed or read internationally and is published by a.o. 3am Magazine, Zeno Press, Ma Bibliothèque, Chris Airlines, HOAX, PaperWork Magazine. In addition to her own practice Katharina works on editorial, curatorial and educational projects.

Alanna McKnight holds a PhD in Communication and Culture from Toronto Metropolitan University, Toronto. She has been researching the intersection of fashion and labour in nineteenth-century Toronto, Canada for the past 15 years. Her upcoming book engages in an extended case study of the manufacturing and consumer centres of Toronto during this moment of history to argue that corsets are a site of feminist agency—a stark contradiction to common media portrayals of the garment. Her academic work is enriched by her former career as a theatre costumer, and she has been an avid wearer and maker of corsets for over 20 years.

Jana Melkumova-Reynolds is Assistant Professor of Sociology at the London School of Economics and Political Science where she convenes the MSc Culture and Society programme. She has lectured and supervised students' research at Chelsea College of Arts, Central Saint Martins, London College of Fashion and Parsons Paris. Her research is underpinned by feminist and queer epistemologies and methodologies, and her interests include time and temporalities, cultural production, material and visual culture, and disability studies. She is currently working on a book that focuses on subjectivity, affect and knowledge in the world of fashion intermediaries. She is also developing an ethnographic and participatory movement-based research project that will investigate cultural imaginaries and practices which conjure queer-crip utopias. Her work has appeared in *Fashion Theory* journal and in edited collections including *Dangerous Bodies* (Palgrave Macmillan, 2023), *Routledge Handbook of Fashion Studies* (Routledge, 2021), *Bodies in Flux* (Brill, 2019) and others.

Christopher M. Rudeen is a doctoral candidate in the Department of the History of Science at Harvard University with a secondary field in Studies of Women, Gender, and Sexuality. His research focuses on the ways in which nontraditional materials and practices are used for constructing and healing the self. His dissertation, 'Treating Clothes: Dress and the Sciences of Subjectivity', explores the ways in which clothing was studied in the mind sciences during the twentieth century to produce an objective study of selfhood and define disciplinary boundaries. He is also interested in other related projects at the intersection of clothing and the human sciences, including thinking about 'Rest in Peace' T-shirts as technologies of group therapy and the methodologies of Mass-Observation. His work has been published in *Fashion Studies Journal* and the *Journal of the History of the Behavioral Sciences.*

Ellen Sampson is an artist and material culture researcher whose work uses film, photography, and writing to explore the relationships between bodies, memory and garments, both in museums and archives, and in everyday life. She is Senior Research Fellow in Design at Northumbria University and was previously a Curatorial Fellow at The Costume Institute of the Metropolitan Museum of Art, and Professorial Fellow at UCA. Her book *Worn: Footwear Attachment and the Affects of Wear* was published by Bloomsbury in 2020.

Dawn Woolley is an artist and a research fellow at Leeds Arts University. She completed an MA in Photography (2008) and PhD by project in Fine Art (2017) at the Royal College of Art. Recent solo exhibitions include 'Consumed: Stilled Lives' bildkultur Gallery, Stuttgart (2022); Perth Centre for Photography, Australia (2021); 'Dance for Good & Exercise Your Rights' Public Space One gallery, Iowa City (Hard Stop 2020); 'Visual Pleasure', Hippolyte Photography Gallery, Helsinki, Finland (2013); Vilniaus Fotografijos Galerija, Lithuania (2012); and Ffotogallery, Cardiff (2011). Recent publications include: *Consuming the Body: Capitalism, Social Media and Commodification* (London: Bloomsbury, 2023); 'The Quantified Self, The Ideology of Health and Fat', in *The Body Productive* (London: Bloomsbury, 2023); and 'The Dissecting Gaze: Fashioned Bodies on Social Networking Sites', in *Revisiting the Gaze: Feminism, Fashion and the Female Body* (London: Bloomsbury, 2020).

List of Figures

CHAPTER 1

Wearable Objects and Curative Things

Dawn Woolley, Fiona Johnstone,
Ellen Sampson, and Paula Chambers

1.1 Introduction

Canes, crutches, leg braces and walking frames incorporated into contemporary dance-based performances; wearable artworks made by a mother for a daughter conveying the tensions of chronic illness and familial care; a fitness tracking watch redeployed to critique the neoliberal discourse of health as a consumer choice; an 'electric' corset; an office chair; a charm bracelet; a fashionable hat that signifies the wearer's 'madness'; an artificial silk that claims to harness the 'healing' powers of the sun; and a luxury fashion range featuring anti-smog masks, gas detectors and other personal protection devices designed to help the wearer navigate a toxic urban environment.

D. Woolley (✉) • P. Chambers
Leeds Arts University, Leeds, UK
e-mail: dawn.woolley@leeds-art.ac.uk; paula.chambers@leeds-art.ac.uk

F. Johnstone
Institute for Medical Humanities, Durham University, Durham, UK
e-mail: fiona.r.johnstone@durham.ac.uk

E. Sampson
School of Design, Northumbria University, Newcastle upon Tyne, UK
e-mail: ellen.sampson@northumbria.ac.uk

D. Woolley et al. (eds.), *Wearable Objects and Curative Things*, Palgrave Studies in Fashion and the Body,
https://doi.org/10.1007/978-3-031-40017-9_1

This interdisciplinary volume mobilises an object-centred approach to explore a set of entanglements between art and fashion and health and medicine. Addressing a rich range of 'wearable' artefacts, from mobility aids to clothing and accessories to digital health tracking devices, its theoretical framework has been inspired by the work of materialist thinkers that include Sherry Turkle, Bruno Latour and Jane Bennett. The political theorist Jane Bennett extends the body materialism of Merleau-Ponty, Foucault, Irigaray and Butler (among others) to consider the vitality of non-human objects.[1] Building on Bruno Latour's notion of things as *actants*, Bennett proposes that objects exert a 'thing power materialism'; that is, objects are not merely passive and inert matter, but active relational agents that are able 'to animate, to act, to produce effects dramatic and subtle'.[2] Bennett explicitly links this materialist framework to questions of human health and wellbeing, arguing that human flourishing can only be realised through recognising the shared materiality and interconnectedness of all things, both human and non-human.[3] This volume responds to Bennett's call to 'take seriously the vitality of (nonhuman) bodies',[4] addressing objects—and more specifically, wearable objects—as 'things that matter' in the exploration of human health and its wider contexts.

Sherry Turkle—who like Bennett, Latour and others recognises objects as active life presences with world-making properties—observes that material things are both 'goods-to-think with' (neatly drawing attention to the intersections of materiality and consumer capitalism) and 'good-to-think-with'; that is, helpful tools for intellectual enquiry.[5] This volume uses wearable objects as things to think with, drawing attention to the rich intersections between human health and wearable materiality. As Bruno Latour has argued, things 'bind us all together in matter of concern': a focus on material artefacts offers a useful hermeneutic tool for bringing together scholars and practitioners from a range of disciplines around a

[1] Jane Bennett, 'The Force of Things: Steps toward an Ecology of Matter', *Political Theory* 32, no.3 (June 2004), 347–372. See also Jane Bennett, *Vibrant Matter: A Political Ecology of Things*. Durham and London: Duke University Press, 2010.

[2] Bruno Latour, (2005) *Reassembling the Social. An Introduction to Actor-Network Theory*, Oxford: Oxford University Press; Bennett, 'The Force of Things', 351.

[3] Bennett, *Vibrant Matter*, 12–13.

[4] Bennett, *Vibrant Matter*, viii.

[5] Turkle, *Evocative Objects*, 2007, 9.

shared intellectual enquiry.[6] Accordingly, this volume uses 'things' to bring together three broad disciplinary fields: art and design practice, fashion studies, and medical and health humanities: to our knowledge, this is the first time that these fields have been brought into conversation within a single volume. This reflects the disciplinary backgrounds of the four editors of this book: Dawn Woolley and Paula Chambers are artists and researchers who specialise in consumer culture and feminism; Ellen Sampson is an artist and material culture researcher with a particular interest in the relationship between bodily experience and the worn artefact; and Fiona Johnstone is an art historian whose work focuses on the intersections between visual culture and medical and health humanities. Our collaboration has been stimulated by a shared interest in the materiality of 'things': Woolley and Chambers are co-conveners of the Thing Power research group at Leeds Arts University; Sampson is co-director of The Fashion Research Network; and at time of writing Johnstone had recently finished directing a visual medical humanities project called *Thinking Through Things*.[7] This shared interest led to an online symposium hosted by Leeds Arts University in February 2021 (in the middle of the UK's second Covid-19 lockdown), which was accompanied by a series of artists' poster campaigns displayed in commercial advertising spaces across Leeds.[8] Unpacking the relationships between wearable objects and human health, and exploring how artists and designers are creatively responding to and rethinking these relationships, the symposium brought together historians, sociologists, fashion researchers, philosophers, designers, art historians, artists, creative writers and practitioners, and more. Several of the papers

[6] Latour and Weibel, 'From Realpolitik to Dingpolitik. Or, How to Make Things Public.' In *Making Things Public:*

Atmospheres of Democracy, edited by Bruno Latour and Peter Weibel, 14–41. Cambridge, MA: MIT Press, 2005.

[7] The Thing Power research group comprises academics from a variety of creative disciplines who examine things as sources of social value, loci of emotional experience, powerful and empowering tools, and agents capable of disrupting dominant discourses. The Fashion Research Network (www.fashionresearchnetwork.com) is co-founded and co-chaired by Ellen Sampson. The collaborative project Thinking Through Things: Object Encounters in the Medical Humanities (http://nnmh.org.uk/thinking-through-things/), supported by the Northern Network for Medical Humanities Research and Wellcome Trust, was led by Fiona Johnstone from 2019–2021.

[8] Artists' poster campaigns included Mystical Apparatus by Dawn Woolley; Office Exercises by Lucie Armstrong; and Lacking Charm by Paula Chambers, and was commissioned by Dr Catriona McAra (then curator at Leeds Arts University) and Dawn Woolley.

originally presented at the symposium find their final form in this book, which includes academic essays, artists' and designers' statements and art writing; other texts have been commissioned especially for the volume. The objects explored in these pages might be placed in a number of overlapping ontological categories: some are explicitly medical objects, and others are art objects or consumer goods. All, however, are social agents, capable of exerting affect and influence on the subjects they encounter (or at least having been marketed to the prospective consumer as having the ability to do so). Neither independent of, nor entirely dependent upon, the bodies of their human co-conspirators, these 'curative things' (a deliberately provocative title which will be elaborated upon shortly) are here offered the opportunity to 'speak', drawing attention to the increasingly permeable boundaries between different categories of wearable objects.

Our understanding of the key term 'wearable object' deserves clarification here. In the most straightforward sense, a 'wearable object' might denote anything that can be worn on, supported by or facilitated by the body: clothes, jewellery, glasses, bags and hats are all obvious examples of objects that interact with the human form and respond to the wearer's movements and being-in-the-world. In this book, however, we deliberately activate an expanded understanding of the term 'wearable' to encompass both objects worn on or by the body (clothing, footwear and accessories) and objects which function as prosthetic extensions to the body. There is an established history of artists working with wearable objects in an experimental way that broadens the notion of the wearable beyond the most obvious examples of clothes and accessories, often by deliberately drawing attention to the interactions of the body with the world around it. For example, Rebecca Horn's *Finger Gloves* (1972) are performative bodily extensions that enable creative interactions with subjects, objects and spaces, whilst simultaneously interrupting normative everyday social relations. Horn's work brings to mind the anthropologist Alfred Gell's formulation of art works as active social agents (rather than symbolic representations or visual codes); capable of materialising networks of social relations, artworks have a power to assert influence that can be thought of as performative (in the Butlerian sense of bringing something into being).[9]

More recently, and particularly relevant to the concerns of this present volume, the US-based artist Panteha Abareshi has eloquently articulated their own lived experience of chronic illness through processes, actions

[9] Alfred Gell, *Art and Agency: An Anthropological Theory* (Oxford: Oxford University Press, 1998); Judith Butler, *Bodies That Matter* (London and New York: Routledge, 1993).

and objects across sculpture, film and performance. In Abareshi's 2021 performance work, *Methods of Care for the Precarious Body*, objects commonly used in medical contexts, such as protective gloves, back support and neck brace, are donned by the artist in response to a series of increasingly intrusive instructional texts. In a series of sculptural works titled collectively *This is Not a Body* (2022), Abareshi creates poignant assemblages of the wearable objects of chronic illness: prosthetic legs and feet, crutches, casts for broken limbs, and various wires and tubing associated with invasive medical care. These works both evoke and require the body's presence, in a way that implies the relational 'thingliness' of new materialism rather than the subject/object dichotomy of medical prosthesis. Similar observations might be made of the collapsed crutches, canes and techno-prosthetic appendages incorporated into installations by the UK-based artist Jesse Darling and US-based artist Carolyn Lazard: like Abareshi, both Darling and Lazard use these objects to question and disrupt, rather than celebrate, the uncritical techno-fetishism that frequently frames material practices of bodily extension.[10]

A number of recent curatorial projects have brought together contemporary artworks with wearable artefacts from medical collections, often forcing a reconsideration of the arbitrariness of different object categories. For the show *The Body Extended: Sculpture and Prosthetics* (2016), the Henry Moore Institute in Leeds exhibited works by artists including Rebecca Horn and Louise Bourgeois alongside objects sourced from medical museums, including a painted metal facial prosthesis made by the classically trained sculptor Anna Coleman Ladd for servicemen disfigured in the First World War (borrowed from the Anthony Wallace Archives of the British Association of Plastic, Reconstructive and Aesthetics Surgeons). (A similar juxtaposition was made in *The Milk of Dreams*, curated by Cecilia Alemani for the 2022 Venice Biennale, where Ladd's facial prosthesis, accompanied by documentary photographs of wounded servicemen wearing the masks, was displayed alongside sculptural works by Horn and other artists.) The 'portrait masks' created by Ladd and others were tailor-made for the recipient; carefully crafted, these were precious aesthetic objects in their own right, akin perhaps to a valuable watch or a bespoke hat.[11] Understood as both artwork and medical object, Ladd's

[10] Giulia Smith, 'Chronic Illness as Critique: Crip Aesthetics Across the Atlantic', *Art History* 44, no. 2 (2021): 286–310.

[11] Suzannah Biernoff, 'The Rhetoric of Disfigurement in First World War Britain', *Social History of Medicine* 24, no. 3 (2011): 666–685; 680.

facial prosthesis draws attention to the complex inter-relationships between creative practice, clinical care and embodied experience.[12]

Indelibly associated with fantasies about the utopian potentiality of the technologically enhanced post-human body, the prosthetic (as an epistemological concept, if not necessarily an ontological object) has had an extraordinary hold on the cultural imagination of the late twentieth and early twenty-first centuries.[13] Consider, for example, the prosthetic legs of Aimee Mullins, a Paralympian athlete and double amputee who has collaborated with fashion designers, photographers and artists. Mullins has been photographed doll-like in smooth limbs and crinoline cage by Nick Knight for an issue of *Dazed and Confused* guest-edited by Alexander McQueen in 1998; modelled intricately carved ashwood legs on the catwalk for McQueen's Spring/Summer collection in London in 1999; and donned a variety of prosthesis (including a pair of cat legs that nod to her carbon-fibre 'Cheetah' running blades) for the final episode of Matthew Barney's *Cremaster* cycle in 2002. Paradigmatic 'wearable objects' that connect art and fashion with health and medicine, Mullin's legs have attracted commentary from scholars in a range of disciplines, including visual cultural studies, fashion studies and medical humanities.[14] Significantly for this volume, and as Laina Burton and Jana Melkumova-

[12] See Suzannah Biernoff, *Portraits of Violence: War and the Aesthetics of Disfigurement* (Ann Arbor: University of Michigan Press, 2017) for a discussion of Ladd's work in relation to aesthetics and medicine.

[13] On prosthetic culture as a discourse that often overlooks the material reality of prosthesis, see Vivian Sobchack, 'A Leg to Stand On: Prosthetics, Metaphor, and Materiality.', in *The Prosthetic Impulse: From A Posthuman Present to a Biocultural Future*, ed. Marquard Smith and Joanna Morra (Cambridge, Mass.: MIT Press, 2006), 17–41.

[14] On the tensions and contradictions of the prosthetic metaphor in relation to Aimee Mullins, see Marquard Smith, 'The Vulnerable Articulate: James Gillingham, Aimee Mullins, and Matthew Barney', in *The Prosthetic Impulse: From a Posthuman Present to a Biocultural Future*, ed. Marquard Smith and Joanna Morra (Cambridge, Mass.: MIT Press, 2005), 45–72; Olga Vainshtein, '"I Have a Suitcase Just Full of Legs Because I Need Options for Different Clothing": Accessorizing Bodyscapes', *Fashion Theory* 16, no. 2 (2015): 139–69; Luna Dolezal, 'Representing Posthuman Embodiment: Considering Disability and the Case of Aimee Mullins', *Women's Studies* 46, no. 1 (2017): 60–75; Laini Burton and Jana Melkumova-Reynolds, '"My Leg Is a Giant Stiletto Heel": Fashioning the Prosthetised Body', *Fashion Theory* 23, no. 2 (2019): 195–218; Luna Dolezal, 'Disability as Malleability: The Prosthetic Metaphor, Merleau-Ponty and the Case of Aimee Mullins', in *Medial Bodies between Fiction and Faction: Reinventing Corporeality*, ed. Denisa Butnaru (Bielfeeld: Verlag, 2020), 125–45; Anne Farren & Andrew Hutchison (2004) Cyborgs, New Technology, and the Body: The Changing Nature of Garments, *Fashion Theory*, 8, no.4, 461–475.

Reynolds point out, bodies like Mullins' invoke the intimate interconnectedness of human and non-human matter: 'such a body does not wear fashion—it becomes fashion'.[15]

Fashion studies is the second major disciplinary field represented with this volume. Within fashion studies the material and embodied turns have reoriented the field both towards bodily practices of wearing and the complex agencies embodied in the things we wear. Building on theorists of the body such as Maurice Merleau-Ponty and Michel Foucault, fashion scholars have long recognised dress as an embodied practice.[16] Since Entwistle's *Fashioning the Body* considerable work has been undertaken on the bodily experience of dress and of dressing.[17] However, the more recent sensory and emotional turns in fashion studies have led to a renewed focus on the ways clothes make wearers 'feel' and thus on well-being and on garments' 'therapeutic' histories and potentials.[18] For example both the work of Renate Stauss on 'Therapy of Fashion'[19] amongst psychiatric patients in 1960s and the recent exhibition 'Mirror Mirror—Fashion & the Psyche' at MoMu in Antwerp and Dr. Guislain psychiatric Museum in Ghent explored the complex interconnections between fashion, psychology, self-

[15] Burton and Melkumova-Reynolds, '"My Leg Is a Giant Stiletto Heel": Fashioning the Prosthetised Body', 9. See also Malcom Barnard's observation that "We are happy to think about fashion and clothing as prostheses: something that is not us but which we add to ourselves and without which we would consider ourselves incomplete" in Malcom Barnard, *Fashion Theory: An Introduction* (Abingdon and New York: Routledge, 2014), 16; cited in Burton and Melkumova-Reynolds, 3.

[16] See for example: Joanne Entwistle, 'Fashion and the Fleshy Body: Dress as Embodied Practice,' *Fashion Theory* 4, no.3 (2000): 323–347; Lucia Ruggerone, 'The Feeling of Being Dressed: Affect Studies and the Clothed Body,' *Fashion Theory* 21, no.5 (2017): 573–593; and Lleywellyn Negrin, 'Fashion as an embodied art form,' in Estelle Barrett & Barbara Bolt (eds.), *Carnal Knowledge: Towards a 'New Materialism' Through the Arts.* (London: I.B. Tauris, 2013).

[17] See for example Hilary Davidson, 'The Embodied Turn: Making and Remaking Dress as an Academic Practice,' *Fashion Theory* 23:3 (2019): 329–362; Sophie Woodward, *Why Women Wear What They Wear* (London: Berg, 2007); and Ilya Parkins, '"You'll Never Regret Going Bold": The Moods of Wedding Apparel on a Practical Wedding,' *Fashion Theory* 25, no.6 (2021): 799–817.

[18] See for example Sara Chong Kwan, 'The Ambient Gaze: Sensory Atmosphere and the Dressed Body,' in *Revisiting the Gaze: The Fashioned Body and the Politics of Looking* (London: Bloomsbury, 2020); and Lucia Ruggerone 'The Feeling of Being Dressed: Affect Studies and the Clothed Body', *Fashion Theory* 21, no.5 (2017): 573–593.

[19] Renate Stauss, 'Passing as Fashionable, Feminine and Sane: "Therapy of Fashion" and the Normalization of Psychiatric Patients in 1960s US,' *Fashion Theory* 24, no.4 (2020): 601–637.

image and identity formation. The idea of 'therapeutic' dress again comes into play in scholarship which addresses the role of uniforms in medical settings, such as Susan Hardy & Anthony Corones' 'Medical clothing as character making or ethopoietic'[20] and Huber's work on the ritualised nature of the white coat.[21]

In parallel a body of practice-led design-based scholarship has emerged which explores the role of fashion and dress as aids to wellbeing, as treatment, or assistive and adaptative devices.[22] In particular these design-led approaches explore the potential of new materials to alter and improve wearers' embodied experiences, and foreground the central role that dress plays in our negotiations with the material world. The ways that clothing and fashion aid these bodily and cultural negotiations is further developed in work on the fashionable pursuit of 'health' and its intersections with wealth and cultural capital including Emma Markiewicz's work on hair in the eighteenth century;[23] Martin's work on cosmetics in nineteenth-century France;[24] and Charpy's research on nineteenth-century rubber clothing.[25] Perhaps of particular relevance to this volume is a body of work which explores the increasing number of ways in which the body is fashioned not only through dress but through cosmetic surgery, medical

[20] Susan Hardy & Anthony Corones, 'Dressed to Heal: The Changing Semiotics of Surgical Dress,' *Fashion Theory*, 20, no.1 (2016): 27–49; Susan Hardy & Anthony Corones, 'The Nurse's Uniform as Ethopoietic Fashion', *Fashion Theory*, 21:5, 523–552.

[21] S. J. Huber, 2003, 'The White Coat Ceremony: Contemporary Medical Ritual', *Journal of Medical Ethics,* 29 (2017): 364–366.10.1136/jme.29.6.364

[22] See for example Jenny Tillotson, 'Scentsory Design: A "Holistic" Approach to Fashion as a Vehicle to Deliver Emotional Well-being,' *Fashion Practice* 1, no.1 (2009): 33–61; Chanmi Hwang, Lindsay McCoy & Michele R. Shaw, 'Redesigning Maternity Hospital Gowns', *Fashion Practice,* 14, no.1 (2022): 79–98, Kerri McBee-Black, '"Making Life Easier": A Case Study Exploring the Development of Adaptive Apparel Design Innovations from a User-Centered Approach,' *Fashion Practice* 14, no.2, (2022): 203–224; and Maria Tsakalidou, 'Analysing Anthropometric Measurement and Body Shape Data to Incorporate Body Asymmetry, due to Scoliosis, into Improved Clothing Sizing Systems,' *Fashion Practice* 9, no.3, (2017): 398–424.

[23] Emma Markiewicz, 'Performing Health and Beauty in Eighteenth-Century England: The Significance of Hair in the Creation of Appearances,' *Fashion Theory* 22, no.6, (2018): 617–640.

[24] M. Martin, *Selling Beauty: Cosmetics, Commerce, and French Society, 1750–1830.* Baltimore: Johns Hopkins University Press, 2009.

[25] Manuel Charpy, 'Craze and Shame: Rubber Clothing during the Nineteenth Century in Paris, London, and New York City,' *Fashion Theory* 16, no.4, (2012): 433–460.

treatments and devices.[26] Meredith Jones observes that cosmetic surgery is being realigned away from the medico-beauty industry and towards the fashion industry, and this realignment is influencing the aesthetics and marketing of cosmetic procedures, and the availability and normalisation of them.[27] These intersections between health-related design practices and medical humanities scholarship are similarly nascent; accordingly this volume draws these disciplinary fields together in dialogue for the first time. Stimulated by recent fashion scholarship addressing embodiment,[28] the senses,[29] materiality,[30] and the post-human,[31] this volume takes a materialist, object-based approach to a broad range of contemporary and historical wearable objects including clothing, headwear, jewellery, textiles, implants, prostheses, medical and fitness devices and physical aids. By affording these wearables critical cross-disciplinary attention, this volume acknowledges and articulates the complexity of ways in which human beings and thing-hood entangle, and in doing so generates fresh perspectives on embodiment and human health.

The third disciplinary field represented within this volume is the medical and health humanities. A relatively new field, the medical humanities encompass 'a series of intersections, exchanges, and entanglements between the biomedical sciences, the arts and humanities, and the social sciences'.[32] Whilst highly interdisciplinary in nature, to date the medical

[26] See for example Luciana Ugrina, 'Celebrity Biometrics: Norms, New Materialism, and the Agentic Body in Cosmetic Surgery Photography,' *Fashion Theory* 18, no.1 (2014): 27–44; and Florentina C. Andreescu, 'Covering over Trauma with a Fetishized Body Image: The Invasive Imaginary and Cosmetic Surgery,' *Fashion Theory* 18, no.1 (2014): 7–26.

[27] Meredith Jones, 'Cosmetic Surgery and the Fashionable Face,' *Fashion Theory* 16, no.2 (2012): 199.

[28] Lleywellyn Negrin, 'Fashion as an embodied art form,' in Estelle Barrett & Barbara Bolt (eds.), *Carnal Knowledge: Towards a 'New Materialism' Through the Arts* (London: I.B. Tauris, 2013); and Lucia Ruggerone, 'The Feeling of Being Dressed: Affect Studies and the Clothed Body,' *Fashion Theory* 21, no.5 (2017): 573–593.

[29] Joanne B. Eicher, 'Dress, the Senses, and Public, Private, and Secret Selves,' *Fashion Theory*, 25, no.6 (2021): 777–797.

[30] Bethan Bide, 'Signs of Wear: Encountering Memory in the Worn Materiality of a Museum Fashion Collection,' *Fashion Theory*, 21, no.4 (2017): 449–476 and Yeseung Lee, *Seamlessness: Making and (Un)Knowing in Fashion Practice*, Bristol: Intellect, 2016.

[31] Anneke Smelik, 'Fractal Folds: The Posthuman Fashion of Iris van Herpen,' *Fashion Theory* 26, no.1 (2020): 5–26.

[32] Anne Whitehead and Angela Woods, 'Introduction', in *The Edinburgh Companion to the Critical Medical Humanities*, ed. Anne Whitehead and Angela Woods (Edinburgh: Edinburgh University Press, 2016), 1.

and health humanities have barely engaged with fashion studies at all. And whilst contemporary art practice has recently undergone a 'turn to health',[33] it is only recently that medical humanities have begun to engage in-depth with arts practices and histories.[34] If a 'first wave' of medical humanities tended to regard art practice in a primarily instrumental way as useful for arts-in-health interventions and the training of doctors in 'soft' skills like empathy, a second 'critical' wave has begun to make space for art as a valid form of knowledge-production.[35] Many of the objects explored in this volume deliberately problematise the notion of health as a quantifiable object of study; few (if any) are concerned with producing measurable health outcomes. Almost all draw our attention to the broader cultural and historical contexts that shape understandings and experiences of health, illness and disability.

This volume is intended to be a starting point in bringing these different fields together: we hope other scholars and practitioners will be able to make use of it, to deepen and strengthen the relations between these three areas.

1.2 About This Book

Our editorial approach to this volume has been multi-disciplinary, drawing on and shaped by the editorial team's diverse areas of expertise and methodological approaches, in material culture, psychoanalytic and sensory approaches to the dressed body (Sampson), contemporary art history, the medical humanities and fine art (Johnstone), consumer cultures and commoditisation of health (Woolley) and feminist theory and feral objects (Chambers). Contributions take a variety of disciplinary approaches:

[33] Bárbara Rodríguez Muñoz, 'Introduction', in *Health*, ed. Bárbara Rodríguez Muñoz, Documents of Contemporary Art (London and Cambridge MA: Whitechapel Gallery and the MIT Press, 2020), 13.

[34] Fiona Johnstone, 'Manifesto for a Visual Medical Humanities', *Medical Humanities* (blog), 31 July 2018, https://blogs.bmj.com/medical-humanities/2018/07/31/manifesto-for-a-visual-medical-humanities/. Stella Bolaki, *Illness as Many Narratives: Arts, Medicine and Culture* (Edinburgh: Edinburgh University Press, 2016); and Rachael Allen, 'The Body Beyond the Anatomy Lab: (Re)Addressing Arts Methodologies for the Critical Medical Humanities', in *The Edinburgh Companion to the Critical Medical Humanities*, ed. Anne Whitehead and Angela Woods (Edinburgh: Edinburgh University Press, 2016), 186–208.

[35] On first and second wave medical humanities see Whitehead and Woods, 'Introduction'; 3–5.

whilst several essays address historical case studies, others explore how contemporary artists and designers are creatively responding to and rethinking human-object relations.

Daniel Miller advocates for the importance of material culture as the stuff through which we experience being-in-the-world.[36] Miller proposes a theory of the humility of objects, through which he frames an understanding of what constitutes 'things' as the objects or stuff of material culture that exist 'not through our consciousness or body, but as an exterior environment that habituates and prompts us'.[37] Miller theorises the humility of objects as their unexpected capacity to fade out of focus yet remain peripheral to our vision in ways that determine our behaviour and identity. The curative things discussed in the chapters of this book are often objects that have been overlooked or obscured; here they have been facilitated to 'speak' in various ways by the contributing authors through academic and art practice research strategies.

As an interdisciplinary editorial team, we have elected not to organise the chapters by object type or methodological approach in order to avoid reinforcing the disciplinary boundaries that often hamper the study of such objects. Instead, the chapters are grouped into sections that bring together traditional academic writing with creative and practice-based contributions (including photography, film and performative texts). These sections are organised around four gerund verbs: Collaborating, Covering, Controlling, and Communicating. Each verb describes the ways in which the objects addressed in that section might act upon, with, and for, their human co-collaborators. The boundaries between these sections are intentionally porous, and many of the (deliberately undisciplined) objects in this book might comfortably straddle more than one category.

The first section, **Collaborating**, addresses how wearable objects and bodies work together. Jana Melkumova-Reynolds' chapter 'On Crutches, Choreography and (Crip) Care: Curative Objects and Palliative Things in Two Performance Pieces' is an analysis of two choreographed dance works which incorporate medical assistive devices. Borrowing from actor-network theory, phenomenology, disability and queer theory, Melkumova-Reynolds questions the use and intention of medical assistive devices as alternately curative objects and palliative things. The curative object she

[36] Daniel Miller, *Material Culture and Mass Consumption* (Oxford: Blackwell Publishers, 1987), 85–108.

[37] Miller, *Material Culture and Mass Consumption*, 5.

proposes implies a binary of vulnerability and mastery; the palliative thing however is relational, entangled and enabling. Emily Beaney's 'Breaking the Fall' is an artist's text that details the collaboration between the artist and artist's mother, through the production of wearable artworks presented through a film work. The artwork, film and collaborative processes materialise relationships, both familial and material, conveying the tensions, tenderness and entanglements of illness and familial caring experiences. The chapter is interspersed with still images from the film which eloquently portray the wearable as touch-based knowledge and mediator of affect. Alison L Goodrum's chapter 'Sitting Pretty: A Dress History of the L-Shaped Frame, the Side-Saddle Habit and the Design of Adaptive Wearables' takes as its starting point the phenomena of waist-up dressing to explore how the seated body acts upon fabric and how fabric acts upon the seated body, and how the principals of side-saddle tailoring can be reimagined as an inclusive design ethos of seated fashion for wheelchair users. Using an analysis of the design, cut, fit and function of the specialist kit for side-saddle horse riding, Goodrum explores the interplay between artefact and touch, balance and physicality. In 'The Itches: Embodiment and Distributed Meaning in the Age of Technological Entanglement', Sonia Bernac proposes prosthesis as more than bodily extensions, but rather as objects that disrupt the boundaries of the body through processes of distributed sensing. This chapter questions an understanding of the body as a sum of its diverse parts with specialised functions, and troubles the distinctions between natural and artificial, the organic and the inorganic. Bernac proposes prostheses as a specific form of encounter, an embodied exchange, an attachment formed *with* the corporeal body.

Section Two, **Covering**, explores anxieties around the exposure of the body; the potential consequences of exposure; and strategies of mitigation. Christopher M. Rudeen's contribution 'Securing a Place in the Sun: Clothing, Exposure, and Health' presents an analysis of Celanese, an artificial silk fabric permeable to ultraviolet light within the context of the specific anxieties of the white middle classes in Britain in the early twentieth century. Marketed as a health-giving product that allowed for tanning whilst clothed, Rudeen proposes that Celanese indexed moral implications of public nudity, in addition to broader concerns of race and class. Andrew Groves' chapter 'Palliative Prototypes or Therapeutic Functionality? Examining C.P. Company's Urban Protection Range' addresses anxieties about the future and the role of technology materialised through wearables that cross the line between fashion and art. This chapter analyses ten objects from the Urban Protection Range, considering the garments as multifunctional protective barriers between the wearer and a hostile urban environment and in response to perceived physical and psychological threats posed by ecological, environmental, and digital disasters. In 'Skin and Textile Interaction and the Future of Fashion as Therapeutics', textile designer Rosie Broadhead discusses biomaterials and skin microbiome-friendly clothing in relation to her bio-design project *Skin II—Probiotic Clothing*. Contextualising the complex ecosystem of the human body as cross-species entanglement, a process of interaction and intra-action between skin and textile in clothing, this chapter explores the health benefits of encapsulating probiotic bacteria into the fibres of clothing.

Section Three, **Controlling**, explores how objects and the wider contexts through which they are encountered suggest a range of disciplinary techniques for the (self-)production of 'healthy' bodies. Dawn Woolley's 'Desire Lines: Quantified-Self-Portraits Produced with a Fitness Tracking Watch' is an analysis of self-tracking as embodied archive. In neoliberal societies that equate health with good citizenship and moral worth self-tracking devices can be understood as objects of bodily measurement and control. Woolley subverts the self-optimising intention of these devices by tracking mundane domestic activities and chores, re-presenting the data produced through a series of hand cut lino prints, thereby critiquing the body's abstraction into numbers as materialised through the bodily management of self-quantification. In 'Health, Elegance and Comfort: The Shocking History of Electric Corsets' Alana McKnight investigates the ambivalent understanding in the late Victorian period of corsetry and its relationship to women's bodies and physical health. McKnight presents the 'electric' corset as a fraudulent object with pseudo-scientific claims marketed to capitalise on anxieties about women's health, as a cure-all for physical and mental illness at a time when women's bodies and natural functions were widely pathologised. Lucie Armstrong's 'Office Exercises' is an artist's text that contextualises a series of photographic works developed in response to a personal experience of the mundanity and repetitive nature of office work. Armstrong analyses her intention for these images as a subtle parody of the physical impact on health of the office-type workplace environment, and as a critique of workplace wellness posters and narratives, strategies intended to mitigate against the reproduction of neoliberal narratives.

The final section, **Communicating**, expands upon ideas around how objects or things respond to the body in ways that might be protective, restrictive or expressive. 'Votives and Charm Bracelets: Materialising

Health-Related Experiences through "Sacred" Objects' is an artist's text by Garry Baker in which the connection between everyday human existence and psychical or spiritual experience materialises as a physical artefact acting as an intermediary. This chapter focuses on two projects undertaken by the author in which the relationship between the interior and exterior of the body as a conjoined set of forms was visualised through the production of images and objects to heal rather than cure, to assist in the psychological task of dealing with a challenging life experience. In Katharina Ludwig's creative text '(Ad)dressing wounds—a trauma in Seven Act(or)s' metaphorical considerations of the hole or wound are presented as a performance script of a play without a play. Fictionalised characters in this script were developed from ideas first introduced in *Woundlickers* as presented at the *Curative Things: Medicine/Fashion/Art* Symposium. In Ludwig's text language becomes an abstract body, not a thing as such but a body with linguistic wounds as textual holes. The final chapter in this volume, Anna Jamieson's 'Crazy Jane Hats and Maria Medallions: Consuming, Collecting and Containing Love's Madness', explores the commercialisation of female insanity through consumer goods in the late eighteenth century. Through a detailed analysis of the ambiguities inherent in the two objects of this chapter's title, Jamieson contextualises these wearable objects as associative symbols that linked their wearers or owners to the sought-after emotional qualities that convention evoked, the cultural phenomena of the exhibition of a mild form of nerves as a signifier of one's virtue, of fidelity and a refined sensibility.

One notable omission, particularly for a book which originated from a symposium held during a pandemic lockdown, is a discussion of masks and masking. This omission is conscious: there are a number of forthcoming volumes which specifically address masks, masking and the pandemic and much had been written about them both in fashion studies,[38] the broader humanities and social sciences[39] and the press. We have therefore elected

[38] See for example Joshua M. Bluteau, 'Undercover—From Necessity to Luxury: The Evolution of Face Coverings during COVID-19,' *Fashion Theory* (2022) online only (https://doi.org/10.1080/1362704X.2022.2129138); Caroline Kipp & Ana María Rule, 'Masks for This Medical Moment. July 7, 2020,' *The Journal of Modern Craft* 14, no1 (2021): 5–11; and Caroline Kipp & Kate Kretz, 'Masks, Art, Protection, and Politics. July 15, 2020,' *The Journal of Modern Craft* 14, no.1 (2021): 19–24.

[39] See for example Sara Beth Keough, 'Masks And Materiality In The Era Of Covid-19,' *Geographical Review,* 111, no.4 (2021): 558–570: Emi Kanemoto & Sasha Allgayer, 'Masks across borders: etiquette, threat and prevention,' *Journal of Applied Communication Research,* 50, sup.1, (2022): S24–S32; and Jennifer Beth Spiegel, 'The viral politics of masks: pandemic resistance and ontological performance,' Text and Performance Quarterly 42, no.2, (2022): 111–125.

to signpost these many excellent existing projects rather than broach a complex and still emerging area of scholarship without being able to give it the space and attention that it deserves.

1.3 Curative Things

The chapters in this book address a collection of wearable objects that we have provocatively categorised as 'curative', a charged term that requires careful unpacking. Etymologically, cure is closely related to care, with both derived from the Latin verb *curare*, to take care of. Within this present volume the historical entanglements between cure and care are alluded to in Katharina Ludwig's creative text '(Ad)dressing wounds' via the fictional figure of the Wound Dresser (described as a doctor, surgeon or medical worker):

> He [the Wound Dresser] knows that the term *cure* derives from the Latin *curare—to care*, and to cure therefore doesn't necessarily denote to heal. Rather it means to mind, to *treat*, to *attend* to wounds and comprises many acts of care. He doesn't consider himself a healer but much rather a specialist of wound care.[40]

Well-practised in 'cauterising, purging and blood-letting' and knowledgeable about 'the balance of fluids such as blood, phlegm, bile and black bile', the Wound Dresser is an allegory for a pre-modern medicine defined by a dominant paradigm of a humoral body that was open, porous and in flux.[41] In Michel Foucault's well-known formulation, the pre-modern clinical encounter was defined by a community-based, dialogic exchange of knowledge: in Ludwig's text, the embodied and oral quality of this encounter is literalised in the tongues of the Wound Lickers.[42] Foucault defines the rise of modern medicine in the eighteenth century in terms of

[40] Katharina Ludwig, '(Ad)dressing Wounds', this volume, 305.

[41] On the humoral body, see Gail Kern Paster, *The Body Embarrased: Drama and the Discipline of Shame in Early Modern England* (New York: Cornell University Press, 1993), 1–22; and Nancy Sirasi, *Medieval and Early Renaissance Medicine* (Chicago: University of Chicago Press, 1990), 104–5.

[42] Michel Foucault, *The Birth of the Clinic*, trans. A.M. Sheridan (London: Routledge, 1989).

a shift from a holistic and experiential understanding of health (suggested by the question 'What is the matter with you?') to a focus on localised bodily symptoms ('Where does it hurt?') and the aetiology of disease.[43]

Historians of medicine have characterised the development of modern medicine as a shift from care to cure.[44] Modern medicine has been described as 'cure-fixated', focussed on treating the disease rather than attending to the person as a whole.[45] For this reason, within healthcare contexts scholars have often found it useful to make a distinction between practices of care (used to describe activities such as washing, feeding or dressing wounds, done to make the patient more comfortable) and bio-medical interventions intended to have a curative effect. However, for the philosopher Annemarie Mol, writing in 2008, these older distinctions between cure and care no longer make sense.[46] Mol notes how in contemporary healthcare practice, activities designated as care and cure overlap; furthermore, because many diseases are now chronic in character, 'cure' does not aim at recovery, but at making life more liveable: cure has effectively become a form of care.

Disability rights activists have pointed out how curative medicine is frequently shaped by ableist assumptions about what is 'normal', 'natural', desirable or liveable in relation to health and embodiment.[47] In *Brilliant Imperfection*, Eli Clare observes that the ideology of cure always invokes a fantasy of restoration, a return to an idealised former body-mind entity. This paradigm follows a logic of diagnosis and eradication: a particularised 'trouble' is recognised and removed, either from an individual body-mind

[43] Foucault, xxi.

[44] Charles E. Rosenberg, *The Care of Strangers: The Rise of America's Hospital System* (Baltimore: Johns Hopkins University Press, 1995); Charles E. Rosenberg and Janet Golden, eds., *Framing Disease: Studies in Cultural History: Health and Medicine in American Society* (New Brunswick, N.J.: Rutgers University Press, 1992).

[45] Roy Porter, 'The Patient's View: Doing Medical History from Below', *Theory and Society* 14, no. 2 (1985): 193.

[46] Annemarie Mol, *The Logic of Care: Health and the Problem of Patient Choice* (Abingdon and New York: Routledge, 2008), 1.

[47] For example, see Robert McRuer, 'Critical Investments: AIDS, Christopher Reeve, and Queer / Disability Studies', *Journal of Medical Humanities* 23, no. 3–4 (2002): 221–37; Robert McRuer, 'A "Last Stand" Against Cure', *Ragged Edge Online*, 2006, n.p.; Eunjung Kim, *Curative Violence: Rehabilitating Disability, Gender, and Sexuality in Modern Korea* (Durham, N.C.: Duke University Press, 2017).

(e.g. an infected appendix) or from the world at large (e.g. cancer, AIDS).[48] Whilst the elimination of life-threatening conditions and illnesses might benefit some people in some ways, the ideology of cure also has the potential to commit violence and damage, turning people into medical objects and pathologising lived experience. As Clare and others have pointed out, 'cure' has also been mobilised in relation to categories such as heteronormativity, gender conformity, and neurodiversity. In short, cure is complicated: it both 'saves lives and ends lives, propels eradication and promises us that our body-minds can change. It is a tool in the drive to normalize humans, to shrink the diversity of shape, form, size, and function among us'.[49] The notion of cure is also profoundly and problematically individualistic, locating disability and ill-health as damage to individual body-minds, rather than attending to the wider social and cultural contexts of health.[50]

Alison Kafer's notion of 'curative time' is helpful in capturing the temporality of the curative. Within a dominant cultural paradigm of curative time, the only way in which the disabled mind or body can be understood is in terms of its movement towards a cure or towards normalisation. Cure, in this context, not only signals the elimination of impairment, 'but can also mean normalizing treatments that work to assimilate the disabled mind/body as much as possible'.[51]

In her chapter in this book, Jana Melkumova-Reynolds draws on Alison Kafer's notion of the 'curative imaginary' as a social mindset that can only understand disability in terms of a normalising paradigm of intervention that is always future-focussed. She posits the palliative as an opposing conceptual model denoting the use of care to alleviate symptoms, rather than eliminate the cause of the disease (or 'the trouble' to use Eli Clare's vocabulary). She sees the curative and palliative paradigms as occupying fundamentally different relationships to time, drawing out the essentially 'queer' character of palliative time, which is not future-focussed, but based on the here and now. Ultimately, Melkumova-Reynolds chooses to read her selected objects as both curative and palliative. If curative objects promise

[48] Eli Clare, *Brilliant Imperfection: Grappling With Cure* (Durham and London: Duke University Press, 2017), 71.

[49] Clare, *Brilliant Imperfection: Grappling With Cure*, 70.

[50] Clare, *Brilliant Imperfection: Grappling With Cure*, 15.

[51] Alison Kafer, *Feminist, Queer, Crip* (Bloomington & Indianapolis: Indiana University Press, 2013), 19.

to help us to become 'better' versions of ourselves, palliative things enable cloaking, dwelling and being-with.

Several chapters reinvigorate the relationship between cure and care. For her film *Breaking the Fall*, the artist Emily Beaney puts on a series of increasingly eccentric garments. Some of these objects—for example, a cloth cap similar to those used to affix electrodes to the head for an electroencephalogram (EEG)—suggest the medical monitoring of a chronic condition (in this particular case, the artist's epilepsy), blurring care and cure. These garments have been handmade by the artist's mother, who in the film assists her daughter in dressing: fluffy and fantastical, these objects literalise the mother's desire to wrap her child in cotton wool. These 'curative things' do not offer a cure in a biomedical sense, but offer a material expression of medical and familial care. In a similar way, the artist Garry Barker writes about his use of charm bracelets to articulate people's health-related narratives. Again, these objects do not aim at a biomedical cure, but are concerned with externalising internal somatic experience. 'Therapeutic' in some senses, these items complicate an arts-for-health paradigm, in that, whilst they have a therapeutic function (perhaps invoking the curative paradigm of the 'talking cure') this is not their primary purpose.

1.4 Capitalist Cures

The conceptual reach of the curative extends beyond the strictly medical into almost every area of daily life: as Clare notes, 'encounters with the ideology of cure can be as daily as a cosmetic cream'.[52] The obligation to self-improvement sold by the wellness market, the beauty business and the fitness industry is an integral part of curative culture and its relationship with capitalism. In neoliberal societies health is viewed as a personal responsibility, a sign of successful self-care and good citizenship.[53] The association of good health with good citizenship conceals the social inequalities relating to gender, class, disability, sexuality, and race that contribute to health inequalities.[54] Like structural inequality, health inequality

[52] Clare, *Brilliant Imperfection: Grappling With Cure*, 80.

[53] Julie Guthman, Weighing In: Obesity, Food Justice, and the Limits of Capitalism (Berkeley, CA: University of California Press), 2011.

[54] Paul Ernsberger, 'Does social class explain the connection between weight and health?', in Esther Rothblum and Sondra Soloway (eds), The Fat Studies Reader (New York: New York University Press, 2009); 25–36.

is intersectional and cumulative, and stress caused by poverty, discrimination, and oppression can lead to anxiety, depression, insecurity, and low self-esteem, which can lead to chronic health conditions.[55] However, neoliberal societies continue to position 'the individual as an isolated physical unit making rational choices in a good-enough environment'.[56] Medical and wellness practices are commoditised, reinforcing the notion that health problems and their solutions are consumer choices. Some of the things in this book reproduce or subvert notions of personal responsibilisation for health. In relation to her photographic series *Office Exercises* Lucie Armstrong focuses on the office chair as a site of discomfort and control via wellness initiatives that aim to prolong the worker's ability to undertake sedentary work. She notes that workplace wellness initiatives neoliberalise the workforce by making them compliant with the notion that being 'fit for work' is a personal responsibility. Dawn Woolley used her fitness tracking watch as a collaborative tool to create self-portraits that draw attention to hidden labour such as care and cleaning, that tend to be the responsibility of marginalised people and may impede pursuits of health. Rather than reinforce the idea that health is equally accessible to anyone who is able to buy a self-tracking device, Woolley aims to subvert the devices' individualistic, competitive imperative.

Other chapters examine things that provide a sense of control for the consumer through the commodification of specific health fears. These garments present the prevention or cure of illnesses, often caused by the environment and society, as an individual choice achieved via the consumption of commodities. For example, Andrew Groves discusses C.P. Company's Urban Protection Collection of menswear as calling forth anxiety about environmental contamination and exhaustion in contemporary life, whilst presenting the garments as curative in relation to that anxiety. In a manner that anticipates neoliberal ideology, Alanna McKnight discusses how electric corset advertisers in the late nineteenth century highlighted fears around the health of female bodies in relation to the increasing speed of life in modernising Victorian societies. The corset can be viewed as both curative and beautifying; a compressive garment that supports the body

[55] Lucy Aphramor and Jacqui Gingras, 'Helping people change: promoting politicised practice in the health care professions', in Emma Rich, Lee F. Monaghan and Lucy Aphramor (eds), Debating Obesity: Critical Perspectives (New York: Palgrave Macmillan, 2011); 192–218.

[56] Emma Rich, Lee F. Monaghan and Lucy Aphramor, 'Introduction: contesting obesity discourse and presenting an alternative', ibid., 1–35; 19.

and fashionable underclothing that produces a desirable silhouette through constriction.

In contemporary advertising 'health' and 'beauty' are often conflated, enabling products associated with the improvement of appearance to be promoted in a manner that is not overtly objectifying. Rosalind Gill describes Nike's 'just do it' campaigns as fetishisations of fitness that enrol women in a 'regime of disciplinary power in which they become morally responsible for disciplining their own bodies, and where beauty work is redefined in terms of health and pleasure'.[57] By camouflaging beauty standards as health standards, adverts promote beauty as a desirable attribute that can be achieved by consuming commodities, and pre-emptively counter complaints about sexism and objectification.

Some of the things in this book blur boundaries between fashion accessory and curative talisman. In Anna Jamieson's discussion of the elusive Crazy Jane Hat and Maria Medallion, the objects enabled society women to be associated with mild forms of mental illness that were romanticised in the late eighteenth and early nineteenth century. These objects may be viewed as commoditised anxiety, marketed to incite worry, and then sold to overcome it, as in the case of C.P. Company's Urban Protection Collection. However, the variety of consumer items featuring figures symbolising love's madness, demonstrate that signs of illness (though not the illnesses themselves) were fashionable accessories. Garry Barker's votive objects also materialise immaterial bodily sensations and emotions, and his charm bracelet sculptures straddle the line between fashion and healing. As symbolic containers of pain and worry they function as protective amulets, and may also be valued as fashionable objects that align the wearer to forms of spirituality that are popular in contemporary consumer culture. These multiple affordances and meanings enrich the objects rather than devalue them.

Sonia Bernac warns that oppositional or antithetical categories such as care-oppression and necessity-vanity can be applied to and problematised by prosthetic objects because they 'always negotiate, conflate, or transgress these polarities'.[58] The objects in this book are 'ontologically disruptive' because they reside at the intersection of art, fashion and medicine, often repurposing or extending the expected uses of objects to challenge

[57] Rosalind Gill, *Gender and the Media*, 7th edn (Cambridge: Polity Press, 2013); 86–87.

[58] Sonia Bernac, 'The Itches: embodiment and Distributed Meaning in the Age of Technological Entanglement', this volume, 103–104.

preconceived ideas about health. For example, Jana Melkumova-Reynolds shows how crutches, as mobility aids and performance props used by contemporary dancers, can reinforce notions about the limits of bodies and extend the assumed capabilities of disabled bodies. The crutch is enabling and expressive, functional and creative. The characters of the Woundlicker, Woundaddresser and Sutress in Katharina Ludwig's creative text also explicate and conflate dualities, through the notion of absence—a hole—as a thing. Noting that garments are holes and edges brought together through stitches and seams, Ludwig draws connections between stitched holes and wounds in order to challenge the equation of wholeness with health or cure. The whole, healthy body, idealised and idolised in capitalist societies is an erroneous, fantasy object. It is an elusive object that would be undesirable to capitalism because it would no longer require cure via consumption.

* * *

The categories of medical wearable and fashion object increasingly overlap, with these complex artefacts playing an ever-expanding role in our lives. Ageing populations, medical and technological advances, changes in the dissemination of data and trends, and lives lived (in part) online have contributed to an environment in which fashion objects and practices are increasingly presented as indicative of or contributing to health, and bodies, medical objects and procedures are understood in the context of fashionability, cultural capital and trend. Thus, the boundaries between art, fashion and medicine are increasingly permeable and there is an evident need to address both the histories and current manifestations of these connections and inter-relations.

The disparate objects in this book are worn on, used by, and collaborate with bodies. By placing things at the centre of each chapter and structuring the book around what the things do, this book follows Bennett's suggestion that we should view people-thing assemblages as horizontal juxtapositions in which properties are exchanged between both parties, and not as a hierarchical structure in which the subject acts upon an object. Things mould behaviours and modify emotions. Whether curative, palliative or placebo, these are vibrant things full of affect.

References

Allen, Rachael. 'The Body Beyond the Anatomy Lab: (Re)Addressing Arts Methodologies for the Critical Medical Humanities.' In *The Edinburgh Companion to the Critical Medical Humanities*, edited by Anne Whitehead and Angela Woods, 186–208. Edinburgh: Edinburgh University Press, 2016.

Andreescu, Florentina C. 'Covering over Trauma with a Fetishized Body Image: The Invasive Imaginary and Cosmetic Surgery.' *Fashion Theory* 18, no.1 (2015): 7–26.

Aphramor, Lucy and Gingras, Jacqui. 'Helping people change: promoting politicised practice in the health care professions.' In *Debating Obesity: Critical Perspectives,* edited by Emma Rich, Lee F. Monaghan and Lucy Aphramor, 192–218. New York: Palgrave Macmillan, 2011.

Barnard, Malcom. *Fashion Theory: An Introduction*. Abingdon and New York: Routledge, 2014.

Bennett, Jane. 'The Force of Things: Steps toward an Ecology of Matter.' *Political Theory* 32, no.3 (Jun., 2004): 347–372.

Bennett, Jane. *Vibrant Matter: A Political Ecology of Things*. Durham and London: Duke University Press, 2010.

Bide, Bethan. 'Signs of Wear: Encountering Memory in the Worn Materiality of a Museum Fashion Collection.' *Fashion Theory* 21, no.4 (2017): 449–476.

Biernoff, Suzannah. 'The Rhetoric of Disfigurement in First World War Britain.' *Social History of Medicine* 24, no.3 (2011): 666–685.

Biernoff, Suzannah. *Portraits of Violence: War and the Aesthetics of Disfigurement*. Ann Arbor: University of Michigan Press, 2017.

Bluteau, Joshua M. 'Undercover—From Necessity to Luxury: The Evolution of Face Coverings during COVID-19.' *Fashion Theory* (2022). Online only: https://doi.org/10.1080/1362704X.2022.2129138.

Bolaki, Stella. *Illness as Many Narratives: Arts, Medicine and Culture*. Edinburgh: Edinburgh University Press, 2016.

Burton, Laini and Melkumova-Reynolds, Jana. '"My Leg Is a Giant Stiletto Heel": Fashioning the Prosthetised Body.' *Fashion Theory* 23, no.2 (2019): 195–218.

Butler, Judith. *Bodies That Matter*. London and New York: Routledge, 1993.

Charpy, Manuel. 'Craze and Shame: Rubber Clothing during the Nineteenth Century in Paris, London, and New York City.' *Fashion Theory* 16, no.4 (2012): 433–460.

Chong Kwan, Sara. 'The Ambient Gaze: Sensory Atmosphere and the Dressed Body.' In *Revisiting the Gaze: The Fashioned Body and the Politics of Looking*. London: Bloomsbury, 2020.

Clare, Eli. *Brilliant Imperfection: Grappling with Cure*. Durham and London: Duke University Press, 2017.

Davidson, Hilary. 'The Embodied Turn: Making and Remaking Dress as an Academic Practice.' *Fashion Theory* 23, no.3 (2019): 329–362.

Dolezal, Luna. 'Disability as Malleability: The Prosthetic Metaphor, Merleau-Ponty and the Case of Aimee Mullins.' In *Medial Bodies between Fiction and Faction: Reinventing Corporeality*, edited by Denisa Butnaru, 125–45. Bielfeeld: Verlag, 2020.

Dolezal, Luna. 'Representing Posthuman Embodiment: Considering Disability and the Case of Aimee Mullins.' *Women's Studies* 46, no.1 (2017): 60–75.

Eicher, Joanne B. 'Dress, the Senses, and Public, Private, and Secret Selves.' *Fashion Theory* 25, no.6 (2021): 777–797.

Entwistle, Joanne. 'Fashion and the Fleshy Body: Dress as Embodied Practice.' *Fashion Theory* 4, no.3 (2000): 323–347.

Ernsberger, Paul. 'Does social class explain the connection between weight and health?' In *The Fat Studies Reader*, edited by Esther Rothblum and Sondra Soloway, 25–36. New York: New York University Press, 2009.

Farren, Anne and Hutchison, Andrew. 'Cyborgs, New Technology, and the Body: The Changing Nature of Garments.' *Fashion Theory* 8, no.4 (2004) 461–475.

Foucault, Michel. *The Birth of the Clinic*. Trans. A.M. Sheridan. London: Routledge, 1989.

Gell, Alfred. *Art and Agency: An Anthropological Theory*. Oxford: Oxford University Press, 1998.

Gill, Rosalind. *Gender and the Media*. 7th edn. Cambridge: Polity Press, 2013.

Guthman, Julie. *Weighing In: Obesity, Food Justice, and the Limits of Capitalism*. Berkeley, CA: University of California Press, 2011.

Hardy, Susan and Corones, Anthony. 'Dressed to Heal: The Changing Semiotics of Surgical Dress.' *Fashion Theory* 20, no.1 (2016): 27–49.

Hardy, Susan and Corones, Anthony. 'The Nurse's Uniform as Ethopoietic Fashion.' *Fashion Theory* 21, no.5 (2017): 523–552.

Huber, S. J. 'The White Coat Ceremony: Contemporary Medical Ritual.' *Journal of Medical Ethics* 29 (2003): 364–366.https://doi.org/10.1136/jme.29.6.364

Hwang, Chanmi, McCoy, Lindsay and Shaw, Michele R. 'Redesigning Maternity Hospital Gowns.' *Fashion Practice* 14, no.1 (2022): 79–98.

Johnstone, Fiona 'Manifesto for a Visual Medical Humanities', *Medical Humanities* (blog), 31 July 2018, https://blogs.bmj.com/medical-humanities/2018/07/31/manifesto-for-a-visual-medical-humanities/.

Jones, Meredith. 'Cosmetic Surgery and the Fashionable Face.' *Fashion Theory* 16, no.2 (2012): 193–209.

Kafer, Alison. *Feminist, Queer, Crip*. Bloomington & Indianapolis: Indiana University Press, 2013.

Kanemoto, Emi and Allgayer, Sasha. 'Masks across borders: etiquette, threat and prevention.' *Journal of Applied Communication Research* 50:sup1 (2022): S24–S32.

Keough, Sara Beth. 'Masks and Materiality in The Era Of Covid-19.' *Geographical Review* 111, no.4 (2021): 558–570.

Kern Paster, Gail. *The Body Embarrased: Drama and the Discipline of Shame in Early Modern England.* New York: Cornell University Press, 1993.

Kim, Eunjung. *Curative Violence: Rehabilitating Disability, Gender, and Sexuality in Modern Korea.* Durham, N.C.: Duke University Press, 2017.

Kipp Caroline and Rule, Ana María. 'Masks for This Medical Moment. July 7, 2020.' *The Journal of Modern Craft* 14, no.1 (2021): 5–11.

Kipp, Caroline and Kretz, Kate. 'Masks, Art, Protection, and Politics. July 15, 2020.' *The Journal of Modern Craft* 14, no.1 (2021): 19–24.

Latour, Bruno and Weibel, Peter. 'From Realpolitik to Dingpolitik. Or, How to Make Things Public.' In *Making Things Public: Atmospheres of Democracy*, edited by Bruno Latour and Peter Weibel, 14–41. Cambridge, MA: MIT Press, 2005.

Latour, Bruno. *Reassembling the Social. An Introduction to Actor-Network Theory.* Oxford: Oxford University Press; 2005.

Lee, Yeseung. *Seamlessness: Making and (Un)Knowing in Fashion Practice*, Bristol: Intellect, 2016.

Markiewicz, Emma. 'Performing Health and Beauty in Eighteenth-Century England: The Significance of Hair in the Creation of Appearances.' *Fashion Theory* 22, no.6 (2018): 617–640.

Martin, M. *Selling Beauty: Cosmetics, Commerce, and French Society, 1750–1830.* Baltimore: Johns Hopkins University Press, 2009.

McBee-Black, Kerri. '"Making Life Easier": A Case Study Exploring the Development of Adaptive Apparel Design Innovations from a User-Centered Approach.' *Fashion Practice* 14, no.2 (2022): 203–224.

McRuer, Robert. 'A "Last Stand" Against Cure', *Ragged Edge Online*, 2006. http://www.raggededgemagazine.com/departments/closerlook/001144.html. [Accessed 20 February 2023.]

McRuer, Robert. 'Critical Investments: AIDS, Christopher Reeve, and Queer / Disability Studies.' *Journal of Medical Humanities* 23, no.3–4 (2002): 221–37.

Miller, Daniel, (1987) *Material Culture and Mass Consumption.* Oxford: Blackwell Publishers, 1987.

Mol, Annemarie. *The Logic of Care: Health and the Problem of Patient Choice.* Abingdon and New York: Routledge, 2008.

Negrin, Lleywellyn. 'Fashion as an embodied art form.' In *Carnal Knowledge: Towards a 'New Materialism' Through the Arts*, edited by Estelle Barrett & Barbara Bolt, 141–154. London: I.B. Tauris, 2013.

Parkins, Ilya. '"You'll Never Regret Going Bold": The Moods of Wedding Apparel on a Practical Wedding.' *Fashion Theory* 25, no.6 (2021): 799–817.

Porter, Roy. 'The Patient's View: Doing Medical History from Below.' *Theory and Society* 14, no.2 (1985): 175–198.

Rich, Emma, Monaghan, Lee F. and Aphramor, Lucy. 'Introduction: contesting obesity discourse and presenting an alternative'. In *Rethinking Obesity,* edited by Lee F. Monaghan, Emma Rich and Andrea E. Bombak, 1–35. Abingdon and New York: Routledge, 2022.

Rodríguez Muñoz, Bárbara. 'Introduction.' In *Health (Documents of Contemporary Art)*, edited by Bárbara Rodríguez Muñoz, 12–19. London and Cambridge MA: Whitechapel Gallery and the MIT Press, 2020.

Rosenberg, Charles E. *The Care of Strangers: The Rise of America's Hospital System.* Baltimore: Johns Hopkins University Press, 1995.

Rosenberg, Charles E. and Janet Golden (eds.). *Framing Disease: Studies in Cultural History: Health and Medicine in American Society.* New Brunswick, N.J.: Rutgers University Press, 1992.

Ruggerone, Lucia. 'The Feeling of Being Dressed: Affect Studies and the Clothed Body.' *Fashion Theory* 21, no.5 (2017): 573–593.

Sirasi, Nancy. *Medieval and Early Renaissance Medicine.* Chicago: University of Chicago Press, 1990.

Smelik, Anneke. 'Fractal Folds: The Posthuman Fashion of Iris van Herpen.' *Fashion Theory* 26, no.1 (2020): 5–26.

Smith, Giulia. 'Chronic Illness as Critique: Crip Aesthetics Across the Atlantic.' *Art History* 44, no.2 (2021): 286–310.

Smith, Marquard. 'The Vulnerable Articulate: James Gillingham, Aimee Mullins, and Matthew Barney.' In *The Prosthetic Impulse: From a Posthuman Present to a Biocultural Future*, edited by Marquard Smith and Joanna Morra, 45–72. Cambridge, Mass.: MIT Press, 2005.

Sobchack, Vivian. 'A Leg to Stand On: Prosthetics, Metaphor, and Materiality.' In *The Prosthetic Impulse: From A Posthuman Present to a Biocultural Future*, edited by Marquard Smith and Joanna Morra, 17–41. Cambridge, Mass.: MIT Press, 2006.

Spiegel, Jennifer Beth. 'The viral politics of masks: pandemic resistance and ontological performance.' *Text and Performance Quarterly* 42, no.2 (2022): 111–125.

Stauss, Renate. 'Passing as Fashionable, Feminine and Sane: "Therapy of Fashion" and the Normalization of Psychiatric Patients in 1960s US.' *Fashion Theory* 24, no.4 (2009): 601–637.

Tillotson, Jenny. 'Scentsory Design: A "Holistic" Approach to Fashion as a Vehicle to Deliver Emotional Well-being.' *Fashion Practice* 1, no.1 (2009): 33–61.

Tsakalidou, Maria. 'Analysing Anthropometric Measurement and Body Shape Data to Incorporate Body Asymmetry, due to Scoliosis, into Improved Clothing Sizing Systems.' *Fashion Practice* 9, no.3 (2017): 398–424.

Turkle, Sherry. *Evocative Objects: Things We Think With.* Cambridge, MA: MIT Press, 2007.

Ugrina, Luciana. 'Celebrity Biometrics: Norms, New Materialism, and the Agentic Body in Cosmetic Surgery Photography.' *Fashion Theory* 18, no.1 (2014): 27–44.

Vainshtein, Olga. '"I Have a Suitcase Just Full of Legs Because I Need Options for Different Clothing": Accessorizing Bodyscapes', *Fashion Theory* 16, no.2 (2015): 139–69.
Whitehead, Anne and Woods, Angela. 'Introduction'. In *The Edinburgh Companion to the Critical Medical Humanities*, edited by Anne Whitehead and Angela Woods, 1–31. Edinburgh: Edinburgh University Press, 2016.
Woodward, Sophie. *Why Women Wear What They Wear*. London: Berg, 2007.

Dawn Woolley

Things, as opposed to objects, are relational and caught up in a process of being and becoming.[1] Some of the things we possess increase our capacities and sense of self. For example, during transitional phases in life, possessions can play an important role in stabilising and maintaining one's sense of self. In psychoanalysis, objects may enable an infant or child to negotiate the transition between dependence and independence.[2] The symbolic self-completion thesis, a psychological theory, suggests that low self-esteem caused by a sense of incompleteness can be alleviated by the acquisition of objects, particularly for a cherished collection.[3] Russell Belk calls this 'self-plus-possessions' identity the 'extended self'.[4] He argues that the ability to control an object and be controlled by an object causes the object to be viewed as a part of the self. This suggests that objects and people impose identity characteristics on each other, and that extension is a mutual and collaborative process.

In 'Sitting Pretty: A Dress History of the L-Shaped Frame, the Side-Saddle Habit and the Design of Adaptive Wearables', Alison L Goodrum

[1] Martin Heidegger, 'The Thing', *Poetry, Language, Thought,* New York: Harper Perennial, 2001.

[2] D.W. Winicott, 'Transitional Objects and Transitional Phenomena', *International Journal of Psychoanalysis,* 34:2 (1953), 89–97.

[3] Robert A. Wicklund, and Peter M. Gollwitzer, *Symbolic Self Completion*, Hillsdale, NJ: Lawrence Erlbaum Associates, 1982.

[4] Russell Belk, Possessions and the Extended Self, *Journal of Consumer Research*, 15:2, (1988) 139–168, 140.

considers the way that fabric interacts with the body when seated in chairs and wheelchairs or riding side-saddle. From the mid-nineteenth to mid-twentieth century, female equestrians were expected to sit side-saddle. Clothing not designed for this purpose was uncomfortable and potentially dangerous: voluminous skirts could frighten the horse and get caught on the saddle if the rider fell, causing them to be dragged along the ground. They also bunched, creased, and rubbed causing discomfort. However, specifically designed side-saddle garments became collaborating things within an entangled activity in which 'multiple layers of horseflesh, saddle leather, habit fabric and human sinew operate in dynamic combination, pressing against, responding to, and impacting on, each other to form a partnership that is corporeal, material, tactile and sensual in mix'.[5] Goodrum notes that how we sit is 'infused with political doctrine and … systems of cultural etiquette'.[6] In the global North, sitting is coded differently for women and men, signifying the amount of space they are permitted to inhabit. In the Victorian period, dress styles, such as crinoline cages and bustles further inhibited seating postures for women. In *Queer Phenomenology*, Sara Ahmed writes that some objects are readily available to us or come into view when we choose a particular path or orientation.[7] These choices in direction and bodily movement are also affected by social expectations and restrictions. In relation to Edmund Husserl's writing table Ahmed asks, if this is the site where his thoughts unfold, what are the conditions that have made the table available to him? In answer she hypothesises that a wife keeps the table clean and children's hands away from its papers. Husserl is able to orientate himself towards the table, the productive platform for his thoughts, because he is also able to turn away from family life and the reproductive space of the kitchen table. Bodies are shaped by the types of objects that are available to them, including objects that support gendered roles relating to intellectual labour, care, and leisure. Ahmed writes that queer phenomenology 'turns the tables' by turning or retuning us towards other objects.[8]

The tables are turned and returned on assistive apparatus in the dance performances discussed in Jana Melkumova-Reynolds' chapter 'On

[5] Alison L Goodrum, 'A Dress History Of The L-Shaped Frame, The Side-Saddle Habit And The Design Of Adaptive Wearables', this volume, 87.

[6] Goodrum, 'A Dress History Of The L-Shaped Frame', 80.

[7] Sara Ahmed, *Queer Phenomenology: Orientations, Objects, Others*, Durham and London: Duke University Press, 2006, 116.

[8] Ahmed, *Queer Phenomenology*.

Crutches, Choreography and (Crip) Care: Curative Objects and Palliative Things in Two Performance Pieces'. In *bODY rEMIX*, the mobility aids and medical props are 'rigid, uncooperative, reluctant to negotiate': they impede the performers or encourage antagonistic actions between them.[9] The performers attempt to master and control the prosthesis, presenting them as a burden that must be overcome. In *The Way You Look (at me) Tonight*, however, Melkumova-Reynolds, interprets the use of crutches by performer Claire Cunningham as a collaborative entanglement in which the crutches activate a 'relational space' and 'ongoing processes of entanglement with other bodies and things, and must be thought of as constituting, and being constituted by, the webs of relations and intra-actions they are enmeshed in'.[10] They are 'enablers and enactors' that turn the tables on common conceptions of mobility aids because they do not aim for mastery or minimise vulnerability and dependency.

The crutches in Cunningham's performance also mediate her interactions with audience members as she pauses and hovers before lightly touching down on an arm or leg. The crutches become an 'instrument of care' in allowing the performer to attune her attention to the potential participant.[11] Touch and attunement are similarly employed in Emily Beaney's 'Breaking the Fall' to 'convey the tensions, tenderness and entanglements of illness and familial caring experiences'.[12] Beaney notes that touch, unlike vision, brings objects close to the body, increasing our sense of involvement with them and responsibility to them. Medical imaging technologies and diagnostic terms have a distancing effect. They universalise experiences of illness while minimising the importance of 'the embodied, personal and social qualities of illness'.[13] Beaney's performance props combine soft, cushioning material, with hard constraining structures and intrusive, tangling headwear to convey the complexities of participating in diagnosis, treatment, and practices of care. Medical devices are decentred, allowing the ill body to form collaborative entanglements with materials, through which a variety of knowledge may be shared.

In their contradictory functions as enablers and obstacles, the things in Goodrum, Melkumova-Reynolds and Beaney's chapters demonstrate the

[9] Jana Melkumova-Reynolds, 'On Crutches, Choreography And (Crip) Care: Curative Objects And Palliative Things In Two Performance Pieces', this volume, 45.

[10] Melkumova-Reynolds, 'On Crutches, Choreography And (Crip) Care', 54.

[11] Melkumova-Reynolds, 'On Crutches, Choreography And (Crip) Care', 52.

[12] Emily Beaney, 'Breaking the Fall', this volume, 60.

[13] Beaney, 'Breaking the Fall', 70.

'contextual flickering' described by Sonia Bernac in her materialist investigation of prostheses. In 'The Itches: embodiment and distributed meaning in the age of technological entanglement' Bernac notes that body-prosthetic entanglements are not a relationship between two distinct entities but are 'complex anatomies of new hybrid-emergent selves' 'complicating ideas of the whole and the fragment'.[14] New capabilities and processes emerge through our entanglements with things. For example, cochlear implants stimulate the auditory nerve rather than amplify sound vibrations like standard hearing aids 'creating an entirely different way of processing sound in people with profound hearing impairments'.[15] As Bernac notes, contemporary prostheses often exceed the effectivity and lifespan of the bodily circuits or organs they replace or enhance, and may even produce entirely new capabilities and senses through these emergent assemblages.

Jane Bennett describes assemblages as ad hoc groupings of diverse 'vibrant materials' and 'living, throbbing confederations' acting in alliance and sometimes against each other.[16] The power relations are unequal but no 'central head' governs the assemblage, and like the cochlear implant and auditory nerve, the grouping produces emergent properties that act in ways that isolated components cannot. Bennett writes: 'Each member or proto-member of the assemblage has a certain vital force, but there is also an effective proper to the grouping as such: an agency *of* the assemblage'.[17] Assemblages are greater than the sum of their parts, and can help and hinder, like the crutches, riding clothes, prostheses, and materialities of care described in the chapters that follow. In paying close attention to these collaborating things, we can experience 'a fuller range of the nonhuman powers circulating around and within human bodies'.[18] Viewing things as collaborators within non-hierarchical assemblages offers an opportunity to decentralise the reductive notion of the ideal human that is modelled on a male subject without illness or disability. However, as Bernac notes, technological entanglements can lead to an outsourcing of decision-making and a suspension of ethics that reinforce discriminatory ideals and oppression. Collaborative things can extend our powers to harm as well as heal.

[14] Sonia Bernac, 'The Itches: embodiment and distributed meaning in the age of technological entanglement', this volume, 102 and 105.

[15] Bernac, The Itches, 110.

[16] Jane Bennett, *Vibrant Matter: a political ecology of things*, Durham: Duke University Press, 2010, 23.

[17] Bennett, *Vibrant Matter*, 24.

[18] Bennett *Vibrant Matter*, ix.

References

Ahmed, Sara. *Queer Phenomenology: Orientations, Objects, Others*. Durham and London: Duke University Press, 2006.

Belk, Russell. Possessions and the Extended Self. In *Journal of Consumer Research*. 15:2 (1988), 139–168.

Bennett, Jane. *Vibrant Matter: A political ecology of things*. Durham: Duke University Press, 2010.

Heidegger, Martin. 'The Thing'. In *Poetry, Language, Thought*. New York: Harper Perennial, 2001.

Wicklund, Robert A. and Peter M. Gollwitzer. *Symbolic Self Completion*. Hillsdale, NJ: Lawrence Erlbaum Associates, 1982.

Winicott, D.W. Transitional Objects and Transitional Phenomena. In *International Journal of Psychoanalysis*, 34:2 (1953), 89–97.

CHAPTER 2

On Crutches, Choreography and (Crip) Care: Curative Objects and Palliative Things in Two Performance Pieces

Jana Melkumova-Reynolds

For G. F.

Snapshot 1: two tall, slim, long-limbed, impossibly athletic, nearly nude female dancers with sleek hairdos enter stage right. They are, quite literally, joined at the hip: a leg brace is holding together the right leg of one and the left leg of the other, making their (already perfectly coordinated, though odd and peculiar) movements flow with even more synchronicity and rhythmic precision. From the left, enters another, equally lean woman, clad in suggestive underwear which consists of thin strips of white material similar to those that constitute the leg brace worn by the two other dancers. Her outfit—a harness bra and harness panties—looks like it has come

J. Melkumova-Reynolds (✉)
London School of Economics and Political Science, London, UK
e-mail: Y.M.Reynolds@lse.ac.uk

D. Woolley et al. (eds.), *Wearable Objects and Curative Things*, Palgrave Studies in Fashion and the Body,
https://doi.org/10.1007/978-3-031-40017-9_2

straight out of the medical BDSM fetish scene; bandage meets bondage. She is using a medical walking cane that is too short for her tall frame, which is further amplified by her pointe shoes. The cane hinders rather than helps her movement, and she theatrically struggles with it: due to its shortness it gets in the way of her maintaining her balance; the awkward angles it forces her body into interfere with her balletic uprightness. After a series of grotesque and uncomfortable moves, she relinquishes it. Immediately, her virtuoso technique becomes apparent as she performs a sexually charged, animalistic dance at the two barres that have been placed in the middle of the stage by two male dancers while she was grappling with the cane. Even now, her dance is far from smooth; her vigorous, sharp moves suggest anguish, contorting her body in poses that invoke the iconographies of hysteria, and yet they are way more controlled and less painful to watch than her interaction with the cane was.

Snapshot 2: a boyish, petite woman wearing jeans, a loose T-shirt and a pixie haircut, is moving on crutches around the performance floor, populated with sparsely seated members of the audience—some in chairs, some in wheelchairs, some on cushions—and a tall male dancer lying on the ground. Something about her physique, other than the crutches, suggests a non-normative body; it might be her unusual torso-to-legs proportion, the inward turn of her feet, or the intensely focused attention she pays to the ground while moving. I will allow myself to cite Julia Watts Belser's beautifully detailed description of this part of the performance rather than trying to write it anew:

> [The female dancer] Claire moves fluidly among the audience on stage, her steps fast and light, the music up-tempo and staccato. As she approaches Jess [the male dancer], she plants her crutches to either side of his legs, then levers her body up, lands her feet upon his knees. She lingers there for a moment, then spins off her perch, tucking herself into a curl, her body held horizontal by the crutches, one breath of perfect suspension before she sweeps her leg into a slow, deliberate curve that brings her feet back to the ground. She approaches again, spiralling her way through another portion of the audience [...] Crutches allow her to hover in the air [...] The next time she spins, she brings her feet into contact with a member of the audience, alighting on someone's knees, touching down against a woman's crossed arms.[1]

[1] Julia Watts Belser, 'Improv and the angel: Disability dance, embodied ethics, and Jewish Biblical narrative', *Journal of Religious Ethics* 47:3 (2019) 443–469, 461.

The first snapshot describes a scene from *bODY_rEMIX/gOLDBERG_vARIATIONS*, a ballet (to use the term utilised on the project's website) staged by French Canadian choreographer Marie Chouinard and performed by the dancers from her dance company. The second snapshot captures a score in *The Way You Look (at me) Tonight*, a 'dance-based performance project' by San Francisco-based choreographer and performer Jess Curtis and Scottish artist Claire Cunningham.[2] Both performances incorporate medical assistive devices: in *bODY_rEMIX* this includes a range of objects such as canes, crutches, leg braces, rollators and walking frames (all used by dancers without visible disabilities), while in *The Way You Look...* both the disabled dancer, Claire Cunningham, and at several points her able-bodied partner, Jess Curtis, use extendable crutches.

Prosthetic and assistive devices have been utilised by both disabled and non-disabled artists over the last two decades in increasingly creative and novel ways. This use has been celebrated as a means of resignifying objects that had previously been construed, and read, as medicalised, undesirable or even degraded. As performance theorist Bree Hadley notes, 'symbols associated with the disabled body are being reappropriated and recontextualised not just by disabled artists, but by other artists, too, as positive symbols of difference'.[3] Such 'positive' reinscribing of new meanings on medical items through their use in arts and culture has been discussed at length by scholars from a variety of fields.[4] The current chapter, however, moves beyond the semiotic reading of assistive devices and considers their use through material-semiotic and non-representational lenses. That is, rather than analysing what crutches and other medicalised props *stand for* in these performance pieces, I aim to elucidate what they *do*. Borrowing from an actor-network theory approach to material culture, I am interested in objects' and things' actancy and their capacity to 'authorise, allow,

[2] Jess Curtis, '"The Way You Look (at me) Tonight": Touch Tours, Haptic Practices, and Sensory Strategies', in *Thinking Touch in Partnering and Contact Improvisation: Philosophy, Pedagogy, Practice*, ed. Malaika Sarco-Thomas, 10–26, Cambridge: Cambridge Scholars Publishing, 2020, 10.

[3] Bree Hadley, *Disability, Public Space Performance and Spectatorship: Unconscious Performers*, London: Palgrave Macmillan, 2014, 152.

[4] For discussions about the use of prostheses in photography, fashion and visual arts, see Laini Burton and Jana Melkumova-Reynolds, '"My leg is a giant stiletto heel": Fashioning the prosthetised body', *Fashion Theory: Journal of Dress, Body and Culture*, 23:2 (2019) 195–218; Jana Melkumova-Reynolds, '"Let me be your stimy toy": Fashioning disability, cripping fashion', in *Dangerous Bodies: New Perspectives on Fashion and Transgression*, eds. Royce Mahawatte and Jacki Willson, London: Palgrave Macmillan, 2023.

afford, encourage, permit, suggest, influence, block, render possible, forbid, and so on', as well as—in fact, more than—in their signifying power.[5]

Conceived as a response to the title and theme of this volume, this chapter considers how medical devices used in contemporary dance and performance are configured, in some cases, as curative and in others, as palliative; in some cases, as things, and in others, as objects. It enquires how, by affording different entanglements—between bodies, things/objects, space and other bodies—crutches and other medical devices in the two performances produce different temporalities, corporealities, subjectivities and ontologies. My readings are informed by queer and crip theories, phenomenology, psychoanalysis and by my own embodied experiences, both of dance and dance training (albeit as an amateur) and of using an assistive device—in my case, a back brace (albeit a lot less consistently than my doctors would have wished for).

I begin with defining some of the key concepts I use in my analysis. I then turn to a close reading of the use of crutches in the two performance pieces through the lens of these conceptual frameworks, demonstrating how such use construes different paradigms of embodiment, (dis)ability and relationships between bodies and objects/things.

2.1 Curative/Palliative

In her seminal book *Feminist, Queer, Crip*, disability theorist Alison Kafer discusses 'a curative imaginary' which is 'an understanding of disability that not only expects and assumes intervention but also cannot imagine or comprehend anything other than intervention'.[6] Such an imaginary is predicated on the idea of disability—or indeed any disease—as a problem to be resolved or, at the very least, mitigated. In this normalising paradigm, a 'cure' for a disabled or diseased body/mind is something that is sought by default. The logic of a curative imaginary, then, is that of human perfectibility.

It is not difficult to see how this logic implies a certain temporality, one that Kafer refers to as 'curative time' where 'the only appropriate disabled mind/body is one cured or moving toward cure'.[7] 'Moving toward' is an important feature of the curative imaginary whose defining characteristic

[5] Bruno Latour, *Reassembling the Social*, Oxford: Oxford University Press, 2005, 72.

[6] Alison Kafer, *Feminist, Queer, Crip*, Bloomington: Indiana University Press, 2013, 27.

[7] Kafer, *Feminist*, 28.

is the injunction to progress, to aim—and work—towards overcoming, or at least *mastering*, the disease at some point in the future. Such an imaginary relies, to use Sara Ahmed's term, on 'promissory forms of happiness'[8]; on the idea that 'happiness is what you get if you reach certain points'.[9] In a curative imaginary, being 'well'—a mastery of the body, of the self and, ultimately, of the real—is (1) Attainable (2) Desirable (3) Not yet achieved.

The conceptual opposite of the curative model of care within medicine is the palliative model where care is aimed to alleviate symptoms, rather than remove the cause of the disease. To use Ahmed's language again, this model eschews the 'promise of happiness' and instead operates from the premise that there is no cure for the condition in question. In a sense, the palliative model is an instantiation of Heideggerian 'Being-towards-death',[10] just like the curative model can be seen as a form of 'being-towards-happiness'—or, perhaps more appropriately for the purposes of this chapter, 'being-towards-mastery'. Rather than striving to make the subject fundamentally 'better' in the future, palliative care focuses on making their lived experience (ultimately, of living towards death) more tolerable in the present.

The time paradigm of palliative care is clearly different from that of the curative model because it is not underpinned by the idea of progress. In its refusal of futurity, palliative time shares many similarities with queer time as conceptualised by queer theorists such as Lee Edelman: eschewing 'the constraining mandate of futurism' and embracing the idea that there may be 'no future', it moves beyond the familiar tropes of purposeful linear development and growth, allowing for stillness and repetition.[11] In her poignant meditation on time and care, psychoanalyst Lisa Baraitser invites her reader 'to think of how we might attempt to take care of time when it seems to pool, dammed up by a foreclosed future that no longer brings [a] promise'.[12] In this passage, she is not talking about palliative time as such, and yet her discussions of 'time's suspension—modes of waiting, staying, delaying, enduring, persisting, repeating, maintaining, preserving and remaining—that produce felt experiences of time not passing', which she

[8] Sara Ahmed, *The Promise of Happiness*, Durham: Duke University Press, 2010, 160.

[9] Ahmed, *The Promise*, 26.

[10] Martin Heidegger, *Being and Time*, Oxford: Blackwell Publishing, 1962.

[11] Lee Edelman, *No Future: Queer Theory and the Death Drive*, Durham: Duke University Press, 2004, 4.

[12] Lisa Baraitser, *Enduring Time*, London: Bloomsbury, 2017, 12.

uses to refer to temporalities of other forms of care, could be productive to think with about the temporal modalities of palliation, too.[13]

Etymologically, the term 'palliate' is thought to originate from Latin 'palla' (a garment) and 'pallium' (a cloak).[14] 'The word 'pallium' was used to refer to a garment worn by Greeks made from wool, flax, or cotton'.[15] Another linguistic tradition traces it to the proto-Indo-European word 'pelte' which means to 'shield', and some advocates prefer this interpretation as they find the concept of 'cloaking' to be ridden with the negative connotations of 'covering up' or 'masking'.[16] Thus, medical humanities scholar David Morris contends that palliative care 'shields the patients from assault of symptoms' and offers 'security amid circumstances full of risk and uncertainty'.[17] Such a reading, he maintains, is richer and more conducive to a recognition of the importance of palliative care than its association with 'cloaking'. What Morris seems to overlook here, however, is how vital cloaking itself can be—one only has to think of security blankets and their role in comforting the child, or the use of emergency blankets in first aid.

In this chapter, I would like to think of objects and things as curative or palliative. Curative objects/things aim to 'cure' us, that is, to make us better. They are our aids in the projects of self-mastery and self-improvement, there to propel us towards our desired aims and goals. In Ahmed's terms, they are 'happy objects'—objects that 'become happiness pointers, as if to follow their point would be to find happiness [...] in directing ourselves toward this or that object, we are aiming somewhere else: toward a happiness that is presumed to follow'.[18] Assisting us in our quest for the 'good life', curative objects/things are telos-oriented and, in the original sense of the word, prosthetic: the term 'prosthesis', derived, via late Latin *prostheticus*, from ancient Greek *prosthetikós*, 'adding; repletive; giving additional

[13] Baraitser, *Enduring Time*, 12.

[14] Salimah H. Meghani, 'A concept analysis of palliative care in the United States', *Journal of Advanced Nursing*, 46: 2 (2004) 152–161, 155.

[15] Meghani, A concept analysis, 155.

[16] David B. Morris, The cloak and the shield: A thumbnail history of palliation, *Illness, Crisis and Loss*, 6 (1998) 229–232, 231.

[17] Morris, The cloak, 231.

[18] Ahmed, *The Promise*, 26.

power', has the idea of extending, building up and developing embedded in its etymology.[19]

Conversely, palliative objects/things do not aim to change us into better versions of us, nor to aid our progress; they are non-teleological. They step in to shroud us, comfort us, stay with us while we are living through pain, anguish and rupture; to care for us without attempting to cure us. One of the etymological traditions links the word 'palliate' to 'pall', a cloud (as in 'cast a pall').[20] A cloud floats, hovers over,[21] dwells, cloaks. I propose to think of palliative things as those that enable and enact hovering, cloaking, dwelling, and being-with.

2.2 Objects/Things

Before I move on to the analysis of the two performances, I need to disentangle another dichotomy that the current volume's title invites us to consider, that of objects and things. The scholarship that draws a distinction between these two terms builds on Martin Heidegger's essay *The Thing*. Heidegger differentiates between objects and things by suggesting that an 'object' is 'that which stands before, over against, opposite us' whereas the thing 'stands forth', which 'has the sense of stemming from somewhere, whether this be a process of self-making or of being made by another'.[22] An object, in other words, is static, finished, and opposed to the subject (and, possibly, to other objects), while a thing is processual and relational—it is a 'bearing-upon, a concern'.[23] Its processual nature is expressed in Heidegger's proposition that 'a thing things' in a 'worlding world'.[24]

[19] Henry George Liddell and Robert Scott, *A Greek–English Lexicon*, Oxford: Clarendon Press, 1940. Available at http://www.perseus.tufts.edu/hopper/text?doc=Perseus:text:1999.04.0057:entry=prosqetiko/s (accessed 15 February 2023).

[20] Elliot Vredenburg, 'Notes toward a meteorology of the cloud', *Surveillance & Society*, 13:2 (2015) 283–291.

[21] Lisa Baraitser, drawing on the work of Maria Puig de la Bellacasa, mentions 'hovering' as one of the temporal modes of care in a recent interview—see Laura Kemmer, Annika Kühn and Vanessa Weber, 2021, Pandemic times. A conversation with Lisa Baraitser about the temporal politics of COVID-19, *Ephemera: Theory & Politics in Organization*, 21:1, 21–30.

[22] Martin Heidegger, 'The Thing', *Poetry, Language, Thought* (trans. A. Hofstadter. New York: Harper & Row, 1971).

[23] Heidegger, 'The Thing', 173.

[24] Heidegger, 'The Thing', 178

Building on Heidegger's ideas, anthropologist Tim Ingold proposes to think of things as 'gatherings of forces'.[25] He uses the tree as an example of such a gathering: can we really think of a tree, he asks, without including the bark, the creatures that live in the bark, the algae and lichens that cover it, or the currents of the wind that form its 'character'? In other words, 'What is tree and what is not-tree? Where does the tree end and the rest of the world begin?'[26] In a similar vein, he continues, a building cannot be easily disentangled from its environment: 'Rainwater drips through the roof where the wind has blown off a tile, feeding a fungal growth that threatens to decompose the timbers, the gutters are full of rotten leaves', and both human and non-human inhabitants (insects, rodents, pets) constantly come and go.[27] For this reason, to Ingold, 'not unlike the tree, the real house is a gathering of lives, and to inhabit it is to join in the gathering, or in Heidegger's terms, to participate with the thing in its thinging'.[28] A thing, then, is an assemblage of multiple simultaneous, overlapping or conflicting, open-ended processes, 'goings-on'.

Because a thing is emergent, processual and relational, it constitutes other things (including bodies) as such, too. An object presupposes a subject that stands before it, observes it or acts upon it—that is, exercises mastery over it[29]; but a thing summons other forms of relating. Ingold notes that '[t]o observe a thing is not to be locked out but to be invited in to the gathering' that it is.[30] I believe the philosopher Michael Polanyi refers to a similar way of relating to things when he speaks about 'indwelling', that is, experiencing things by 'pour[ing] ourselves into them',[31] 'dwelling' in them, 'depriv[ing] them of their character as external objects'.[32] (The term 'pouring' will become pertinent to my analysis later in this chapter). The collapse of the subject-object dichotomy, invoked here, is a fundamental feature of flat ontologies—that is, ontologies that

[25] Tim Ingold, 'Bringing things to life: Creative entanglements in a world of materials', *Realities Working Papers*, 15 (2010) 2–14, 4.

[26] Ingold, 'Bringing things to life', 4.

[27] Ingold, 'Bringing things to life', 5.

[28] Ingold, 'Bringing things to life', 5.

[29] For a discussion of 'projects of mastery' see, for instance, Leo Bersani, 'Sociality and Sexuality', *Is the Rectum a Grave? and other essays*, London and Chicago: University of Chicago Press, 2010, 102–119.

[30] Ingold, 'Bringing things to life', 4.

[31] Michael Polanyi, 'Sense-giving and sense-reading', *Philosophy: The Journal of the Royal Institute of Philosophy*, 42:162 (1967) 301–325, 303.

[32] Polanyi, 'Sense-giving and sense-reading', 304.

do not privilege any actors/objects over others.[33] In such ontologies, the focus is not individual actors, subjects or objects, but on relations and processes of mutual constitution between various actants in a network (or, to use Ingold's term, meshwork). Things, in the sense defined above, belong in, and produce, flat ontologies, while objects enunciate the more classical subject-object ontologies.

Now that these terms have been defined, however briefly and crudely, I will proceed to consider prosthetics as curative or palliative objects or things.

2.3 Crutches and *Agōn*: *bODY_rEMIX/gOLDBERG_vARIATIONS*

Since the late 1970s, Marie Chouinard has been known for her viscerally moving, provocative, deeply sensual and often troubling performances. These may feature 'the reanimation of the human body via technology and prosthetics; a playful reinscription of the aesthetics and traditions of classical ballet; [...] metamorphosis underpinning the shocking, transgressive, and explicit; a hesitation between the animalistic and the otherworldly'.[34] After over a decade as a solo performer and choreographer, in 1990 she founded Compagnie Marie Chouinard, which went on to become an internationally acclaimed dance company. *bODY_rEMIX/gOLDBERG_vARIATIONS*, premiered at Venice Biennale in 2005, comprises two acts of 45 minutes each, in which ten contemporary dancers (who undertook pointe training for the performance) perform physically vigorous and increasingly intense and bizarre vignettes that involve their interaction with each other, two barres, a clothes rack and an array of medical devices and other props. This is accompanied with a musical score by acousmatic composer Louis Dufort comprising extracts from a 1981 recording of Glenn Gould's rendition of *Goldberg Variations* by Johann Sebastian Bach, interspersed with cut-up, slowed down or sped up and/or heavily reverberated clips from Gould's radio interview; and, at several

[33] See Jane Bennett, *Vibrant Matter*, London and Durham: Duke University Press, 2010; Graham Harman, *Immaterialism: Objects and Social Theory*, Cambridge: Polity Press, 2016; Latour, *Reassembling the Social*.

[34] Alanna Thain, The in-tensions of extensions: Compagnie Marie Chouinard's 'bODYrEMIX/gOLDBERG VARIATIONS', *differences: A Journal of Feminist Cultural Studies*, 19/1 (2008) 71–95, 80.

points, the surreal 'distorted grunts, groans and breaths' emitted by one of the dancers who carries a microphone in her mouth.[35] The show has toured Asia, Europe and North America and received numerous accolades. It has also been praised by scholars of performance and dance. Thus, in her compelling and sophisticated analysis, Alanna Thain considers *bODY_rEMIX* as an exercise in transcending the material and opening up the immaterial, virtual dimension of the dancers' bodies, which 'activates the intensive movement of affect as a resonant exploration of the in-between'.[36] Similarly, Hadley suggests that the prostheses used in the show 'challenge the dancers' bodies to go beyond their normal movement habits, to find new movements, new relationships and new modes of being'.[37] I will come back to some of these discussions later in the chapter.

The performance starts with a female dancer wearing a single pointe shoe standing on her pointe-less, bare foot and knocking the other, pointe-wearing foot on the floor forcefully. The knocking is loud, persistent, unremitting; the kind that makes you certain the knocker is prepared to break in if their call goes unanswered. Pointes and other prosthetics in this performance are, indeed, tools for breaking in: into space, into another dancer's kinesphere,[38] and into the audience's comfort zone.

Such breaking in is necessitated by the profoundly agonistic nature of *bODY_rEMIX*. The performance unfolds as an intense struggle of the dancers with both human and non-human adversaries. This combative tenor becomes pronounced early on, in a scene where two male dancers move the two barres that were previously standing side-by-side and position them in a such a way that they enclose the space, turning what was a ballet class-like setup into a space reminiscent of a boxing ring. They face each other for a few long and tense seconds in what looks like a stand-off and proceed to perform a duet bristling with forceful and seductive lunges, chest-butts and headbutts. The trope of a battle—gripping, at times extremely uncomfortable to watch yet impossible to look away from—has a long genealogy within the history of theatre and the performing arts as the cultural imaginary of *agōn*, the ancient Greek term that can be

[35] Hadley, *Disability*, 160.

[36] Thain, 'The in-tensions', 79.

[37] Hadley, *Disability*, 162.

[38] Kinesphere is 'the sphere around the body whose periphery can be reached by easily extended limbs without stepping away from that place which is the point of support when standing on one foot'—see Rudolf Laban, *Choreutics*, London: Macdonald & Evans, 1966, 10.

translated as 'contest' or 'debate'. The ethics and aesthetics of *agōn* underpinned much of ancient Greece's cultural, social and political life and was the cornerstone of ancient theatrical tragedy and spectator sports. The enjoyment of watching *agōn* as entertainment is, needless to say, still deeply entrenched in Western culture, and I have wondered if *bODY rEMIX* was conceived to make the spectator at once aware of their own enjoyment and slightly embarrassed about it.

In *bODY_rEMIX*, the *agōn* onstage often involves a contest between the human and the prosthetic device: we watch the dancer's attempts to tame an uncomfortable cane, to master the rigidity of crutches and the constraints of walking frames that are perpetually too short for the dancers' height and force them into difficult, often untenable positions. The viewer soon comes to resent the medical items onstage because they clearly stand in the way of the dancers' athletic perfection, thus frustrating the spectator's scopophilic desires. The props are the easily identifiable antagonists in the show; a lot of the time they are plot devices in the agonistic encounters staged by Chouinard, turning what might otherwise be a smooth and eminently watchable contemporary ballet into a steeplechase or, as a comment under a video extract of the performance on YouTube puts it, into 'survival horror'.

When they are not 'standing against' the dancers, the medical devices become allies in the performer's battle against the world, which may include other objects or dancers. Thus, there is a disturbing scene where a female dancer approaches another who is lying on the floor, seemingly exhausted, and pokes her chest with a crutch. Soon, they are performing a fight-like dance, lashing out at each other, in turns, with crutches and with pointe shoes, all while maintaining their exquisite gracefulness. This is one of the many instances in the ballet where crutches and pointes assume similar roles; those of slicing through the space, extending into it and aggressively occupying it. Such slicing into and occupying is played out on the sonic level, too: both crutches and pointes are used to produce sharp, penetrating sounds, be it knocking, clanging or stomping. For instance, there is a particularly grotesque and provocative score where a man on crutches enters the stage with a third crutch attached to his waistline like a strap-on dildo. He approaches a clothes rack and violently thrusts against it, his strap-on hitting it with a loud, piercing metallic noise.

Crutches and other assistive devices, then, activate the stage as an agonistic space. At times, they are the drivers of the struggle, creating orientations and spatial conditions that need to be overcome by the dancers; at others, they aid such overcoming. By engaging with them, the dancers enter into fantastical and phantasmagorical assemblages with these items and with each other. These assemblages offer openings for rethinking the human form—on more than one occasion, the way performers are compelled to position themselves in order to use the prosthetics makes them look like insects, birds, or other non-human beings. Importantly, however, there is never any sense of fusion or incorporation between the dancers and the objects; on the contrary, their relationship is reliant on a continuous and riotous (re)production of difference between them.

Chouinard's choice of devices here is interesting: a crutch, both literally and metaphorically, is something that is meant to take on some of the body's weight, to ease the burden inherent in its (uniquely human condition of) uprightness. And yet, except for one scene where a dancer leans back on her crutches to watch her colleague perform a vigorous routine, in *bODY_rEMIX* they are never used for support. In fact, they become less and less crutch-like as the performance progresses. At one point, a male dancer uses a total of five extremely short crutches; two of them are ostensibly used to prop him up (albeit in a surreal, difficult pose), but the others are not: a short crutch is coming out of his mouth, another crutch is strapped to his forehead, and yet another one to his back. He moves around the stage in an awkward diagonal position, as if permanently coming out of a press-up; his movements are permeated by the same anguished and frantic energy that is palpable throughout *bODY_rEMIX*. The shapes he adopts are mainly unrecognisable, even to the eye of an experienced dance spectator. This is one of the most interesting parts of the performance as it does conjure radically different possibilities of the body: the crutches, which are attached to different parts of the dancer's body, noticeably shift his centre of gravity, thus making for a novel relationship with the ground and, by extension, with the rest of the space, and enabling what Thain refers to as 'a different bodily kinestruct'.[39] Ultimately, however, the crutches here continue to *produce* rather than reduce the dancer's struggle, and produce and reaffirm the dancer's alterity to the world, including the crutches themselves.

What, then, are we to make of the role of prosthetics in *bODY rEMIX*? I propose, firstly, that they are best read as objects rather than things. As Ingold explains, drawing on Heidegger, 'an object stands before us as a

[39] Thain, 'The in-tensions of Extensions', 72.

fait accompli, presenting its congealed, outer surfaces to our inspection. It is defined by its very 'overagainstness' in relation to the setting in which it is placed'.[40] This would be an apt description of the use of props in Chouinard's choreography: they stand in the dancers' way, interfering in their spatial explorations and obstructing their movement. They are rigid, uncooperative, reluctant to negotiate. On the few occasions when they are not working against the dancers, they are used to extend the dancer's body and colonise the space around it. In that sense, they help to render dancers' bodies into objects—also determined by 'overagainstness'—as well, enabling them to acquire, however temporarily, what Leo Bersani might call a 'mastery [that] places the subject in the world on the subject's own terms'.[41] Such mastery, in his analysis, belongs to a particular 'relational system' in which '[r]elationality is grounded in antagonism and misapprehension, which means that to meet the world is always to see the world as a place where I am not', and 'the subject is either in danger of being stolen or has already suffered a loss of self'.[42]

Furthermore, they are objects that foster a curative paradigm in which even the most 'abled' body, like those of the muscular and agile dancers of Compagnie Marie Chouinard, is seen as always already disabled. This is particularly apparent in the several scenes where female dancers are seen only wearing one pointe shoe: the pointe-less leg looks vulnerable, too soft, too short, almost lame. Such a body is constantly struggling to assert itself and its position of mastery in relation to the world and to other bodies; it is incomplete and, despite its athleticism, muscularity and stamina, not-quite-there-yet, and therefore permanently on a quest to get 'there'. In another essay, Bersani speaks of the consciousness constantly forming 'affectively motivated projects that essentially oppose us to the world, projects whose satisfaction requires mastery of otherness'.[43] Here, otherness is used not (only) in terms of identity (racial, sexual and other forms of difference) but refers to everything that is 'not-me', which might include one's own body. The dancers in *bODY_rEMIX* are grappling for such mastery throughout the performance. While *bODY_rEMIX* is not,

[40] Ingold, 'Bringing things to life', 4.

[41] Leo Bersani, 'Sociality and Sexuality', *Is the Rectum a Grave? and other essays*, London and Chicago: University of Chicago Press, 2010, 102–119, 110.

[42] Bersani, 'Sociality and Sexuality', 110.

[43] Leo Bersani, 'Psychoanalysis and the Aesthetic Subject', *Is The Rectum a Grave? And Other Essays*, London and Chicago: University of Chicago Press, 2010, 139–153, 149.

as Thain asserts,[44] 'about' disability as such, I would argue it is about the inherent incompleteness of the human that underpins a need to strive for progress, for completeness, for a contained, coherent and commanding subjectivity.

The time of *bODY_rEMIX* is, to use Julia Kristeva's terminology, 'time as project, teleology, linear and prospective unfolding; time as departure, progression, and arrival' which also 'renders explicit a rupture, an expectation, or an anguish'.[45] It is, in other words, a corollary of curative time, of being-towards-cure, or being-towards-mastery. Crutches, canes and other medical devices in the show are *curative objects* insomuch as, even when they do not enact or promise a cure, they enable and underpin the curative paradigm that is central to the performance. Whether helping or hindering the dancers, they are implicated in, and productive of, the 'projects of mastery' that *bODY_rEMIX* conjures, a mastery of the subject over objects.

2.4 Crutches and Care: *The Way You Look (at me) Tonight*

First performed in 2016, *The Way You Look (at me) Tonight* is a multimedia and multi-format project: a dance performance interspersed with abundant, sometimes (seemingly) unscripted, dialogue and philosophical commentary, poetry, video art, interactions with the audience and, at one point, a song performed live. The show is a collaboration between Claire Cunningham, a Scottish dancer, choreographer and performer born with a medical condition which began to require the use of crutches in her teens; Jess Curtis, an American choreographer, dancer and researcher; and Alva Noë, an American philosopher and a member of Curtis's PhD dissertation committee whose work on enactive perception informed many of the project's ideas. Noë's filmed or audio-recorded commentary is present throughout the performance, woven into the soundscape by Matthias Herrmann, which largely consists of slightly distorted and crackling recordings of popular mid-twentieth-century jazz songs and ethereal ambient music, and into video art by Yoann Trellu projected onto three screens. But even outside of Noë's input, philosophical discourse flows freely throughout the show: wandering around the stage in what looks like

[44] Thain, 'The in-tensions of Extensions', 85.

[45] Julia Kristeva, 'Women's time', *Signs*, 7:1 (1981) 13–35, 17.

part contemporary dance, part performance, part meandering, Curtis and Cunningham discuss perceptions and experience of disability, age(ing) and gender, crutches and wheelchairs, and relationships between bodies, other bodies (including non-human and inanimate ones), and the world. These discussions, although fully accessible to a non-academic, are rooted in philosophy and critical theory; Judith Butler, Donna Haraway, Graham Harman and object-oriented ontology all make an appearance, as does Marie Chouinard, in a brief in-joke: at one point, when Cunningham teaches Curtis to use crutches, she reproaches him, jokingly, for not 'cripping up' enough—that is, for not actively performing pain and deformity as is expected from an able-bodied person using medical items associated with disability. 'I wouldn't get into Marie Chouinard's company, then!' Curtis retorts, to a few knowing laughs in the audience. This is clearly a sarcastic reference to the use of prosthetics in *bODY_rEMIX*—Curtis and Cunningham confirmed this reference but were reluctant to discuss it further when I asked them about this response during the Q&A following their performance at The Place in London in 2019.

Audience involvement is a key feature of the show. At the outset, upon entering the performance space, members of the audience are offered the choice of sitting in the centre and therefore being subject to physical contact with the dancers, or sitting a little further afield. As the show unfolds, the audience is invited to participate in various exercises exploring attention and perception. Most importantly, those who choose to occupy seats in the performance space are regularly touched or brushed with by both Curtis and Cunningham, whose dancing and talking occur in very close proximity to the audience.

Crutches feature prominently both in the choreography of *The Way You Look...* (hereon *TWYL*) and in its dialogue. They are discussed at length throughout the performance and at one point become the subject of a dance lesson that Cunningham gives to Curtis (more on this below). Early in the show, in her reflection on crutches, Cunningham cites disability scholar and activist Julia Watts Belser's writing on what she coins as 'queer relatedness'[46] between wheelchair users and their chairs, premised on recognising and celebrating wheelchairs' 'animacy' and the sense of kinship and interanimation that wheelers experience towards them. Cunningham draws parallels with her own relationship with her prostheses:

[46] Julia Watts Belser, Vital wheels: Disability, relationality, and the queer animacy of vibrant things, *Hypatia* 31:1 (2016) 5–21.

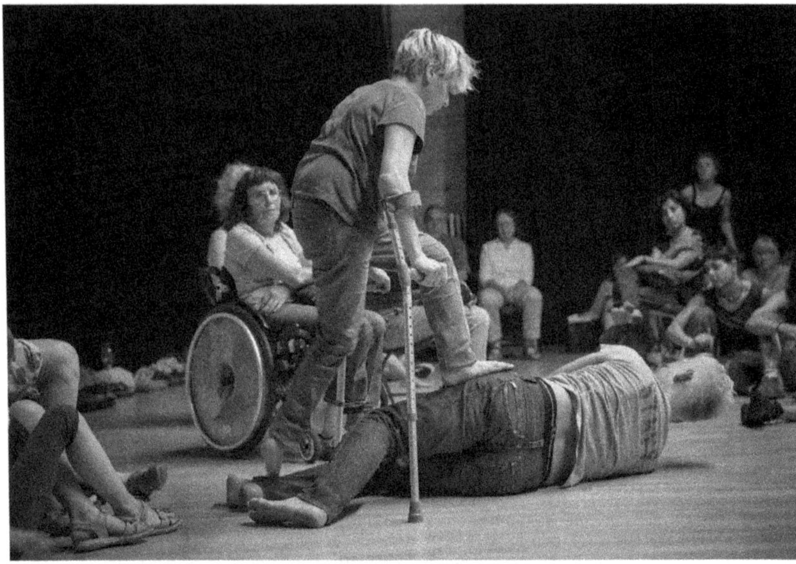

Fig. 2.1 Claire Cunningham and Jess Curtis in *The Way You Look (at me) Tonight*. (Photo by Sven Hagolani)

'I am never really alone', she says, referring to crutches that are both her dance and her life partners.

The use of crutches allows Cunningham to inhabit planes of movement other than the vertical plane characteristic of ballet and the horizontal plane of floor work central to contemporary dance. A lot of the time she is positioned in a liminal state, her body oriented in ways unfamiliar to dance spectators. The logic of her movement is not upright and not bipedal; the crutches make her into a four-legged being (reflected in the playful intertextual title of one of her more recent works, *Four Legs Good*), and her steps are organised accordingly. In interviews, Cunningham reflects on how her embodiment that is premised on having four points of contact with the ground influences her choreography: 'I paid a lot of attention to the ground. I was realising that I was quite geekily obsessed with ground and terrain and that I was noticing the ground a lot, and that it was to do with using the crutches, with having four legs rather than two' (Fig. 2.1).[47]

[47] This interview with Cunningham can be viewed on her website or at https://vimeo.com/453253379.

This 'obsession with ground' is an irreducible part of a particular mode of being-in-the-world that Cunningham describes as follows: 'certain aspects of my attention become very highly tuned that are related to coordinating four feet … I think I became aware of it being a large part of my life—a spatial tension, an attention to terrain'.[48] Watts Belser, in her analysis of the performance, also focuses on the 'quality of perception she [Cunningham] has honed as a crutch user, a mode of motion that requires her to always look down, to assess the landscape, to gauge in an instant where she can safely place a crutch […] Crutch use hones a specific type of knowledge'.[49]

Indeed, a key theme in *TWYL* is the sensory knowing that stems from lived experiences of disability. Although Cunningham and Curtis do not use this term, some disability scholars might call the performance a cripistemological[50] (a portmanteau of crip and epistemology) exercise. *TWYL* is concerned with the phenomenology of disabled modes of moving, feeling and knowing as a complete sensory-perceptual experience and a unique epistemic position. It foregrounds crip subjectivity as a body of knowledge about space, relationships with objects/things, and embodiment itself, and Cunningham's engagement with her crutches is a constant rearticulation and reconfiguring of this body of knowledge. At different points in the performance, the idea of a crip expertise is made explicit in both moving and humorous ways. Such is, for instance, the scene where Cunningham instructs Curtis on how to use crutches, explaining to him how to position his hands on the handles, how to grip them, how to shift his weight and how to navigate the space. A non-disabled performer, Curtis becomes a sensory apprentice to his disabled partner and expresses surprise, unease and then joy as he discovers new modes of moving. This scene places 'a premium on the disabled subject as a knowledge producer';[51] here, crutches subvert the usual positions of the non-disabled person as more proficient (in movement, dealing with material items and generally being-in-the-world) than the disabled person.

[48] https://vimeo.com/453253379 (accessed 15 February 2023).

[49] Watts Belser, 'Improv', 461.

[50] Merri Lisa Johnson and Robert McRuer, Cripistemologies: An Introduction, *Journal of Literary & Cultural Disability Studies*, 8:2 (2014), 127–147.

[51] Tobin Siebers, 'Returning the Social to the Social Model', David T. Mitchell, Susan Antebi, and Sharon L. Snyder eds. *The Matter of Disability: Materiality, Biopolitics, Crip Affect*, Ann Arbor: University of Michigan Press, 2019, 39–48, 47.

However, to assume that the focus here is on Cunningham's mastery of crutches as a means of taming the object world would be to misunderstand the entire ethos of the performance. Despite her proficiency and prowess, the relationship between Cunningham and her crutches is not configured as that of command or mastery. Rather, it is a relationship of (mutual) care. Disability and dance scholars Danielle Peers and Lindsay Eales have once aptly noted that '[t]hose appropriately performing able-bodiedness comfortably *use* technology, and those who fail to perform able-bodiedness (the disabled) are uncomfortably *dependent* upon technology'.[52] Many disability dance projects tend to celebrate the former type of relationship, highlighting disabled dancers' supreme command of wheelchairs or other prostheses. Yet, while this is important for removing the stigma from disability—essentially, by constructing it as super-ability—such projects ultimately reproduce the ableist ideal of a sovereign, empowered subject in command of their body and of the world.

Celebrating dependence (in any form), on the other hand, is no mean feat; it is much more difficult than celebrating mastery, and there is not, as yet, a definitive language for it within contemporary Western culture. As psychoanalyst Adam Phillips writes (emphasis added), 'no one ever says, for example, "he's very good at being dependent on her" [...] Why, if I said I had *an ambition to become more dependent*, would I, at least in this culture, be politically and psychologically disparaged? We can think of success [...] as being related to issues of self-sufficiency'.[53]

The way Cunningham engages with, and talks about, her crutches opens up much-needed ways for rethinking relationships of (inter)dependence as desirable and generative. Much of her language, both kinetic and literal, is informed by contact improvisation (CI), a dance and movement form that both she and Curtis work with. To let the reader grasp the ethos and embodied reality of CI, I will cite a poignant description of one of the key aspects of the technique by choreographer and dance theorist Ann Cooper Albright:

> Starting with two hands, one partner will firmly, yet openly, touch another person on the back or shoulder, kinesthetically "asking" their partner to

[52] Danielle Peers and Lindsay Eales, 'Moving materiality: People, tools, & this *thing* called disability', *Art/Research International: A Transdisciplinary Journal*, 2:2 (2017) 101–125, 112.

[53] Adam Phillips, 'On success', *On Flirtation*, London: Faber & Faber, 1994, 42–59, 53–54.

> pour their weight into the receptacle of their hands. The asking partner can regulate how much weight is given by resisting and pouring back even as they accept the responsibility for the other person's weight. This mutual pouring creates an energetic dialogue that continuously loops between the partners. Eventually, the partners begin to pour their weight back and forth, using different body parts as their physical contact revolves around the space and across their bodies.[54]

As this description suggests, movement within CI is premised on an ethics of care and responsibility; it is about taking, and trusting one's partner(s) to take, the burden/weight of another body, about willingly accepting—in fact, joyfully welcoming—mutual dependence. However, the (most common) way of doing CI described by Cooper Albright only involves human bodies and a 'pouring'—of weight, burden, responsibility—that occurs between them. When such pouring is animated and mediated by another actor (in Cunningham's case, the crutches), this complicates and enlivens things further.

As mentioned earlier, a large part of *TWYL* involves interactions with the audience through touch, and this touch is often mediated and enabled by the crutches. Cunningham approaches members of the audience, pauses next to them to gauge their consent about being touched, lifts herself up on crutches, and lets them hold her in the air momentarily before landing her feet against a viewer's body part. 'When Claire brings her feet against a surface, her touch is light [...] She lands with exquisite precision, with gentleness', notes Watts Belser.[55] Crutches allow her to lean on the audience and share some of her weight with them—but not too much. The audience thus gets to experience a kind of 'light' version of CI: while Cunningham delegates some of her weight to them, it is spread between the crutches and the viewer, making the burden on the latter lower, less heavy. She doesn't break into one's space (unlike Chouinard's dancers); she slowly pours some of herself into it—at least this is how I experienced it as a member of the audience. Another important quality of movement that crutches allow her is that of suspension, or hovering; the precious few seconds she spends pausing in the air, assessing the readiness of the person in front of her to accept her touch. If hovering was invoked earlier as a temporality of care, in *TWYL* it is a prerequisite and even

[54] Ann Cooper Albright, *Engaging Bodies: The Politics and Poetics of Corporeality*, Middletown, CT: Wesleyan University Press, 2019, 242.

[55] Watts Belser, 'Improv', 461.

instrument of care if we were to understand the latter, following Heidegger[56] (and some of the discussions in the performance), as attunement or attention towards someone or something.

In *TWYL*'s choreography, crutches become an instrument of articulating 'qualities of and spatial relations between objects and beings'.[57] Watts Belser cites a conversation with Cunningham where she draws parallels between her attention, and attunement, to the ground and to the bodies of her dance partners: 'a quality of perception she has honed as a crutch user, a mode of motion [...] requires her to always look down, to assess the landscape, to gauge in an instant where she can safely place a crutch. "I'm looking at Jess as landscape" Claire says. "He's terrain"'.[58] Crutches also afford Cunningham a unique way of inhabiting space by dwelling in it: she can be seen leaning on them in almost languid poses or sitting on their handles snugly, creating pockets of cosiness and comfort for herself in the otherwise bare space of the stage. She calls two of the many human-crutch configurations she has invented 'swivel stool' and 'bench stool', and this 'homely' language suggests an intimate ease and familiarity she has with crutches—and, by extension, with the material world: '"I can read the physics of the object that I land on," Claire explains. "I know how to put my weight directly on it and straight through it, without knocking it over. That's a very specific skill I have. When I look at Jess's body, I can read it very fast"'.[59] For her, crutches become tools of emplacement, whereby 'place' can be terrain, the stage, or another person's body.

The final scene of *TWYL* is one of the most poignant in the show. Perched high on her crutches, Cunningham suddenly becomes almost as tall as Curtis as she puts her arms around his neck. Their faces are close; he holds her gently as they rock very slowly to a crackling sound of Jerome Kern and Dorothy Fields' *The Way You Look Tonight*. At a brief glance, the pair's movement looks like a classic slow dance one would associate with courtship. However, it takes more than two bodies, male and female, to sustain it: the swaying engages Cunningham's crutches as much as it does Curtis and herself. It is the crutches that enable the pair to be dancing 'cheek to cheek' (due to their difference in height, among other things),

[56] Heidegger, *Being and Time*.
[57] Curtis, 'The Way', 18.
[58] Watts Belser, 'Improv', 461.
[59] Watts Belser, 'Improv', 461.

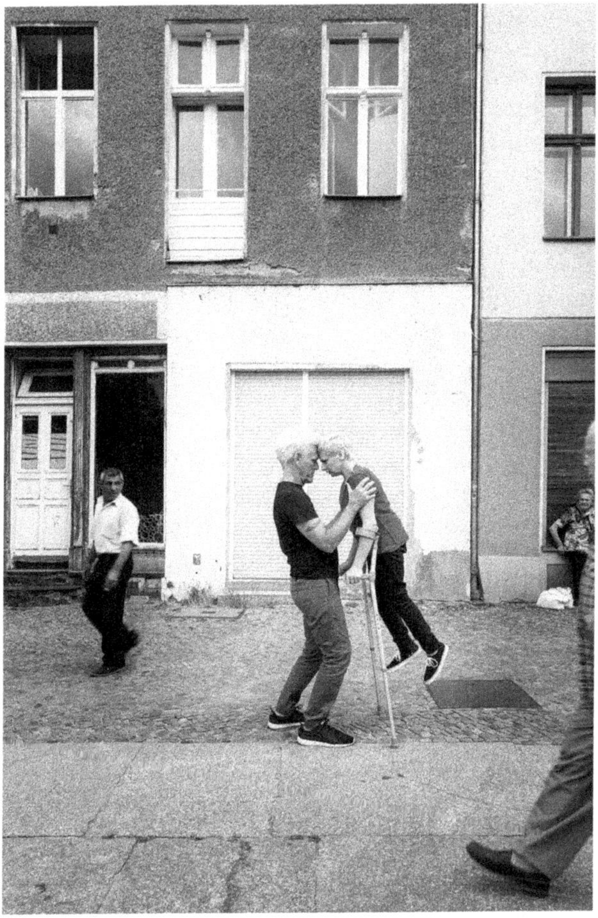

Fig. 2.2 Claire Cunningham and Jess Curtis. (Photo by Sven Hagolani)

and the precarity of Cunningham's perched position necessitates a particularly attentive coordination of motions (Fig. 2.2).

Some viewers may be drawn, by the iconography of the slow dance and the idiosyncratic love song that accompanies it, to read this score in a heteronormative way, as a romantic scene of coupledom that overcomes bodily differences; thus, one of the members of the audience at the performance I attended made a suggestion, during the Q&A, that Cunningham and Curtis are 'so perfect together' that they should 'get married or something' (despite Cunningham openly discussing being asexual and queer and Curtis mentioning his long-term partner, who is obviously not Cunningham, during their onstage dialogue). I find a different reading more productive: I see this dance as a celebration of a different way of being (im)perfect together, one that involves interdependence—including more-than-human interdependence (here, between Cunningham, Curtis and the crutches). The extremely slow—at times, barely perceptible—movements of this sequence invoke the temporality of dwelling, making the scene kindle a 'desire to dwell with disability, a desire which is antagonistic to the normative desire to cure or kill disability'.[60]

Here, I would like to circle back to Albright's discussion of 'pouring' one's weight into another's body in CI. I find it wonderfully resonant with Polanyi's discussion of relationships of indwelling, cited earlier: experiencing things by 'pour[ing] ourselves into them'.[61] It also talks to Ingold's distinction between objects and things: things 'leak', while objects 'present their congealed surfaces for inspection'.[62] Things allow (and possibly invite) pouring while objects do not open up the space for it; things allow indwelling, while objects do not. There is a great deal of 'pouring' throughout *TWYL*, and the final scene, where such slow and careful pouring occurs between Curtis, Cunningham and the crutches, is its epitome.

Crutches, then, activate the space of *TWYL* as a relational space; a space where both bodies and things emerge as 'gatherings', in Heideggerian terms, ongoing processes of entanglement with other bodies and things, and must be thought of as constituting, and being constituted by, the webs of relations and intra-actions they are enmeshed in. To apply the terminology introduced at the outset of this chapter, crutches in *TWYL* are configured as ***palliative things***. They do not summon a 'cure' for the bodies that engage with them, and do not foster relations of mastery. Rather, they enable and enact relationships of interdependence, cooperation and sharing of knowledge, experience, burden, and responsibility. By affording 'indwelling', leaking and pouring between bodies, other bodies and things (such as themselves), they cultivate dwelling, being-with, and hovering; all features of what I earlier defined as palliative time-orientations.

[60] Eliza Chandler, 'Cripping community: New meanings of disability and community', *No More Potlucks, 19*, quoted in Peers & Eales, Moving materiality, 2012, 106.

[61] Polanyi, 'Sense-giving and sense-reading', 303.

[62] Ingold, 'Bringing', 4.

In her analysis of *bODY_rEMIX*, Thain argues that 'the use of prostheses in Chouinard's piece is […] less a reaching out into the world from a centred subjectivity than an exploration of the tensions and lines of movement'.[63] My reading drastically differs from Thain's: I read Chouinard's dancers' agonistic stance as grappling for (if not necessarily a manifestation of) precisely such a 'centred subjectivity', and the use of prostheses as a means of achieving such a subjectivity. If anything, I would use Thain's exquisite formulation to describe the use of prostheses in *TWYL*, which foregrounds, conversely, a decentred subjectivity—that is always already intersubjectivity; a subjectivity premised on interdependence and radical care.

2.5 Conclusion

In her fascinating reflection on dance and Deleuzian ideas of becoming, philosopher Claire Colebrook writes: '[B]ecoming is not a means towards the realisation of some end. Rather, becomings are best seen as counter-actualisations: ways in which the already-constituted actual world always bears a power to become other than it already is'.[64] Later in the piece, she notes that 'dancing—unlike writing a novel that would have an external object of completion—is, at each moment of its actualisation a dance; one does not have to wait until the completion of the performance to produce the dance'.[65] Both dance and becoming, in her account, are non-teleological; becoming is not 'becoming something finite' but an ongoing emergence of new possibilities. Like Heidegger's thing that is thinging in a worlding world, Colebrook's dancing body is 'bodying', without striving to arrive at a final destination, to become-this-or-that.

Crutches in *The Way You Look (at me) Tonight*, in my reading, are enablers and enactors of such non-teleological dance/becoming, while in *bODY_rEMIX/gOLDBERG_vARIATIONS* they permit a different kind of becoming: an end-oriented one, a becoming-masterful. In that sense, as this chapter has argued, in *bODY_rEMIX* they can be read as curative objects: while standing against the dancers or else helping them stand against the world, they are implicated in projects of mastery, articulating

[63] Thain, 'The in-tensions of Extensions', 87.

[64] Claire Colebrook, 'How can we tell the Dancer from the Dance?: The Subject of Dance and the Subject of Philosophy', *Topoi* 24 (2005) 5–14, 5.

[65] Colebrook, 'How can we tell the Dancer from the Dance?', 7–8.

themselves, bodies and subjectivities as 'neatly bounded powerhouses of capacity'.[66] Meanwhile, in *The Way You Look*, they are palliative things that enunciate their own and dancers' bodies' indeterminacy and relationality without attempting to foreclose or bind. They enable ongoing pouring between bodies, things and the world; they call for being-with without securing, for shrouding without enclosing.

I am aware of the potential dangers of a 'palliative' reading of items used in disability dance due to the term's established association with end-of-life care and the implications it has for disability politics. Watts Belser warns against discourses and practices that feed into 'the dominant assumption that people with disabilities are almost/already dead and the oft-voiced claim that people with disabilities would be "better off dead"'.[67] This is not at all my intention when I talk about palliative things: the meanings I attach to the term 'palliative', as outlined earlier, stem from the term's etymology as 'cloaking' and focus on a refusal to follow a curative paradigm. 'Palliative', in my interpretation, is not about envisaging, let alone calling for, death (for people with or without disabilities); rather, it is a corollary of 'crip' and 'queer' in its rebuttal of normalising, progress-oriented, mastery-based ways of thinking, sensing and relating. Palliative things invite the kinds of queer animacies and queer relatedness that Watts Belser conceptualised with reference to wheelchairs and wheelers: relations that 'destabilize the expected notion of the human as sovereign and solitary in relation to inert objects, violating the emotional flatness that is presumed to govern the relations humans have with their owned things', and eschew the imperative to perfect, improve, overcome, or master.[68]

References

Ahmed, Sara. *The Promise of Happiness*. Durham: Duke University Press, 2010.

Baraitser, Lisa. *Enduring Time*. London: Bloomsbury, 2017.

Bennett, Jane. *Vibrant Matter*. London and Durham: Duke University Press, 2010.

Bersani, Leo. 'Psychoanalysis and the Aesthetic Subject'. In *Is The Rectum a Grave? And Other Essays*. London and Chicago: University of Chicago Press, 2010a. 139–153.

Bersani, Leo. 'Sociality and Sexuality'. In *Is the Rectum a Grave? and Other Essays*. London and Chicago: University of Chicago Press, 2010b. 102–119.

[66] Watts Belser, 'Vital wheels', 6.

[67] Watts Belser, 'Vital wheels', 6.

[68] Watts Belser, 'Vital wheels', 9.

Burton, Laini and Jana Melkumova-Reynolds. 'My leg is a giant stiletto heel': Fashioning the prosthetised body. *Fashion Theory: Journal of Dress, Body and Culture*, 23:2 (2019) 195–218.

Colebrook, Claire. How can we tell the Dancer from the Dance?: The Subject of Dance and the Subject of Philosophy. *Topoi* 24 (2005) 5–14.

Cooper Albright, Ann. *Engaging Bodies: The Politics and Poetics of Corporeality*. Middletown, CT: Wesleyan University Press, 2019.

Curtis, Jess. 'The Way You Look (at me) Tonight': Touch Tours, Haptic Practices, and Sensory Strategies. In *Thinking Touch in Partnering and Contact Improvisation: Philosophy, Pedagogy, Practice*, ed. Malaika Sarco-Thomas, 10–26. Cambridge: Cambridge Scholars Publishing, 2020.

Edelman, Lee. *No Future: Queer Theory and the Death Drive*. Durham: Duke University Press, 2004.

Hadley, Bree. *Disability, Public Space Performance and Spectatorship: Unconscious Performers*. London: Palgrave Macmillan, 2014.

Harman, Graham. *Immaterialism: Objects and Social Theory*. Cambridge: Polity Press, 2016.

Heidegger, Martin. *Being and Time*. Oxford: Blackwell Publishing, 1962.

Heidegger, Martin. 'The Thing'. In *Poetry, Language, Thought* (trans. A. Hofstadter). New York: Harper & Row, 1971.

Ingold, Tim. 'Bringing things to life: Creative entanglements in a world of materials'. *Realities Working Papers*, 15 (2010) 2–14.

Johnson, Merri Lisa and Robert McRuer. Cripistemologies: An Introduction. *Journal of Literary & Cultural Disability Studies*, 8:2 (2014), 127–147.

Kafer, Alison. *Feminist, Queer, Crip*. Bloomington: Indiana University Press, 2013.

Kemmer, Laura, Annika Kühn and Vanessa Weber. 'Pandemic times. A conversation with Lisa Baraitser about the temporal politics of COVID-19'. *Ephemera: Theory & Politics in Organization*, 21:1 (2021) 21–30.

Kristeva, Julia. 'Women's time'. *Signs*, 7:1 (1981) 13–35.

Laban, Rudolf. *Choreutics*. London: Macdonald & Evans, 1966.

Latour, Bruno. *Reassembling the Social*. Oxford: Oxford University Press, 2005.

Liddell, Henry George and Robert Scott. *A Greek–English Lexicon*. Oxford: Clarendon Press, 1940. Available at http://www.perseus.tufts.edu/hopper/text?doc=Perseus:text:1999.04.0057:entry=prosqetiko/s (accessed 15 February 2023)

Meghani, Salimah H. 'A concept analysis of palliative care in the United States'. *Journal of Advanced Nursing* 46:2 (2004) 152–161.

Melkumova-Reynolds, Jana. '"Let me be your stimy toy": Fashioning disability, cripping fashion'. In *Dangerous Bodies: New Perspectives on Fashion and Transgression*, eds. Royce Mahawatte and Jacki Willson. London: Palgrave Macmillan, 2023.

Morris, David B. 'The cloak and the shield: A thumbnail history of palliation'. *Illness, Crisis and Loss*, 6 (1998) 229–232.

Peers, Danielle and Lindsay Eales. 'Moving materiality: People, tools, & this *thing* called disability'. *Art/Research International: A Transdisciplinary Journal*, 2:2 (2017) 101–125.

Phillips, Adam. 'On success'. In *On Flirtation*. London: Faber & Faber, 1994. 42–59.

Polanyi, Michael. Sense-giving and sense-reading. *Philosophy: The Journal of the Royal Institute of Philosophy*, 42:162 (1967) 301–325.

Siebers, Tobin. 'Returning the Social to the Social Model'. In David T. Mitchell, Susan Antebi, and Sharon L. Snyder eds. *The Matter of Disability: Materiality, Biopolitics, Crip Affect*. Ann Arbor: University of Michigan Press, 2019. 39–48.

Thain, Alanna. 'The In-tensions of Extensions: Compagnie Marie Chouinard's *bODYrEMIX/gOLDBERG VARIATIONS*'. *differences: A Journal of Feminist Cultural Studies* 19:1 (2008) 71–95.

Vredenburg, Elliot. 'Notes toward a meteorology of the cloud'. *Surveillance & Society*, 13:2 (2015) 283–291.

Watts Belser, Julia. 'Vital wheels: Disability, relationality, and the queer animacy of vibrant things'. *Hypatia* 31:1 (2016) 5–21.

Watts Belser, Julia. Improv and the angel: Disability dance, embodied ethics, and Jewish Biblical narrative. *Journal of Religious Ethics* 47:3 (2019) 443–469.

CHAPTER 3

Breaking the Fall

Emily Beaney

Illness disrupts. It forces us to recognise and question how the mind and body engage with others and everyday life. Illness is an embodied, personal and social experience, yet there is a need for knowledge of how everyday experiences of illness can be expressed outside of medical institutions.[1] Jayjit Sarkar suggests that 'thinking through the ill body' provides new ways of seeing resulting from illness.[2] Phenomenological and affect-based approaches to this creative contribution explore the complexities and possibilities of illness as a way of seeing and knowing, regarding the ill body as a centre of knowledge. Seeking to critically and creatively account for embodied knowledge and everyday acts of care by examining experiences of illness and caring practices within our mother-daughter relationship, *Breaking the Fall* emerged as a collaboration with my mother, Cherrie

[1] Havi Carel, *Phenomenology of Illness* (Oxford: Oxford University Press, 2016), 3.

[2] Jayjit Sarkar, *Illness as Method: Beckett, Kafka, Mann, Woolf, and Eliot* (Wilmington, DE: Vernon Press, 2019), x.

E. Beaney (✉)
University of Edinburgh, Edinburgh, UK

D. Woolley et al. (eds.), *Wearable Objects and Curative Things*, Palgrave Studies in Fashion and the Body,
https://doi.org/10.1007/978-3-031-40017-9_3

Beaney.[3] In a short experimental film following the creation of wearable artworks, my mother narrates shifting dynamics of care as she engages in processes of material embodiment. Desaturated images record contrasting qualities of light and texture as my body responds to the comfort and discord, control and care, of the wearables through movement. Together we engage in a process of representation and, ultimately, power reclamation. This artist's text contains written reflection, analysis and documentation of our practice-based research, responding to embodied knowledge of illness and care in the familial context.

The filmic narrative of *Breaking the Fall* is guided by my mother's voice reflecting upon the nuances of our relationship. Close-up and textural shots communicate with the senses as the imagery opens with my mother's hands, sewing, making and feeling. Her voiceover identifies illness as our point of departure from traditional caring relationships, relaying her struggles with my diagnosis and her need to control and protect despite a breakdown in communication between us. The camera follows my movements dressed in wearable embodiments of my mother's making. Footage depicts my body's response to soft layers of fabric that threaten to overwhelm, to tangled bonds of medically inflexed headwear and to a confining metal structure placed on me by my mother. In the film I push against the restrictions and, as the visual motion builds, my mother reveals her fear that my illness will take me away to a point of no return. The film ends as I free myself from the structure and bonds. *Breaking the Fall* offers no single resolution; instead, it seeks to convey the tensions, tenderness and entanglements of illness and familial caring experiences. Enacted between the two of us, I frame and film using static or slow-moving cameras and the footage is desaturated in post-production to both draw links with and counter, a clinical, surveying aesthetic. Sharing this work largely online in exhibitions and conferences enables access for those unable to attend in-person public screenings; however, connecting with audiences in the domestic home environment also seeks to further highlight the everyday qualities of the body in illness.

Jean Luc Nancy called for radical approaches to representing the body: 'Let there be writing, not about the body, but the body itself. Not bodihood, but the actual body. Not signs, images, or ciphers of the body, but

[3] Johanna Hedva, 'Sick Woman Theory,' in *Health*, ed. Bárbara Rodríguez Muñoz (London: Whitechapel Gallery, 2020), 140.

still the body'.[4] Similarly, *Breaking the Fall* seeks to produce embodiments of illness experience through methods of making, considering the body as a process, in terms of how it affects and is affected.[5] Creative practices here enable the non-verbal body to become an articulation of illness, conveying the personal and social realities of care at home. Designed to reflect hidden narratives of illness experience, this creative contribution seeks to reveal more than a diagnosis.

One has the capacity to affect and be affected through illness and care. Collaborative approaches to this research practice consider how the duality of care relates to the affective relationship between the self/other 'in the capacities to act and be acted upon'.[6] Contextualised within the familial setting, *Breaking the Fall* attends to how illness—in this case, my epilepsy—impacts upon my mother, and how I, in turn, am affected by this impact. It is a dynamic and intertwined relationship. Whilst the potential for radical kinship is examined within the context of our relationship, this study ultimately reveals the capacity for entanglement in caring contexts.[7] The collaborative process explores proximity through practice, whilst gaining distance through critical reflection. Such an exploration reveals how ethical relations can be materialised, as our relationship is made tangible in the creative and collaborative paths taken.[8]

Phenomenological enquiry into how the body is lived, the ways in which it becomes known and moves in and out of consciousness, materially situate our lived experiences and draw attention to sensory perception. Though Maurice Merleau-Ponty identifies a receding of this embodied consciousness in everyday contexts when motor intentionality is achieved, disruptions to everyday flow caused by long-term illness necessitate recalibrations of how bodies engage with the world.[9] As evidenced by Sara Ahmed, bodily orientation towards others and objects is often influenced

[4] Jean Luc Nancy, *Corpus*, trans. Richard A. Rand (New York: Fordham University Press, 2008), 9.

[5] Melissa Gregg and Gregory J. Seigworth, 'An Inventory of Shimmers,' in *The Affect Theory Reader*, ed. Melissa Gregg and Gregory J. Seigworth (Durham: Duke University Press, 2010), 3.

[6] Gregg and Seigworth, An Inventory of Shimmers, 1.

[7] Hedva, 'Sick Woman Theory,' 140.

[8] Walea Beshty, 'Toward an Aesthetics of Ethics' in *Ethics*, ed. Walead Beshty (London: Whitechapel Gallery, 2015), 19.

[9] Maurice Merleau-Ponty, *Phenomenology of Perception*, trans. Donald A. Landes (Abingdon: Routledge, 2012), 139–140.

by dominant social forces that do not account for embodied difference.[10] This suggests that in order to consider the experiences of our sick and caring bodies, we must deviate from traditional approaches to understanding our situatedness in the world. Utilising and expanding upon phenomenological methodologies, *Breaking the Fall* seeks to explore the ways in which illness realises both limit and new learning.

A phenomenology of affect aims to refine a reading of the senses to include that which is unspoken, cannot be categorised sensorially, or may be interpreted as a subtlety, feeling, or shimmer.[11] Susan Kozel suggests referring to Jean Luc Nancy's instructions for listening as an example of how to conduct a phenomenology of affect.[12] Understanding resonance to be the beginning of sense, Nancy treats the body as a resonance chamber, with the subject as a part of the body that is listening to, or vibrating with, 'beyond meaning'.[13] Kozel suggests that Nancy allows for a transgression of the senses in phenomenology, enabling description of the less clearly defined qualities of experience.[14] Expanding upon Kozel's reading of Nancy's listening, the application of a phenomenology of affect to this research practice attends to shifting intensities of texture, movement and light as affective resonances derived from lived experience are materialised as wearable extensions to the body.

In order to recognise the hidden and affective forces of the body, Sarah Pink recommends sensoriality and collaboration as a method of learning about, understanding and representing the lives of others.[15] Sensory ethnographic methods of enquiry therefore form a foundation for the materialisation of our embodied knowledge. Recorded conversations between my mother and I attended to the senses as we navigated the complexities of illness experience and care within our familial relationship. Nancy's treatment of the body as a resonance chamber was applied when carrying

[10] Sara Ahmed, *Queer Phenomenology: Orientations, Objects, Others* (Durham, North Carolina: 2006), 16.

[11] Roland Barthes, *The Pleasure of the Text*, trans. Richard Miller (London: Jonathan Cape, 1976), 101.

[12] Susan Kozel, 'Phenomenology—Practice Based Research in the Arts,' filmed December 2013 at Stanford University, video, 24:09, http://medea.mah.se/2013/12/susan-kozel-phenomenology-practice-based-research-arts/.

[13] Jean Luc Nancy, *Listening*, trans. Charlotte Mandell (New York: Fordham University Press, 2007), 31.

[14] Kozel, 'Phenomenology'.

[15] Sarah Pink, *Doing Sensory Ethnography* (London: SAGE, 2015), 85–86.

out these sensory conversations by engaging the body in the phenomenological perception of internal and external force relations.[16] An awareness of both internal and external phenomena enabled the research practice to identify and move through sensory processes in the recognition of affective resonances.[17] Specifically, control within care arose as a subject with affective resonances for each of us.

Exploration of these resonances existing between myself and my mother demanded the proximity of bodily engagement offered by practice-based research. Gray and Malins argue we 'learn most through practice, through research, and through reflection on both'.[18] Methods of making sought to generate knowledge through action and reflection, regarding the body as a centre of knowledge. Sensory ethnographic tasks were developed to shift our focus to the body and begin responding to these resonances of control within care.[19] When designing our tasks, I sought to disrupt divisions between self/other, internal/external. Erin Manning's reading of Esther Bick's theory of containment, suggests that perceiving the skin in terms of relation and affective attunement, as opposed to individuation and interaction, may open possibilities for a more fluid sense of self in which one can feel with the world and the other.[20] We therefore began by exploring how the skin as a border or boundary could affect and be affected through touch.[21]

Touch moves beyond the distant objectivity of vision, generating proximity with each other and our life worlds.[22] Porteous comments: 'The non-visual senses encourage us to be involved, and being involved, we may come to care'.[23] Here touch offered a method of representing the radical kinship of care present in our mother-daughter relationship. Attending to affective relations of touch and tactility enacted an ethics of

[16] Nancy, *Listening*, 31.

[17] Nancy, *Listening*, 31.

[18] Carole Gray and Julian Malins, *Visualizing Research: A Guide to the Research Process in Art and Design* (Aldershot: Ashgate, 2004), 1.

[19] Pink, *Doing Sensory Ethnography*, 35.

[20] Erin Manning, 'What if it Didn't All Begin and End with Containment? Toward a Leaky Sense of Self,' *Body and Society* 15 no. 3 (September 2009): 34.

[21] Constance Classen, 'Women's Touch' in *The Book of Touch*, ed. Constance Classen (Oxford: Berg, 2005), 203.

[22] Edmund Husserl, *The Crisis of European Sciences and Transcendental Phenomenology*, trans. David Carr (Illinois: Northwestern University Press, 1970), 38.

[23] J. Douglas Porteous, *Landscapes of the Mind: Worlds of Sense and Metaphor* (Toronto: University of Toronto Press, 1990), 200.

feeling-with, enabling compassion within the research process in the materialisation of embodied resonances of control/release between both the internal/external body, and between the self/other.[24]

The balance between care and control within a relationship is easily tipped as divisions between self and other entangle. Reflecting upon an affective moment in which my mother expressed a desire to 'wrap me up in cotton wool', her sensory ethnographic task became the practice of identifying materials that embodied the resonances of care and control that she felt. Drawing upon Pink's recommendation to seek out knowledge about the senses and to use the senses as a route to knowledge, we moved around my mother's home, exploring the sensory properties of objects, textures and places.[25] Again, enacting Nancy's concept of the body as a resonance chamber, my mother attuned to the internal vibrations of our sensory conversation and perceived the external resonances of her life-world.[26] Merleau-Ponty argued: 'Our relationship with things is not a distant one: each speaks to our body and to the way we live. They are clothed in human characteristics (whether docile, soft, hostile or resistant) and conversely they dwell within us as emblems of forms of life we either love or hate'.[27] These forms of life dwelling within us could arguably be read as affective energies. Drawing upon such affective energies in relation to her desire to wrap me in cotton wool resulted in the selection of bundles of fine white tulle, soft yarns and banana fibres, netting and wool to work with (Fig. 3.1).

Cultures of touch within my mother's creative practice became apparent. Having trained as a tapestry artist, her processes of making engaged with touch-based knowledge with a specific focus on texture. As noted by Cathryn Vasseleu: 'texture is at once the cloth, threads, knots, weave, detailed surface, material, matrix and frame'.[28] Texture became a useful tool for revealing both intricacies of conflicting surface, and immersive worlds of sensation. My mother cut the material into strips and began to implement a weaving technique. Documenting on film her process, using close-up shots of her hands working with the materials, enabled close

[24] Hedva, 'Sick Woman Theory,' 140.

[25] Pink, *Doing Sensory Ethnography*, 4.

[26] Nancy, *Listening*, 31.

[27] Maurice Merleau-Ponty, *The World of Perception*, trans. Oliver Davis (London: Routledge, 2004), 63.

[28] Cathryn Vasseleu, *Textures of Light: Vision and Touch in Irigaray, Levinas, and Merleau-Ponty* (London: Routledge, 1998), 11–12.

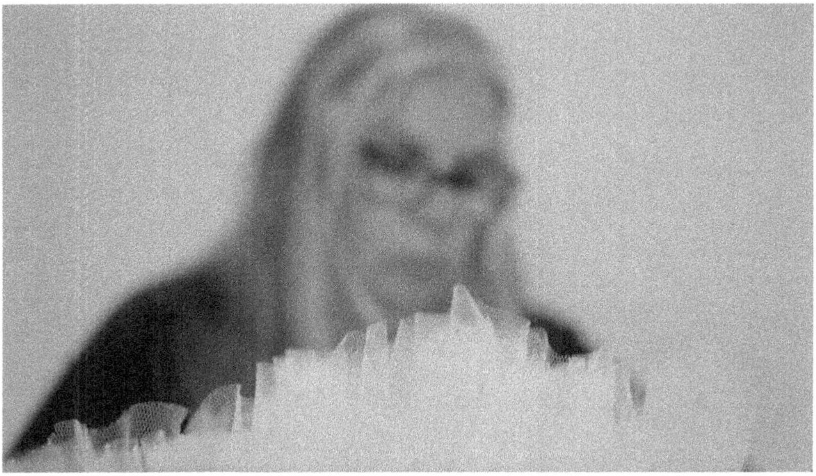

Fig. 3.1 Emily Beaney, Breaking the Fall (Black and white still of folds of white tulle in the foreground. Cherrie sits behind the mound of fabric, eyes down, with her head tilted in a soft focus) 2020. (Film, 10:45 minutes)

examination of how the various surfaces and textures interacted (Fig. 3.2). Drawing upon Kozel's reflection on affect as 'an exchange of forces between people, or between people and objects, the outer world or structures', this practice considered how the materials used in the constructed reality could act as mediators of affect within a material embodiment.[29] As she continued weaving and knotting the fabric, she created a mass of undulating layers that surrounded the central form of the body. The expanse of fabric seemed to reveal the extensiveness of her care as it overwhelmed the body.

The material embodiment that emerged from this practice and the body's appearance of being overwhelmed by it, demonstrated a need for the embodiment and body to sit in direct relation to each other to reveal a sense of excess (Fig. 3.3). We began to form a wearable embodiment of illness experience, focusing upon care and control, a work of creative non-fiction, transgressing boundaries between art and non-art, aesthetic and ethic, artifice and authenticity.[30] My own affective energies were integrated

[29] Kozel, 'Phenomenology.'

[30] Maria Lind and Hito Steyerl, 'Reconsidering the Documentary and Contemporary Art' in *The Green Room*, ed. Maria Lind and Hito Steyerl (Berlin: Sternberg Press, 2008), 16.

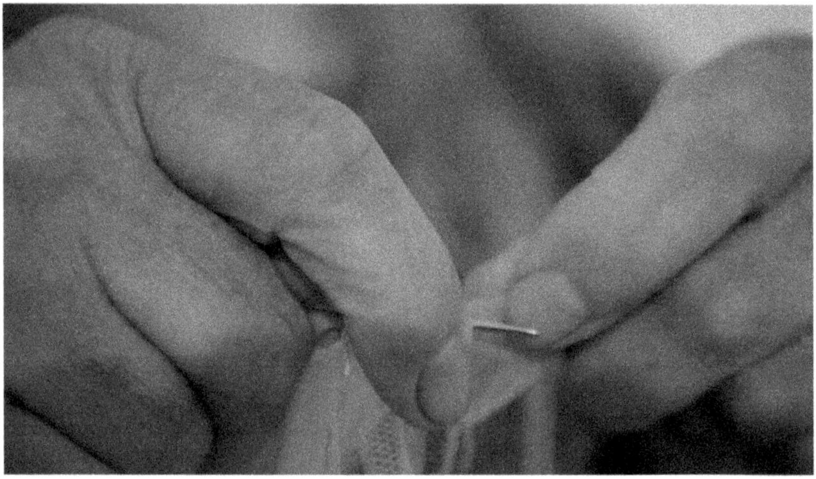

Fig. 3.2 Emily Beaney, Breaking the Fall (Black and white still of Cherrie's hands in close-up, stitching the white tulle) 2020. (Film, 10:45 minutes)

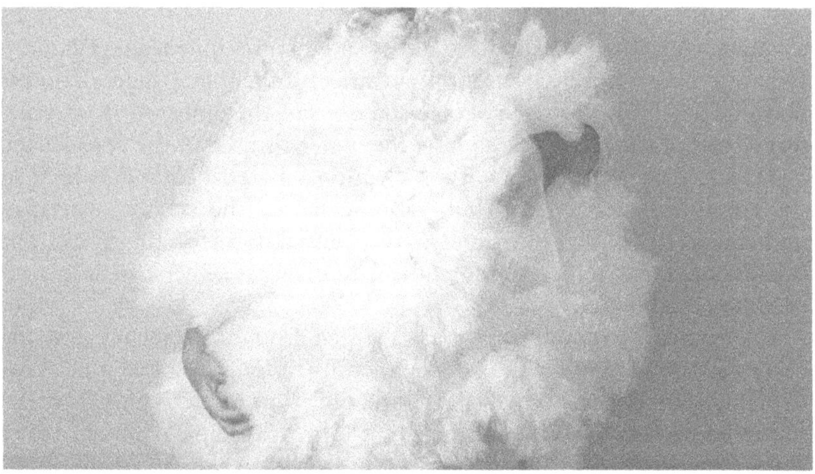

Fig. 3.3 Emily Beaney, Breaking the Fall (Black and white still of Emily's hands feeling their way through a mass of fabrics emanating from her torso) 2020. (Film, 10:45 minutes)

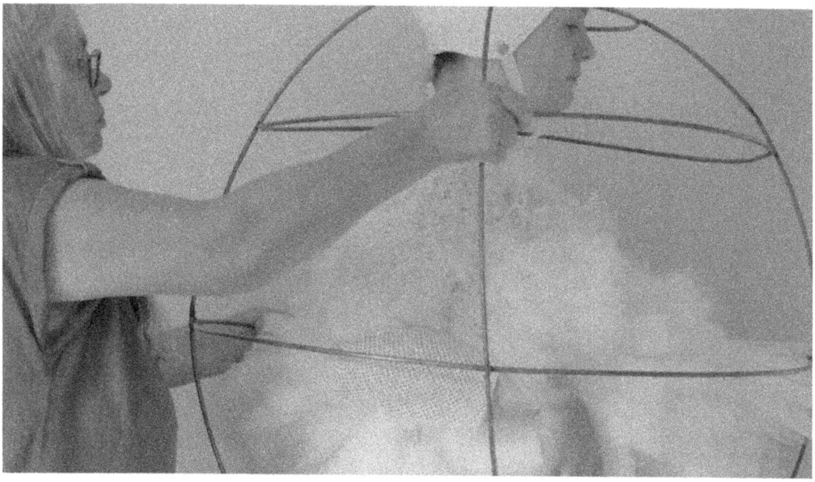

Fig. 3.4 Emily Beaney, Breaking the Fall (Black and white still image of Cherrie and Emily in profile. The shape of the daughter is surrounded by the mass of soft, white materials as the mother places a spherical metal cage over her form) 2020. (Film, 10:45 minutes)

into my mother's embodied contributions by embedding into the practice resonances of being both greatly cared for, but also restricted and controlled. Seeking to create an embodiment that could depict layers of affective experience within complex realities, the same process of attuning to internal and external resonances was used when selecting metal rods to embody restriction. The rigid metal was shaped and welded together to produce a spherical cage to be placed over the tulle, echoing and containing the wearable form my mother had created (Fig. 3.4).

Reflecting upon the wider context of these perceived resonances of control within care, it also proved useful to note that there were other affecting forces outside of our mother-daughter relationship that intensified perceived resonances of control. These were primarily identified as the affective forces of medical institutions. Medical forms of imaging used to monitor long-term health conditions such as epilepsy, often evidence disease only, using technologies that negate the body as a centre of knowledge. Diagnostic terms too, indicate a universalised concept of a disease that can carry value judgements which may negatively impact a person in

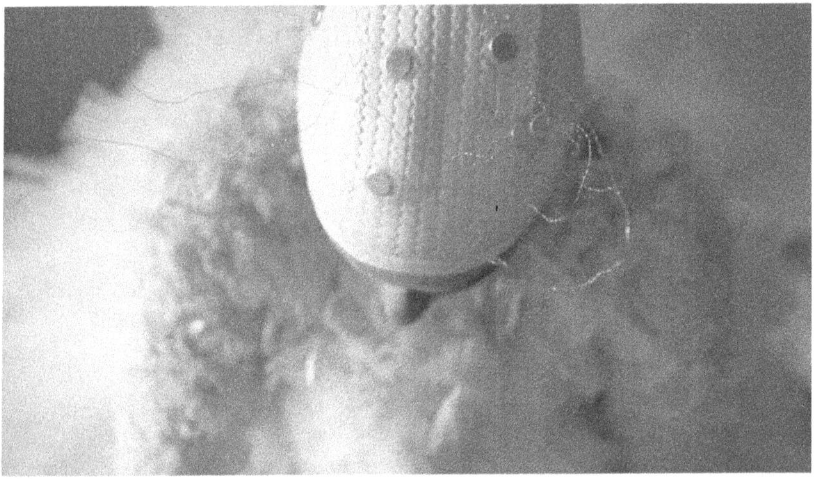

Fig. 3.5 Emily Beaney, Breaking the Fall (Black and white still of the top of Emily's bowed head wearing a white cap with tangled metal discs and wires attached) 2020. (Film, 10:45 minutes)

society.[31] Aiming to restore personal and social agency over illness by validating embodied perceptions as expressions of knowledge, resonances of intrusive medical cultures and feelings of being perceived as a medical object were integrated into the wearable embodiment. A wearable magnetic cap was produced that magnetically drew in metal electrode-like discs attached to wires. The design of the tight-fitting white rubber cap sought to be suggestive of the EEG test, in which a cap is used to place wired electrodes on the head to analyse brain waves in epilepsy. The wearable's multiple magnetics and wires tangled and twisted, with discs clasping onto one another before snapping off the cap if the head deviated from its static position. The magnetic element that was introduced to the EEG-like cap embodied control within care by literally manifesting entanglements of force relations invested in the body. However, the wearable also embodied the long-term affective resonances of continual monitoring within chronic health conditions such as epilepsy by materialising points of connection to external agencies with which the body appears bound (Fig. 3.5).

[31] Peter Conrad and Kristin K Barker, 'The Social Construction of Illness: Key Insights and Policy Implications,' *Journal of health and social behavior* 51, no. 1 (March 2010), 69.

When worn, movement enhanced the tactile nature of the wearable embodiment, highlighting touch through texture, light and contrasting hard, metallic surfaces against soft tulle and skin. Alongside the footage of my mother weaving the textile, we filmed the motions of my mother dressing me and then my body moving in the wearable pieces we had created. The process entailed the translation of haptic perception (a combination of both seeing and feeling touch), to haptic visuality.[32] Marks' theory of haptic visuality argues that images can engage the viewer tactilely, defining a kind of knowledge based on touch. The processes of wearing and viewing the embodiments in motion evidenced that affective moments within these tactile experiences could be intensified by attending to light and movement to create shimmer. Theorists refer to affective shimmers as moments captured within processes of stretching, fluctuating intensities.[33] Seigworth and Gregg speak of the 'shimmering relays between the everyday and affect'.[34] By stretching and highlighting textures through shifting intensities of light and movement, we sought to generate such moments of affective shimmer. These were captured on film in flashes of highlight as my mother used a sewing needle to stitch the tulle together, when the metal cage was placed over the body and when the electrode-like discs attached themselves to my magnetic cap. Motions of being dressed further generated affective moments of engagement between the skin of the self/other and the embodied forms (Fig. 3.6).

Movement, light and texture played a key role in creating tension between the soft and hard, thereby embodying imbalances within our caring relationship and contributing to affective shimmers of fluctuating entanglements and tension. These haptic explorations revealed that the interplay between texture, light and movement in wearables could be utilised to attend to both the subtleties and excesses of lived experience. Affect-based methodologies have been criticised as unsustainable, arguing that the formulation of affect as an excess, sits in contrast to the domestic.[35] Barthes' theory of neutrality disputes this, stating that such methodologies demand 'a hyperconsciousness of the affective minimum, of the microscopic fragment of emotion … which implies an extreme

[32] Laura U. Marks, *Touch: Sensuous Theory and Multisensory Media* (Minneapolis: University of Minnesota Press, 2002), 3.

[33] Barthes, *The Pleasure of the Text*, 101.

[34] Gregg and Seigworth, 'An Inventory of Shimmers,' 21.

[35] Margaret Wetherell, 'Affect and Discourse: What's the Problem?' *Critical Psychology* 6, no. 4 (December 2013): 349.

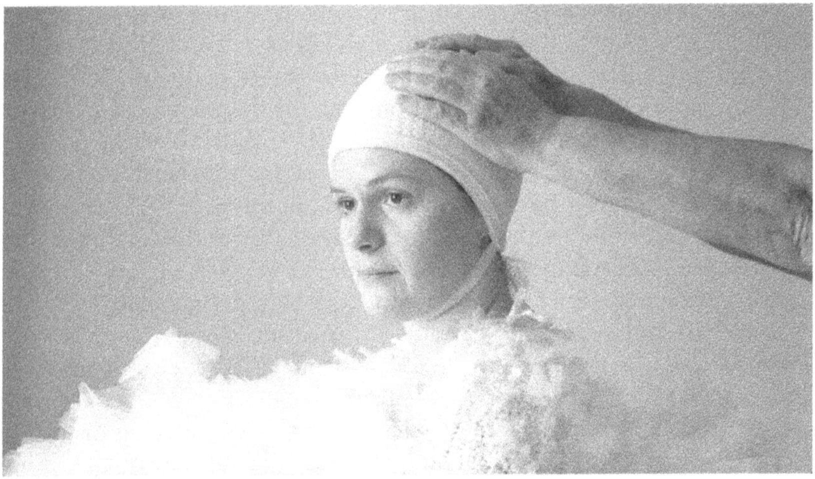

Fig. 3.6 Emily Beaney, Breaking the Fall (Black and white still of Emily in profile. Cherrie's hands sit softly upon her the cap on her head as the mass of materials surround the body) 2020. (Film, 10:45 minutes)

changeability of affective moments, a rapid modification, into shimmer'.[36] The affect-based concept of a shimmer was therefore drawn upon within this research practice to embed affect within the everyday. Such an approach to affect enabled this research to highlight affective moments moving and living within the everyday world's shimmerings.[37]

As power is directed away from the everyday and towards the medical institution as a source of knowledge, the embodied, personal and social qualities of illness experience continue to go unnoticed.[38] *Breaking the Fall* challenged these dominant power structures by generating a shift in representation through forms of expression that recognise the ill body as a centre of knowledge. Utilising a phenomenology of affect, this research has attended to the shimmers of moments felt, yet hidden, in everyday lived experiences of illness, enabling the perception of both internal and external affective relations.

By placing emphasis on the affective potential of illness phenomena, this creative contribution works towards a new means of representation

[36] Barthes, *The Pleasure of the Text*, 101.

[37] Gregg and Seigworth, 'An Inventory of Shimmers,' 21.

[38] Carel, *Phenomenology of Illness*, 3.

that is inclusive of historically unnoticed everyday modes of care.[39] The collaboration with my mother juxtaposed realities and constructed realities of illness and care through creative practice and interplay between the self and other. The focus on touch and tactility that emerged informed the subsequent construction of wearable embodiments. Through material exploration, our practices of creating the wearable embodiments and the act of wearing them, we articulated the move from internal process to external wearable. *Breaking the Fall* therefore revealed embodied knowledge through material embodiments. Lived experiences of care and illness were extended onto the physical and filmic body's surface, thereby manifesting entangled relations of care and control.

The embodied and everyday context as a site of learning is highlighted here as *Breaking the Fall* intervenes in the wider management of chronic illness by foregrounding the affective potential of sustaining and investing in communities of care outside of the medical institution. Adopting an (ill) body-centred approach to the research practice, utilising theories of affect, enabled the representation of both tension and tenderness within a caring relationship. Moments of intensity within these force relations were captured throughout in the manipulation of texture, movement and light as a methodological focus, contributing to understandings of how a phenomenology of affect can reveal shimmers of bodily knowledge relating to experiences of illness and care in the domestic setting and how this methodology may further extend to account for the affective experiences of audiences' internal resonances conversing with the filmic rhythms. In acknowledging these relations, *Breaking the Fall* attends to the unnoticed/unseen/unheard illness experiences of the everyday, thereby contributing towards a form of expression that places power in the body and the lived.

References

Ahmed, Sara. *Queer Phenomenology: Orientations, Objects, Others*. Durham, North Carolina, 2006.

Barthes, Roland. *The Pleasure of the Text*. Translated by Richard Miller. London: Jonathan Cape, 1976.

Beshty, Walead. 'Toward an Aesthetics of Ethics.' In *Ethics*, edited by Walead Beshty, 19 (London: Whitechapel Gallery, 2015), 12–24.

Carel, Havi. *Phenomenology of Illness*. Oxford: Oxford University Press, 2016.

[39] Hedva, 'Sick Woman Theory,' 140.

Classen, Constance. 'Women's Touch.' In *The Book of Touch*, edited by Constance Classen, 203–208. Oxford: Berg, 2005.

Conrad, Peter and Barker, Kristin K. 'The Social Construction of Illness: Key Insights and Policy Implications.' *Journal of Health and Social Behavior* 51, no. 1 (March 2010): 67–79.

Gray, Carole and Malins, Julian. *Visualizing Research: A Guide to the Research Process in Art and Design*. Aldershot: Ashgate, 2004.

Gregg, Melissa and Seigworth, Gregory J. 'An Inventory of Shimmers.' In *The Affect Theory Reader*, edited by Melissa Gregg and Gregory J. Seigworth, 1–25. Durham: Duke University Press, 2010.

Hedva, Johanna. 'Sick Woman Theory.' In *Health*, edited by Bárbara Rodríguez Muñoz, 137–140. London: Whitechapel Gallery, 2020.

Husserl, Edmund. *The Crisis of European Sciences and Transcendental Phenomenology*. Translated by David Carr (Illinois: Northwestern University Press, 1970).

Kozel, Susan. 'Phenomenology—Practice Based Research in the Arts.' Filmed December 2013 at Stanford University. Video, 24:09. http://medea.mah.se/2013/12/susan-kozel-phenomenology-practice-based-research-arts/.

Lind, Maria and Steyerl, Hito. 'Reconsidering the Documentary and Contemporary Art.' In *The Green Room*, edited by Maria Lind and Hito Steyerl, 10–27. Berlin: Sternberg Press, 2008.

Manning, Erin. 'What if it Didn't All Begin and End with Containment? Toward a Leaky Sense of Self.' *Body and Society* 15 no. 3 (September 2009): 33–45

Marks, Laura U. *Touch: Sensuous Theory and Multisensory Media* (Minneapolis: University of Minnesota Press, 2002.

Merleau-Ponty, Maurice. *Phenomenology of Perception*. Translated by Donald A. Landes. Abingdon: Routledge, 2012.

Merleau-Ponty, Maurice. *The World of Perception*. Translated by Oliver Davis. London: Routledge, 2004.

Nancy, Jean Luc. *Corpus*. Translated by Richard A. Rand. New York: Fordham University Press, 2008.

Nancy, Jean Luc. *Listening*. Translated by Charlotte Mandell. New York: Fordham University Press, 2007.

Pink, Sarah. *Doing Sensory Ethnography*. London: SAGE, 2015.

Porteous, J. Douglas. *Landscapes of the Mind: Worlds of Sense and Metaphor*. Toronto: University of Toronto Press, 1990.

Sarkar, Jayjit. *Illness as Method: Beckett, Kafka, Mann, Woolf, and Eliot*. Wilmington, DE: Vernon Press, 2019.

Vasseleu, Cathryn. *Textures of Light: Vision and Touch in Irigaray, Levinas, and Merleau-Ponty*. London: Routledge, 1998.

Wetherell, Margaret. 'Affect and Discourse: What's the Problem?' *Critical Psychology* 6, no. 4 (December 2013): 349–368.

CHAPTER 4

Sitting Pretty: A Dress History of the L-Shaped Frame, the Side-Saddle Habit and the Design of Adaptive Wearables

Alison L. Goodrum

4.1 For a Dress History of Sitting: Introduction

Across the UK, the widespread restrictions, multiple lockdown orders and collective withdrawal wrought by COVID-19 (SARS-CoV-2 virus), particularly during the 12 months from March 2020 to March 2021, were both unprecedented and historic. A report on the correlation between sitting and mental health during the COVID-19 lockdowns found that participants were seated for longer periods than usual and that 55 per cent of participants in the study documented an upsurge in their overall time spent sitting daily.[1] As offices and workplaces were mandated to close

[1] Matthew Pears, Susanna Kola-Palmer and Liane Beretta De Azevedo, 'The impact of sitting time and physical activity on mental health during COVID-19 lockdown', *Sports Sciences For Health* 18 (2022) 179–191.

A. L. Goodrum (✉)
Norwich University of the Arts, Norwich, UK
e-mail: a.goodrum@norwichuni.ac.uk

D. Woolley et al. (eds.), *Wearable Objects and Curative Things*, Palgrave Studies in Fashion and the Body,
https://doi.org/10.1007/978-3-031-40017-9_4

during successive lockdowns, home working became commonplace and, with it, novel modes of appearance management followed, which catered for, and reflected, new, virtual, ways of working, of socialising and of being. In turn, this gave rise to a cultural phenomenon known as 'waist-up dressing', which, according to Cochrane, emerged in response to the 'millions now working from home…[it] has become the solution to meetings moving from face-to-face to video platforms'.[2] This act of emphasising one's torso, shoulders, neck, face and hair, and privileging the top half of an outfit for the purposes of online meetings, is pertinent because it offers a useful entry point into the broader theme to be unpacked over the course of the chapter: of a critical consideration of sitting as an embodied, material and social practice that is entwined with discourses and histories of dress.

The discussion presented here seizes upon the currency of waist-up dressing in, and for, contemporary life and uses it to call for a greater appreciation of dress and its complex and sometimes uneasy relationship to sitting and the seated body or the 'L-shaped' frame. The argument forwarded is based on the critical observation that fashion and dress studies (and their attendant practices) have tended to privilege the standing or linear frame, and the aesthetics and experiences associated with it, over the seated or angular. This chapter seeks to problematise and challenge the predominance of the vertical, what Palmer[3] refers to as the 'standing 'I'', pose with particular reference to existing academic work in the dress history canon. Indeed, it makes a call for a dress history of sitting and takes initial steps to answering that same call by mapping some of the key coordinates around which a critical consideration of L-shaped dress and dressing might be constructed. Forming a central reference point in this mapping exercise are histories taken from the equestrian world and the specialist riding kit associated with it, especially that of the curious and complex side-saddle habit for women, which comprised dress objects explicitly designed for, and worn in, a seated horseback position. The chapter presents purposive examples of side-saddle attire drawn from a range of source material (including pattern books, the sporting press,

[2] Lauren Cochrane, 'Zoom! Power shoulders are back thanks to video meetings', *The Guardian*, Dec 11 2020, https://www.theguardian.com/fashion/2020/dec/11/zoom-power-shoulders-back-thanks-video-meetings-waist-up.

[3] Alexandra Palmer, 'Fashion follows form: patterning a relationship between function and fashion', *ROM Magazine* (Summer 2014) 18–23, 20.

personal albums, equestrian instruction manuals and dress artefacts) and selected from a timeline spanning approximately a century, from about 1850 to 1950.[4] Through a synthesis of these sources, the discussion presents and explains the novel cut and innovative construction of historical habit dress, which was a feat of design engineering and creative pattern techniques. In so doing, it highlights a seldom told history of side-saddle riding and the 'elegant Amazons' who rode and offers a critical interpretation of the attendant material culture: of apron skirts, cut-away jackets and leaping head saddles.[5]

Yet, the intention here is to do more than recount archaic and whimsical examples of sitting dress from history for scholarly ends. Rather, the chapter hinges around a practice-based, and potentially impactful, proposition: that historical approaches to the design, construction, wearing and styling of side-saddle attire may be usefully transposed across time, to the present day, in order to apply certain historical techniques, principles and aesthetical sensibilities to inform and enhance the work of current fashion practice and practitioners, particularly those working in the field of adaptive dress for disabilities and, notably, of clothing design for people using wheelchairs. Dress history, it is argued, has transformative potential in this regard, with a greater part to play in creative design, cut and construction. The research presented here grapples with the enduring design challenges bound up in the embodied act of sitting and its related materiality. For it is easy to overlook corporeal agency in the design process, especially since, as Palmer notes, 'designers are trained to create designs with the pull of gravity' on an almost exclusively perpendicular form.[6] When it is clothed and covered in material, the seated body (be it at a Zoom meeting, on a horse or in a wheelchair) in its L-shaped position acts upon fabric and, of course, fabric, too, acts upon the L-shaped body. Gell's work is useful here, reminding us that 'social agency can be exercised relative to "things" and social agency can be exercised by "things"'.[7] In a seated position, both flesh and fibre may crush, chafe, imprint, bunch, crease, fold, crumple,

[4] A great deal of the source material presented here originates from the Collection of the National Sporting Library & Museum, Virginia. I acknowledge and thank the NSL&M and its staff for their continuing support of my research.

[5] Alison Matthews David, 'Elegant amazons: victorian riding habits and the fashionable horsewoman', *Victorian Literature And Culture* 30:1 (2002) 179–210.

[6] Palmer, Fashion follows form, 20.

[7] Alfred Gell, *Art And Agency: An Anthropological Theory*, Oxford: Clarendon Press, 1998, 17.

stretch and sag in unintended, highly individualised and sometimes problematic or unwanted ways. As Sampson points out, 'garments [both] help and hinder intention'.[8] The proposal forwarded here stops short of resolving the hindrances detailed above but instead shines a light on them as part of a larger exploratory exercise that gathers the, somewhat disparate, principles and traditions of dress history with both pattern-cutting practice and with design for disability. This, intentionally, sets up awkward, yet creative, tensions in an attempt to emulate Pullin's conceit in his treatise on disability and design whereby such 'meetings', as he terms them, may become sources of mutual inspiration between 'distant' communities and cultures of practice.[9] In Pullin's case, the distance lies between the artistic iconoclasm of the design school and the rationalist functionality of medical engineering, and he argues for a *rapprochement* of the two. He suggests that 'like antagonistic pairs of muscles, opposing biceps and triceps, these conflicting priorities might seem to work against each other, but together they afford control of force, position and direction'.[10] It is in this spirit of creative collaboration and possibility that this proposition for a dress history of the L-shaped frame is mooted here.

4.2 Sitting Down and Dressing Down: Observations from Recent History

A note should be added at this juncture to acknowledge that sitting does not only take place in a stiffly formal L-shaped pose, nor only on a chair or seat, and that there are all manner of diverse and disparate cultures and practices that favour, or require, a bent-legged, kneeling or squat position for sitting and/or a 'life without chairs'.[11] Cranz reminds us that 'sitting cross-legged' is a Western term sometimes also referred to as the 'Turkish-style' and, even more apt, occasionally known as sitting 'in the tailor-fashion', a turn of phrase that evokes the traditional posture of the tailoring trade in which men perched ergonomically atop their workbenches to sew by hand.[12] And, one only has to conjure up the drawings, paintings and

[8] Ellen Sampson, *Worn: Footwear, Attachment And The Affects Of Wear*. London: Bloomsbury, 2020, 37.

[9] Graham Pullin, *Design Meets Disability*, Cambridge: MIT Press, 2009.

[10] Pullin, *Design Meets Disability*, 303.

[11] Galen Cranz, *The Chair: Rethinking Culture, Body, and Design*, New York: W.W.Norton & Company, 1998, 25.

[12] Cranz, *The Chair*, 27.

albumen prints depicting Pre-Raphaelite muse, Mrs William 'Janey' Morris (1839–1914), hunched over her embroidery among the billowing folds of her crumpled Artistic Dress or ponderously disarranged in a wicker Arts and Crafts chair, to appreciate the physical and material artistry of languishing and relaxation.

The clothed waist, and waistbands, were topics of considerable debate in the global style press during the COVID-19 pandemic. 'Lockdown has brought change' wrote Priya Elan in *The Guardian* in April 2020, noting how 'fashionistas [now] embrace the joys of an elasticated waistline in their working-from-home outfits'.[13] Sweatpants, jogging bottoms and tracksuit trousers (often made from French terry, jersey, fleece or velour fabrics), along with drawstring pyjamas, pull-on yoga pants and stretch leggings were casual items of leisurewear that became popular choices of dress (for both men and women) whilst under governmental directives to stay at home. These garments were favoured because they possessed both material qualities of ease, stretch and elasticity as well as psychic qualities of comfort, consolation and cosiness. Moreover, as unstructured forms, they were particularly well disposed to accommodating the fleshy folds and bodily bulges of a frame bent at the waist into an L-shaped, seated, position. The rise of what are referred to colloquially as 'joggers' or 'trackies' and the broader correlation between videoconferencing and changed behaviours in lifestyle and dress was noted by *Vogue* magazine, which offered the following commentary on sitting and embodied responses to it: 'it's fair to say that this new way of working has us glued to our seats as never before. It's also changed the way we dress for work. Business-in-the-front-party-in-the-back dressing doesn't fly for teleconferencing; instead, the focus is on waist-up dressing'.[14]

The relative informality of homeworking, along with the fact that legs, bellies, buttocks and feet were rendered invisible under the conditions of COVID-19, cossetted away beneath desks and out of sight of digital camera lenses, negated both the need and desire for the tailored, fixed, waistbands so characteristic of office dress such as workwear and suiting. In August 2021, the fashion journalist, Natasha Marsh, contemplated the

[13] Priya Elan, 'No sweat: how track suit bottoms became the height of lockdown fashion', *The Guardian*, Apr 25 2020, https://www.theguardian.com/fashion/2020/apr/25/no-sweat-how-tracksuit-bottoms-became-the-height-of-lockdown-fashion.

[14] Laird Borrelli-Persson, 'Thank Zoom for reviving the waist up look first popularized in the 1930s', *Vogue*, Apr 14 2020, https://www.vogue.com/article/waist-up-dressing-1930s-versus-for-zoom.

shape and form of her post-pandemic wardrobe, describing how she longed to cast off her stretchy and unstructured loungewear and, instead, return to dressing in jeans in recognition of a return to 'normal life'. Yet, she also recalled that the corporeal experience of wearing those jeans was uncomfortable and constraining, to the point of infliction. She describes the traces inscribed on her body by her jeans: 'the indentation they'd leave on my stomach while I sat cramped over a laptop in my 4x4 New York City apartment'.[15] Confined variously by her clothes, by the dimensions of her domestic space and by her urban environs, the layers and scales to Marsh's experience are finely nuanced. Sampson's research on the intricacies between wear, wearing and wearer resonates here: 'just as the body modifies the worn garment…the garment imprints itself on the body…. Through this tactile engagement, the garment becomes part of the bodily self and can function as an additional psychic receptacle, carrying a history of our embodied relationships within it'.[16] Just as the pandemic disrupted the boundaries of work and domestic life, and the spaces of labour and leisure, so too, the materiality of those dual structures were similarly altered and transformed. For several weeks and months, office life was played out virtually, against the backdrop of a private or familial home or dwelling place and at kitchen tables and in spare bedrooms. The clothes worn for this followed suit, reflecting a disrupted lifestyle in which outfits were formed of hybridised elements picked and mixed from across work and weekend wardrobes, from across garments nominally designated as items of daywear and nightwear, and across formal and casual modalities. In a world destabilised by COVID-19, routine dress practices and body techniques were uncoupled from the stabilities and ordering structures of daily rhythms.

4.3 Putting the L-Shape on, and above, the Table: Examples from Dress History

But what of the *upper* body in relation to practices of waist-up dress and dressing? From (former) American First Lady, Hillary Clinton's 'cold shoulder' dress designed by Donna Karan in 1993 through to the epoch-defining shoulder pads of Eighties power dressing, the shoulders and

[15] Natasha Marsh, 'What clothes will you wear when the pandemic is finally over?' *Byrdie*, 2021, 'https://www.byrdie.com/fashion-trends-post-pandemic-5190627.

[16] Sampson, *Worn*, 131–132.

neckline have had many moments in the fashion spotlight. The waist-up phenomenon of lockdown dressing is, then, by no means new or unprecedented, with *Vogue* purporting the trend for adorning the neckline for online conferencing purposes with decorative collars, elaborate trims and jewellery to be a 'revival' of earlier practices.[17] It is, for instance, the 1930s that are recognised by dress historians as being one of the decades most associated with exaggerated shoulders and elaborate necklines, particularly in women's dress of the period. Blackman tells us that the Hollywood actress, Joan Crawford, defined the look in her cinematic role as *Letty Lynton* in 1932, sporting an iconic white evening gown made by MGM's celebrated costume designer, Gilbert Adrian (1903–1959).[18] The gown was remarkable in its striking and voluminous layering of ruffled, white, organza and chiffon, which frothed elaborately around each shoulder cuff of the garment. This technique was intended to encircle the wearer's collar line as a framing device and was used to highlight Crawford's face in her capacity as screen siren and glamorous starlet. The ruffled effect successfully created an inverted triangle shape, with a highly ornamented and pronounced top line narrowing to a sylph-like waist, in typical Thirties style. The dress was to go on to prove immensely influential as a popular design cue and came to represent the signature style of the decade: 'the fashionable silhouette was evolving into a slender, elongated torso with widening shoulders and a neat head with softly waved short hair'.[19] Perhaps most interesting of all, however, is that Blackman goes on to designate the wide-shouldered look, as popularised in *Letty Lynton*, to be a classic example of the contemporaneous practice of 'above the table dressing'.[20] This was an idea promulgated, at least in part, by *Vogue* during 1935 and referred to the high fashion techniques and body management strategies employed by privileged Anglo-American women who inhabited what was termed as 'the restaurant circuit'. When seated at dinner, the lower body and its garments went largely concealed from both public view and the style judgement of fellow diners, so that efforts in design and dressing came to be concentrated on the most visible parts of the body on full display: from upwards of the waist. Suzy Menkes elaborates, referring to the

[17] Borrelli-Persson, 'Thank Zoom for reviving the waist up look first popularized in the 1930s'.

[18] Cally Blackman, *100 Years Of Fashion*, London: Laurence King, 2012.

[19] Blackman, *100 Years Of Fashion*, 13.

[20] Blackman, *100 Years Of Fashion*, 142.

Duchess of Windsor, Wallis Simpson, as an exemplar of the style, 'with her sleek tailored dinner suits, ideal for the new cocktail and nightclub culture, and slightly risqué gowns slithering over a slender body'.[21] As part of their leisured lifestyle, these women had the luxury of sitting and were able to indulge in seated pursuits and entertainments as fashionable spectators, whether that be sunbathing by the pool, going to the theatre or dining out at supper clubs.

Throughout time and across space, sitting has been infused with political doctrine and socially constructed, enfolded with systems of cultural etiquette to be enforced, adhered to, or transgressed. In Western European culture there remains a widely held convention that it is polite and proper for women to sit with knees tightly closed together, with their dress carefully draped about them in a neat arrangement of body and fabric, symbolising goodness, sexual purity and moral fortitude. This is learned and acquired behaviour and girls are imbued with such socially constructed gender techniques from a young age. Men, on the other hand, have been permitted to inhabit space in more expansive and assertive ways, filling a seat with the physical bulk of their body in masterful poses. Leaping back to the Victorian Era, dress histories of both the crinoline and the bustle offer fascinating examples of spectacular forms of fashionable women's dress that contributed to physical and social restrictions along starkly drawn gender lines. Whether dressed in elaborate crinoline cages and corsets from the mid-1800s or the later 'lobster tail' bustles of the 1870s and 1880s, women were both literally and metaphorically bound and confined by their clothing. Corsets, along with heavily layered undergarments, hoops, trains and fabric swags were inhibiting, unwieldy and impacted significantly on the ability of the wearer to adopt the L-shaped position easily or comfortably. The health afflictions arising directly from prolonged corset-, crinoline- and bustle-wearing are well documented, with maladies ranging from disorders of the lungs, rib deformation and damage to female reproductive organs as well as contamination from infectious diseases and threats to life from combustible fabric construction.[22]

[21] Susy Menkes, 'Blithe spirit: the Windsor set: a glimpse of the era before world war II: beauty on the eve of destruction', *International Herald Tribune* Dec 3 2002, https://www.nytimes.com/2002/12/03/style/IHT-blithe-spiritthe-windsor-seta-glimpse-of-the-era-before-world-war.html.

[22] For example, refer to: Steele, *The Corset: A Cultural History*. New Haven: Yale University Press, 2003; and Alison Matthews David, *Fashion Victims: The Dangers of Dress Past and Present*, London: Bloomsbury, 2015.

Eschner's research on the history of the bustle in the late-Victorian period makes explicit links between sitting and suffering, noting how women were compelled to perch daintily, and precariously, on the very edges of chairs when wearing bulky and padded lobster tails, so much so as to be the identified cause of back and muscular pain and postural discomfort.[23] An anonymous correspondent, featured in the *Boston Medical and Surgical Journal* of 1888, elaborated on this concern, branding the bustle 'as a deformity' and condemning the 'really deleterious effects upon its wearer'.[24] Sitting was singled out by the correspondent as particularly problematic for bustle wearers:

> The woman with a bustle can never sit down in a natural position. It is absolutely impossible for her to rest her back against the back of any seat of ordinary construction. I have no doubt some of the severe backaches in women whose duties keep them seated all day are due to, or at least aggravated by, this disability.[25]

The adverse effects of Victorian dress on women's health along with its restrictions on mobility and activity inspired the establishment of social and political reform movements spearheaded by physicians, suffragists, artists and educators. For example, *The Rational Dress Society* was just one of several organisations promoting physical and social freedoms through the adoption of practical and utilitarian clothing for women based on the classical beauty of natural lines and simple contours of the body. Founded in 1881 in London its stated cause was to protest against 'the introduction of any fashion in dress that either deforms the figure, impedes the movements of the body, or in any way tends to injure... health'. [26] Along with reform movements, the sporting arena also acted as a crucible for the development of practical, freedom-inducing, modes of dress for women at this time and the L-shaped, seated, pursuits of cycling and, later, rowing, motoring and aviation gave rise to pioneering and progressive forms of

[23] Kat Eschner, 'Although less deadly than crinolines, bustles were still a pain in the behind', *Smithsonian Magazine*, Apr 21 2017. https://www.smithsonianmag.com/smart-news/although-less-deadly-crinolines-bustles-were-still-pain-behind-180962919/.

[24] Anonymous, 'Bustles', *Boston Medical and Surgical Journal*, Nov 15 1888, 490.

[25] Anonymous, 'Bustles'.

[26] Patricia Cunningham, *Reforming Women's Fashion, 1850–1920: Politics, Health and Art*, Kent, Ohio: Kent State University Press, 2002, 124.

dress that enabled and facilitated women's bodies in action. The discussion continues with one such example of sitting dress borrowed from the history of women in sport: that of side-saddle riders and their specialist equestrian kit, offering a detailed consideration of the ways in which riding in the 'aside' position necessitated innovative responses to the challenges of designing, cutting, making and wearing clothing for the L-shaped frame.

4.4 Riding Aside and Riding Up: Challenges of Designing and Wearing the Side-Saddle Habit

Equestrianism was popular as a leisure pursuit among aristocratic and socially privileged women from the mid-1800s onwards, with Albrecht, Farrell-Beck and Winakor reporting that, by the 1880s, most riding garments were made for recreational activity.[27] Riding for pleasure, exercise and sport was encouraged as a desirable skill and also regarded to be socially conducive, enabling women to exhibit flair and prowess in the saddle whilst also forging and reinforcing membership of, and status within, an exclusive sporting and class faction. Riding, be it park-riding, informal hacking with friends or formal riding-to-hounds under the auspices of an organised hunt club, offered opportunities for diversion, exertion, romantic matchmaking and mastery, and took far more energetic and vigorous forms than most other contemporaneous pastimes available to women. As such, women who rode were often celebrated as 'Amazons' or as 'Dianas' in equestrian texts as well as the specialist sporting and popular press.[28]

The side-saddle ensemble (Fig. 4.1) in the smartly tailored, masculine, tradition was considered 'correct' when it came to proper appearance for a woman in the saddle: what was termed as one's 'turn out'. For side-saddlers, turn out consisted of a tailored habit jacket, waistcoat and silk shirt-waist with a long-length, full, skirt, which was worn over riding breeches. These few garments formed, and even today remain as, the basis of side-saddle attire but a raft of additional intricacies relating to accessorising and styling contributed complexity and nuance to a way of

[27] Juliana Albrecht, Jane Farrell-Beck, and Geitel Winakor, 'Function, fashion, and convention in American women's riding costume', 1880–1930, *Dress* 14 (1988) 56–67, 56.

[28] Matthews David, *Elegant amazons*.

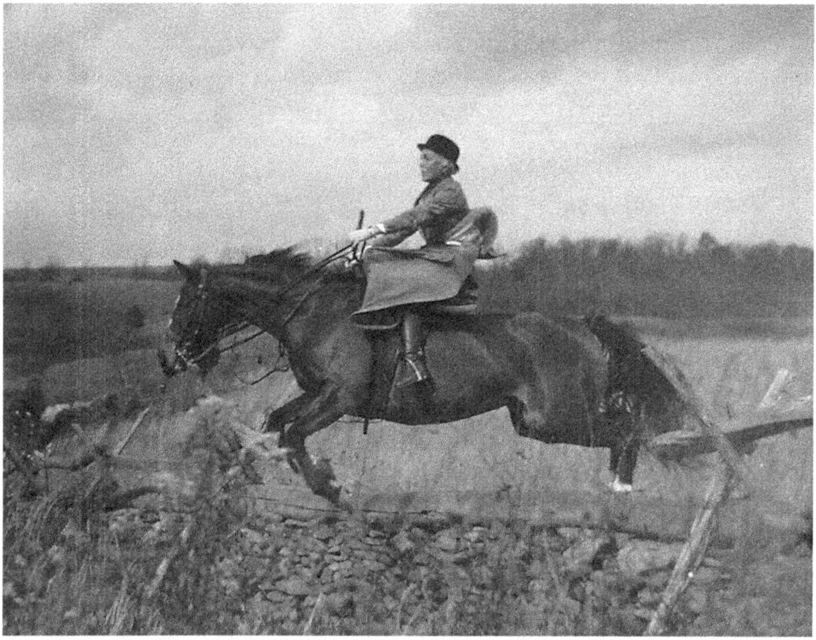

Fig. 4.1 'L.L. on Essie 1948'. Mrs Lucy Howard Linn (née McCormick Blair, 1886–1978) in informal side-saddle turn out. (National Sporting Library & Museum, Virginia)

dressing that was wrought with tradition and protocol. For example, side-saddle riders were expected to wear top hats for formal events and bowlers for informal occasions but seasonal, and climatic, variances also applied, so that in her celebrated treatise, *Riding And Driving For Women* (1912), Belle Beach additionally detailed sailor hats, sombreros and panamas as being among acceptable headgear for Summer.[29] Beach was among a small cohort of women who authored well-respected volumes on both the sport

[29] Belle Beach, *Riding And Driving For Women*, New York: Charles Scribner's, 1912, 127.

and culture of the side-saddle.[30] Between them, they proffered a wealth of, not always consistent and often somewhat stern, advice on the relative merits of different types, styles and ways of wearing all manner of *accoutrements*, including stock ties and cravats, veils, tie pins, gloves, hairstyles, underclothes and boots. Writing in her equestrian instruction and advisory manual of 1913, *Women In The Hunting Field*, Mrs Stuart Menzies devoted an entire chapter to 'dress, complexion and figure' with the following extract providing a taste of her emphatic views:

> Never, never wear patent leather boots or buttoned ones. Patent leather are vulgar and unpardonable, while buttoned are highly dangerous, murderous things. They may catch and prevent you getting your foot out of the stirrup quickly, besides which they are out of keeping and not correct. Again, if there still exists such a thing as elastic-sided boots (I believe I saw a pair on an old lady not long ago), burn them.[31]

Being well turned out was, then, a marker of aptitude as an equestrian, as well as a material signifier of moral fortitude, respectability, and sporting citizenship: of being 'in the know' and having sufficient cultural and economic capital to participate effectively and appropriately in an equestrian world governed by complex codes of body management, self-discipline and material display. The competitive show ring and the hunting field were (and remain as) two equestrian domains governed especially strictly in this regard, with appearances literally being judged in the former and scrupulously policed by the Master and club officials in the latter. On this matter, Mrs Stuart Menzies counselled novices in side-saddle riding thus:

> the unwritten laws and etiquette of the hunting field are rigid. Women have not the same licence in the matter of clothes allowed on other occasions. I

[30] Examples include: Nannie Power O'Donoghue *Ladies On Horseback: Learning, Park-Riding, And Hunting, With Hints Upon Costume, And Numerous Anecdotes*, London: W.H. Allen; Hayes 1903 [1893]. *The Horsewoman: A Practical Guide To Side-Saddle Riding*. London: W. Thacker; E.V.A (Eva) Christy 1907 *Modern Side-Saddle Riding: A Practical Handbook For Horsewomen*. London: Vinton & Co; Diana Sheddon and Violet Apsley 1932, *To Whom The Goddess…: Hunting and Riding For Women*. London: Hutchison and Co; and Doreen Houblon, 1938, *Side-Saddle*. London and New York: Country Life and Charles Scribner's.

[31] A. C. Stuart Menzies, *Women In The Hunting Field*. London: Vinton, 1913, 19.

> would just as soon think of going out hunting with a wreath of flowers in my hair instead of a hat as I would think of going out in any but proper boots.[32]

Habit dress was required to be highly practical and to withstand the esoteric demands of riding on the side, often at speed, possibly across open country and in harsh or changeable weathers. A hunting diary penned by the American side-saddler, Lucy Linn (pictured in Fig. 4.1), during a riding holiday to Ireland in 1948 provides insight as to these rigours: 'the same raw, windy weather with flurries of snow persisted for several days…. Twice we hunted in bitter driving little blizzards which would start and stop and come and go, but never shortened our days in the field by a yard or a minute'.[33] Among a lengthy inventory of requirements, then, riders needed to wear clothing that offered protection from the elements, did not impede their freedom of movement, that facilitated their posture in the saddle and supported the frame of their skeleton, that maintained their dignity when galloping, jumping or taking a tumble, that resisted chafing and that ensured the safety and performance of self and horse in partnership. The discussion continues here by drilling down into two such design challenges peculiar to the side-saddle habit (those of the L-shaped frame and of the hazard of being unseated) in order to build towards a core proposition whereby the ingenuity of the riding habit and the skill of its tailor borrowed from centuries past may usefully be transposed today for inclusive design purposes, benefitting a range of seated communities including people using wheelchairs.

4.5 Design Challenge 1: The L-Shaped Frame

Elizabeth Karr wrote in 1884 that 'the position of a man in the saddle is natural and easy, while that of a woman is artificial, one-sided and less readily acquired'.[34] With side-saddle riding, it is impossible to overlook the influence of the saddle itself on the dress that women wore to practice their sport. Figure 4.2 is instructive in this regard, illustrating (especially in view 'B', without skirt) how the side-saddle functioned in its modern, two-pronged, form, by entwining around the bent legs of the rider in

[32] Stuart Menzies, *Women In The Hunting Field*, 19.

[33] Lucy Linn, *Thirteen Hunts In Ireland: Feb 13 To Mar 13, 1948*. Privately Printed in Chicago, 1948, 22.

[34] Elizabeth Karr, *The American Horsewoman*, Cambridge: The Riverside Press, 1884, iv.

PLATE I

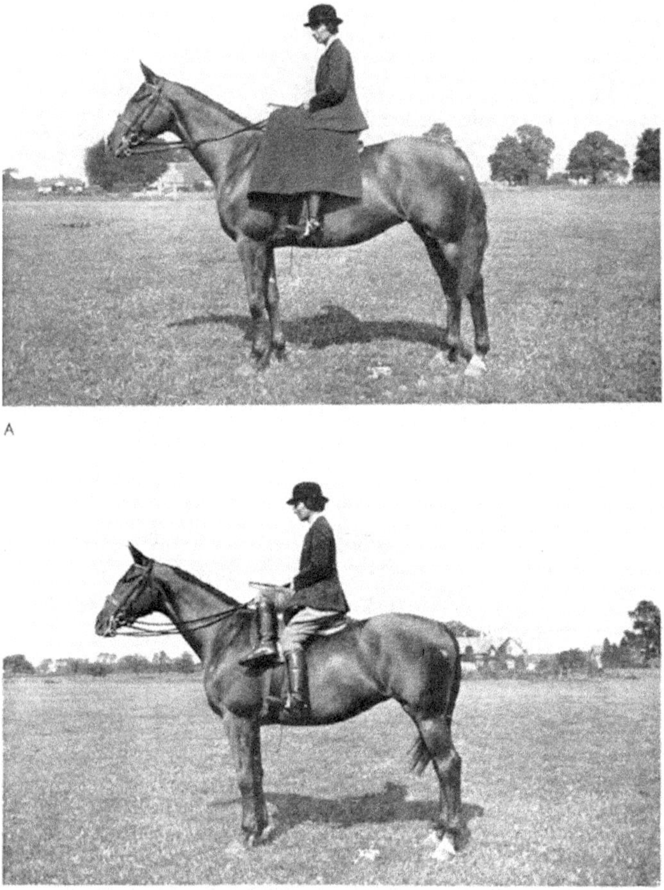

A

B

NORMAL SEAT IN A SIDE-SADDLE

(A) With skirt. (B) Without skirt.

Fig. 4.2 Demonstrating the 'normal seat' in a side-saddle, with skirt (view A) and without skirt (view B). (From Doreen Archer Houblon's *Side-Saddle*, 1938)

seated pose. Chafing of the legs and knees caused by this arrangement was a common complaint and padding in forms ranging from sheepskin fleece to soft chamois was sometimes inserted into the rider's breeches as a protective, makeshift, buffer against the rasping effect of saddle on skin. Mrs Power O'Donoghue was just one of several riding instructors to share her acquired wisdom on this topic, encouraging novices to innovate by 'put[ting] on...soft padding under the right knee and over the left, to prevent the friction of the pommels, which, to a beginner, generally causes much pain and uneasiness'.[35]

One of the most significant developments, signalling a veritable sea-change, in side-saddle history, was the introduction of the lower, down-turned, prong of the saddle that cradled the left thigh, known as the 'leaping head'. The leaping head innovation, which emerged during the 1830s and endures to this day, was considered revolutionary because it allowed women to finesse their leg grip. It offered greater purchase in the saddle, which, in turn, allowed women to press forward with their thigh and body weight against the leaping head in order to maintain traction, supply momentum and, crucially, to go about urging their horse into a leap or jump, as never before.[36] Riding aside is, then, an embodied act and activity whereby the multiple layers of horseflesh, saddle leather, habit fabric and human sinew operate in dynamic combination, pressing against, responding to, and impacting on, each other to form a partnership that is corporeal, material, tactile and sensual in mix. The language and terminology specific to side-saddle riding adds further detail to this discussion of the interplay between artefact, touch, feel and sitting, notably through the key concept of The Seat. To clarify, the seat in this instance refers to more than the actual leather artefact of the side-saddle and is a complex, and technical, referent, encompassing the rider's entire physical presence, being and bearing when sitting in the saddle, and their interplay with it. Beach explains that 'form in riding depends chiefly on the seat, and that in turn depends upon balance and correct position'.[37] Correctness of seat was something that a side-saddle rider had to work to acquire and sustain

[35] Power O'Donoghue, *Ladies On Horseback*, 11–12.

[36] Furthermore, side-saddlers describe the leaping head as offering a particularly secure hold for the legs and body and liken it to riding 'as if in a rocking chair', a metaphor that is especially suited to the broader discussion here on the dress history of sitting and the seated body.

[37] Beach, *Riding And Driving For Women*, 5.

through experience, training and the honing of natural intuition. Karr's book contained a sustained discussion on the topic providing an entire chapter devoted to 'the seat on horseback', which numbered some 30 pages.[38] The seat was about the positioning of the body in the saddle, the movement and sway of the body against it, the distribution of body weight on it, as well as posture, pose and balance. The seat was fundamental to excelling in the saddle and riders would acquire a reputation for, or be judged upon, their possession of a 'good' or 'firm' seat, or not. Being 'unseated' was also a widely used euphemism for falling off one's mount and taking a tumble.

Doubtless, the side-saddle seat was decidedly peculiar, largely because of the asymmetrical, aside, pose that was required to practice its art and which evoked its distinctive character. When mounted, both legs of the side-saddle rider were draped to one side—the left 'near' side—of the horse when mounted and were arranged, bent at the knee, in an angular, L-shaped, and highly unusual, position (refer, again, to Fig. 4.2, view 'B'). This twisted position of the body, along with the uneven distribution of weight in the saddle and skewed hips, pelvis and buttocks had to be accounted for in the design of the side-saddle habit. The L-shaped pose impacted, contorted even, the equestrian body by rounding buttocks, shortening the natural waist and forming flexed layers of muscle as well as a spread of flesh around the seat, the stomach and the lower torso. Riding aside required, then, a buckling of the body, bending it at the waist and, again, at the knees to form, and conform, to the shape and construction of the saddle with its unusual, dual pommel, configuration. The riding habit was tailor-made both to accommodate and to compensate for this, becoming an adaptive item of performance-enhancing, or (in certain instances of bad-fit or poor judgement) performance-diminishing, technical dress. A ready example of this is provided by a particular style of riding jacket known as the 'cut-away', which found favour among equestrian women in the interwar period (as depicted in Fig. 4.3). The style succeeded in removing an excess volume of fabric over the seated rider's abdomen with the express purpose to facilitate sitting: bunching around the waist was reduced by an assistive, pared down, design whilst the hemline and front vent of the jacket was cut to curve and to fall, ergonomically, around the soft contours of the stomach when in the L-shaped pose.

[38] Karr, *The American Horsewoman*, 114–144.

Fig. 4.3 Miss Catharine G Mellick hunting with the Essex Fox Hounds, New Jersey, 1939. (National Sporting Library & Museum, Virginia)

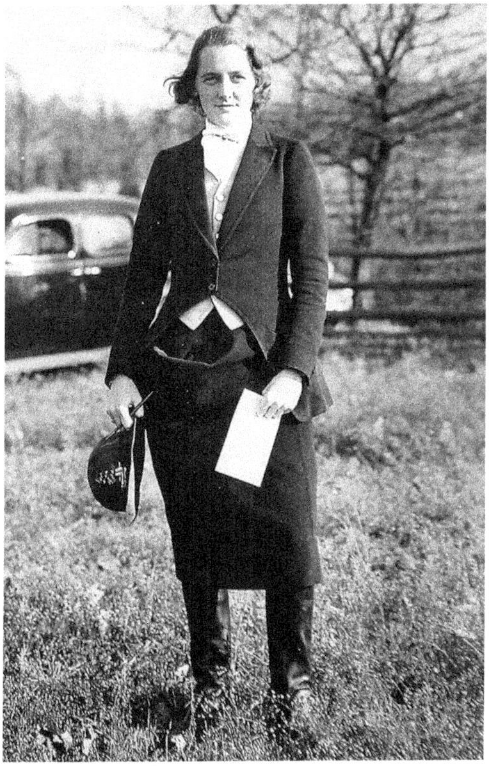

Other assistive cutting strategies extended to the riding breeches that were worn underneath a side-saddler's skirt. It was advised, for example, to have breeches generously cut across the backside and along the seam length of the upper leg to prevent fabric from riding up uncomfortably or embarrassingly around the crotch when sitting in the L-shaped pose. In this regard, Mrs Stuart Menzies advised her readers in 1913 that,

> breeches of the present day are a thing of beauty and a joy for ever, compared with what we used to ride in, but be sure you have them made long enough from the waist to the knee so that they may not catch you anywhere and pull out of place.[39]

[39] Stuart Menzies, *Women In The Hunting Field*, 15–16.

4.6 Design Challenge 2: Unseating

Around the turn of the twentieth century, as equestrian activity became more accessible to women, and more vigorously pursued by them, a number of accidents, or unseatings, occurred involving some high-profile members of the side-saddle community. While falls and tumbles were regarded as part and parcel of riding, the hazard of being dragged was a particular threat to, and a heightened possibility among, practitioners of the side-saddle. An unseated rider might be dragged perilously along the ground by an agitated horse due to the material expanse of their habit skirt becoming accidentally entwined around the protruding prongs of the side-saddle, acting effectively as a clothes hook that 'suspended'[40] or 'hung up'[41] the victim. There were further perils particular to the side-saddle, which were either caused, or exacerbated, by the expansive volume of late-Victorian, styles of habit skirt. For example, if a horse rolled to the near-side and the mounted side-saddler be thrown, a flowing skirt could become trapped underneath the considerable weight of a fallen horse, thereby hindering the rider's escape and risking injury from crushing, trampling and kicking. Mrs. Stirling Clarke, counselled her readers as to this threat, as follows: 'the position and costume of a lady render her comparatively so helpless upon these trying occasions, that I am convinced,—and long experience confirms me in the conviction,—that, as a general rule, the greatest chance of safety consists in her keeping as much as possible in the saddle'.[42] Another hazard came in the form of billowing and the way that the habit skirt had the potential to cause alarm or pose a menace to the horse if caught suddenly by the wind or fly up during a leap. A sudden and erratic movement from a considerable yardage of skirt could startle a horse, causing it to shy or bolt and this threat was considered sufficiently troubling that inexperienced horses were trained in the art of drapery as part of the breaking-in regimen of a side-saddle pony.[43] Hayes, for example, coined the term 'habit-shy' to describe the way in which some uninitiated horses found encounters with the riding skirt to be a source of unease and distress.[44]

[40] Hayes, *The Horsewoman*, 65.

[41] William Kerr, *Riding For Ladies*, New York: Frederick A. Stokes Company, 1891, 64.

[42] J. Stirling Clarke, *The Habit And The Horse: A Treatise On Female Equitation*. London: The Authoress, 1857, 201.

[43] Houblon, *Side-Saddle*, 3.

[44] Hayes, *The Horsewoman*, 440.

At this point in the history of the riding habit, that is, during the 1890s, the habit skirt remained as somewhat flowing and voluminous in style, shape and silhouette. Material evidence to support this is provided through two examples of late-Victorian habits dating from *circa* 1880 to 1890 held by the Collections Resource Centre in Sileby, Leicestershire: one of navy-blue serge with a hem circumference of 96 inches and one of black broad-cloth with a hem of 106 inches.[45] The muted colouring and plainness of these two garments are typical. Riding uniform was governed by simplicity, sobriety and conservatism of taste, and these organising principles endure. Appearing dishevelled or unkempt in the saddle was decidedly taboo and the design of habit dress was engineered and adapted to ensure that smoothness and straightness of garment line were maintained at all costs. 'Never' warned Stuart Menzies 'wear anything that can possibly ruck up, or make crinkles'.[46] In part, such advice prevented against the discomfort and chafing brought on by ill-fitting fabrics and lumpen clothing but there was also an aesthetic driver to looking uncrumpled on horseback: something referred to as a 'cult of smoothness'.[47] Habit-makers went to great lengths, and displayed considerable ingenuity, in attaining and preserving clean silhouettes and perfectly balanced forms. For example, coins or lead shot were sewn into the hems of skirts to give weight and drape to the garment, thereby generating a perfect—and perfectly smooth—'hang'. For, turn-out etiquette insisted that the bottom hem of the habit skirt be aligned exactly parallel to the ground when the rider was mounted (as illustrated in Fig. 4.2, view A). This stipulation was tricky to achieve in practice, especially as the bent legs of the L-shaped frame formed awkward undulations that the skirt needed to cover with effortless perfection. Beneath its outward, unornamented, expanse, then, the habit skirt concealed an internal and elaborate complex of pattern engineering. Among other things, this comprised elastic foot and leg loops to anchor the skirt in place as well as advanced seam and darting technology, which formed an internal cavity of fabric to accommodate the L-shaped arrangement of the seated rider's legs. What is interesting is that, when out of the saddle and standing upright, this cavity innovation gave the skirt a severely

[45] Accession numbers: 82.1960/20 and 155.1956/1. For more on the archives formerly held at Sileby contact Leicestershire Museums Service.

[46] Stuart Menzies, *Women In The Hunting Field*, 17.

[47] Alison Goodrum, A severity of plainness: the culture of female riding dress in America during the 1920s and 1930s, *Annals Of Leisure Research* 15:1 (2012) 87–105, 97.

misshapen appearance so that the design did not translate at all effectively from the angular 'L' to the perpendicular 'I' stance. Rather, it sagged, bunched and puckered with the effect of gravity when the wearer was unmounted and stood up straight. As Mrs Power O' Donoghue noted 'the better shaped a habit-skirt is for riding the more unsightly it looks when seen on a standing figure'.[48]

If smoothness was a governing principle of Victorian equestrian dress, so, too, was safety and the necessity to guard against dragging drove innovation and design advancements in side-saddle attire at this time. In general terms, the volume of the habit skirt gradually came to be pared down so that, by the turn of the century, it was of a more streamlined silhouette (reflecting, too, the general trend in fashions in dress of the day). The side-saddle 'safety skirt' also appeared in answer to dragging concerns, with Alice Hayes renouncing older models of habit skirt as 'death-traps' and 'dangerous'.[49] In his manual, *Riding For Ladies* of 1891, William Kerr espoused the 'clever and smart' virtues of *The Zenith* safety skirt, pronouncing it to be 'an ingenious arrangement which should be universally patronized for its absolute safety, if for no less weighty reason'.[50] Many variations on the safety skirt model of design emerged but, in its earliest of guises, the general principle was that the garment would part company from its wearer in the event of an unseating, and, thereby, avert any threat of dragging, rendering the rider both un-skirted as well as unharmed. Mechanisms to achieve this fast-action removal included fall away seams, press stud-like tab fastenings, and vented false closures. While such designs were effective, offering an augmented standard of safety for riders, the eccentric design concept was also derided as indecent and met with considerable ridicule and scorn. For example, a Leech cartoon, published in *Punch*, 1860, depicted an unseated huntswoman, her white petticoats exposed, watching helplessly as her horse galloped into the far distance, trailing with it her habit skirt: 'Miss Diana slips off at a fence, and is so unfortunate as to leave the better half of her habit on the pommels of her saddle', so the caption went.[51]

[48] Power O'Donoghue, *Ladies On Horseback*, 49.

[49] Hayes, *The Horsewoman*, 92–93.

[50] Kerr, *Riding For Ladies*, 64.

[51] John Leech, *John Leech's Pictures of Life And Character, Volume II*, London: Bradbury, Agnew & Co., 1887, 67.

In light of its shortcomings and defects of design, by the early 1900s the pattern and form of the safety skirt had evolved and been finessed, representing something very much akin to the modern habit skirt of today. It morphed into a far more serviceable apron-style, which removed the problematic, and potentially dangerous, material excess of the underside of the skirt completely (Fig. 4.4). Beach explained the configuration of the apron-style thus: 'the skirt is entirely cut away on the side next to the horse so that, when the rider is mounted, her legs are in direct contact with the saddle'.[52] The emergence of, and increasing popularity for, the safety skirt is traceable through the content of pattern-cutting and tailoring books of the period. For example, *The Standard Work Of Cutting Ladies' Tailor-Made Garments*[53] of 1908 contained a 'safety side-saddle skirt' pattern whilst *The International System Of Ladies' Garment Cutting* (fifth edition),[54] published in 1910, included a selection of some four or five safety patterns for side-saddle riding ranging from a 'pommel clear' through to a 'looped skirt' model (see Fig. 4.4).

4.7 Shapes of Things to Come: Dress History Meets Inclusive and Adaptive Design

The habit skirt, be it apron-style or otherwise, functioned to conceal the lower body of the side-saddle rider and to hide the contours of the legs, thighs, pelvis and buttocks from view, swathing them in a smooth expanse of weighty cloth. There are echoes, here, that return us, full circle, to the opening discussion of waist-up dressing, a more recent moment—or movement—in the history of dress that, somewhat similarly, obscured the lower body from watchful gaze (albeit for vastly different reasons) and, also, highlighted once more the possibilities and pitfalls of designing for the L-shaped frame and dressing for the seated body.

There are, then, design lessons to be learned, revised, reconstructed, inverted and played with when these dress histories of Victorian and/or

[52] Beach, *Riding And Driving For Women*, 110.

[53] S. S. Gordon, *The 'Standard' Work On Cutting Ladies' Tailor-Made Garments: A Complete Treatise On The Art And Science Of Delineating All Garments for Women Made By Tailors*. New York: Mitchell Co., 1908.

[54] J. P. Thornton, *The International System of Ladies' Garment Cutting*. London: The Thornton Institute,1910 (fifth edition).

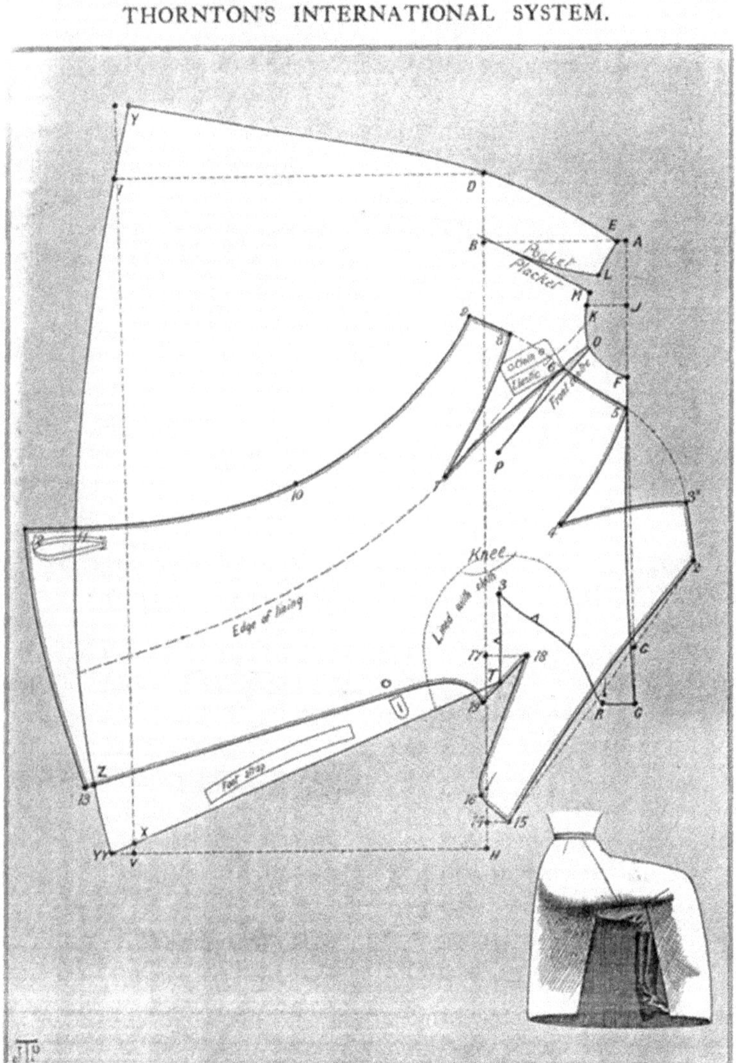

Fig. 4.4 Pattern for 'Lady's Apron Riding Skirt' from Thornton's *International System of Ladies' Garment Cutting* (fifth edition, 1910)

Interwar equestrians 'meet' (to invoke Pullin's language, above)[55] with modern-day product designers, pattern cutters, fashion stylists and creative practitioners.[56] Rather than an outlandish object of little consequence beyond the archive, then, habit dress may be usefully recommissioned and may act as a provocation to creative design, especially in the field of design for disability. Inroads have been made already in this regard with The Royal Ontario Museum's *Fashion Follows Form: Designs For Sitting*[57] exhibition (June 2014 to January 2015), posited here as a touchpaper, providing a curatorial framework through which to ignite both thinking and practice.[58] The exhibition showcased the pioneering work of Canadian fashion designer, Izzy Camilleri and her *IZAdaptive* line of clothing 'for the growing demographic of men and women who use wheelchairs and people living with limited mobility and dexterity'.[59] In *Fashion Follows Form*, designs from Camilleri's contemporary fashion collections were juxtaposed with archive holdings from the eighteenth and nineteenth century: a four-piece wool and velvet side-saddle habit dating from the late 1870s amongst them.[60] The intention was to forge meetings, of both mind and material, across temporal schisms so that the practical challenges of seated life in the modern world might collide with the, usually distant, historical objects of the museum store or display case. When interviewed for the exhibition, Camilleri described her design 'epiphany' as the moment she realised that the guiding principle for accessible fashion was to fit, cut and shape it for a seated, L-shaped, body, creating designs explicitly for the angular pose rather than through the mere alteration of those

[55] Pullin, *Design Meets Disability*.

[56] And, of course, users and/or wearers are also vital stakeholders in the design and development process, too. Interesting examples pertaining both to sitting dress, and to seated makers, are provided by a growing community of grassroots, online, craft collectives and social justice groups (such as *The Sewcialists*, *Seated Sewing* and the social media feed, *#SewnShownSeated*) that advocate for inclusive clothing, the normalisation of the L-shape in fashion and design adaptations to fit and suit people using wheelchairs or with limited mobility. Refer to: https://thesewcialists.com and https://seatedsewing.co.uk.

[57] Royal Ontario Museum, 'Fashion follows form: designs for sitting', 2014, https://www.rom.on.ca/en/exhibitions-galleries/exhibitions/fashion-follows-form-designs-for-sitting.

[58] For an extended review of the exhibition, refer to Rebecca Halliday, Four exhibitions in Toronto. *Fashion Theory: The Journal Of Dress, Body & Culture* 19:4 (2015) 519–539.

[59] IZAdaptive, 'IZAdaptive home', 2022, https://izadaptive.com.

[60] The riding habit in question is held by the Royal Ontario Museum, Canada, accession no: 925.38.19.A-C.

intended for, and manufactured in, the customary upright perpendicular I-shape.[61] Thus:

> she [Camilleri] invented completely new pattern shapes. Seams were carefully placed and pared down, and engineered to avoid abrasion. She incorporated features such as a longer rise in the seat; she eliminated bunching and folds in the lap and she adjusted hems to fall evenly.[62]

Debulking, anti-wrinkling, chafe-resisting: the parallels between the inclusive design ethos of Camilleri's seated fashion for people in wheelchairs, articulated above, and the side-saddle tailoring principles of the traditional habit-maker related over the course of the foregoing chapter, are both striking and instructive. So, too, the references made (above) to Camilleri's 'even hems' and 'lengthy seat' reverberate with the timeworn voices of Mrs Stuart Menzies, of Belle Beach and of Nannie O'Donoghue some 150 years past as they urged, and advised on, correctness of turn out, straightness of line and a well-crafted balance of comfort and style. These echoes float, if unwittingly so, across the corporate rhetoric used by *IZAdaptive* for its online product marketing purposes, and, in so doing, connect a dress history of sitting with current inclusive fashion and design practice for the seated position. The brand's *Junction* trench coat for women offers a particularly compelling example, being marketed on the *IZAdaptive* website as featuring a specially patented 'wheelchair cut' along with design details such as hang, closures and hemming that are evocatively reminiscent of those characterising the historical equestrian apron skirt. The *Junction* coat has:

> a weightier fabric so that it hangs perfectly, and strong magnetic closures for quick fastening when you are in a hurry. Lined with a lustrous pink satin, this coat won't ride up your torso, and it shimmers on the outside and the in. The coat is hemmed to the seat line and doesn't have extra fabric that requires bunching and tucking, so you can roll in style.[63]

What this case study of Camilleri tells us is that there is mileage to be gained in adding voices from dress history both to the conceptual and to the creative work relating to inclusive design and the L-shaped body. The

[61] Palmer, 'Fashion follows form', 20.
[62] Palmer, 'Fashion follows form', 20–21.
[63] IZAdaptive, 'IZAdaptive home'.

time is ripe for a fulsome exploration of a dress history of sitting and for that same project to be collaborative in tenor. If the side-saddle and side-saddle riding have, on occasion, been regarded as anachronisms, then dress history, as a sometimes rarefied and abstracted discipline, has also (if unfairly) come under fire in the past for similar reasons. Doubtless there is room afresh for greater engagement by dress historians in collaborative and applied activity that would shift the discipline into new and impactful registers and forge powerful, and empowering, pathways for both scholarship, practice, and also for advocacy. Just as dress history perspectives, approaches and expertise may enhance the work of creative practitioners and product developers, so, too, may the experimental techniques and traditions of the design studio and workshop bear fruit through which to nourish dress history in, and for, a changed and changing world.

References

Albrecht, Juliana, Jane Farrell-Beck, and Geitel Winakor. 'Function, fashion, and convention in American women's riding costume', 1880–1930. *Dress* 14 (1988) 56–67.

Anonymous. Bustles. *Boston Medical and Surgical Journal*, (Nov 15 1888) 490.

Beach, Belle. *Riding and Driving for Women*. New York: Charles Scribner's, 1912.

Blackman, Cally. *100 Years of Fashion*. London: Laurence King, 2012.

Borrelli-Persson, Laird. 'Thank Zoom for reviving the waist up look first popularized in the 1930s'. *Vogue* (Apr 14 2020) https://www.vogue.com/article/waist-up-dressing-1930s-versus-for-zoom. Accessed 6 Apr 2022.

Christy, E.V.A (Eva). *Modern Side-Saddle Riding: A Practical Handbook for Horsewomen*. London: Vinton & Co, 1907.

Cochrane, Lauren. 'Zoom! Power shoulders are back thanks to video meetings'. *The Guardian*, (Dec 11 2020) https://www.theguardian.com/fashion/2020/dec/11/zoom-power-shoulders-back-thanks-video-meetings-waist-up. Accessed 6 Apr 2022.

Cranz, Galen. *The Chair: Rethinking Culture, Body, and Design*. New York: W.W. Norton & Company, 1998.

Cunningham, Patricia. *Reforming Women's Fashion, 1850–1920: Politics, Health and Art*. Kent, Ohio: Kent State University Press, 2002.

Elan, Priya. 'No sweat: how track suit bottoms became the height of lockdown fashion'. *The Guardian* (Apr 25 2020) https://www.theguardian.com/fashion/2020/apr/25/no-sweat-how-tracksuit-bottoms-became-the-height-of-lockdown-fashion. Accessed 6 Apr 2022.

Eschner, Kat. 'Although less deadly than crinolines, bustles were still a pain in the behind'. *Smithsonian Magazine*, (Apr 21 2017) https://www.smithsonianmag.com/smart-news/although-less-deadly-crinolines-bustles-were-still-pain-behind-180962919/. Accessed 10 Apr 2022.

Gell, Alfred. *Art and Agency: An Anthropological Theory.* Oxford: Clarendon Press, 1998.

Goodrum, Alison. 'A severity of plainness: the culture of female riding dress in America during the 1920s and 1930s'. *Annals of Leisure Research* 15, 1 (2012) 87–105.

Gordon, S. S. *The 'Standard' Work on Cutting Ladies' Tailor-Made Garments: A Complete Treatise on the Art and Science of Delineating All Garments for Women Made By Tailors.* New York: Mitchell Co, 1908.

Halliday, Rebecca. 'Four exhibitions in Toronto'. *Fashion Theory: The Journal of Dress, Body & Culture* 19:4 (2015) 519–539.

Hayes, Alice. *The Horsewoman: A Practical Guide to Side-Saddle Riding.* London: W. Thacker, 1903 [1893].

Houblon, Doreen. *Side-Saddle.* London and New York: Country Life and Charles Scribner's, 1938.

IZAdaptive. 'IZAdaptive home'. https://izadaptive.com. Accessed Mar 7, 2022.

Karr, Elizabeth. *The American Horsewoman.* Cambridge: The Riverside Press, 1884.

Kerr, William. *Riding For Ladies.* New York: Frederick A. Stokes Company, 1891.

Leech, John. *John Leech's Pictures of Life And Character, Volume II.* London: Bradbury, Agnew & Co., 1887.

Linn, Lucy. *Thirteen Hunts in Ireland: Feb 13 to Mar 13, 1948.* Privately Printed in Chicago, 1949.

Marsh, Natasha. 'What clothes will you wear when the pandemic is finally over?' *Byrdie.* https://www.byrdie.com/fashion-trends-post-pandemic-5190627. 2021. Accessed 25 Mar 2022.

Matthews David, Alison. 'Elegant amazons: victorian riding habits and the fashionable horsewoman'. *Victorian Literature And Culture* 30:1 (2002) 179–210.

Matthews David, Alison. *Fashion Victims: The Dangers of Dress Past and Present.* London: Bloomsbury, 2015.

Menkes, Suzy. 'Blithe spirit: the Windsor set: a glimpse of the era before world war II: beauty on the eve of destruction'. *International Herald Tribune* (Dec 3 2002) https://www.nytimes.com/2002/12/03/style/IHT-blithe-spiritthe-windsor-seta-glimpse-of-the-era-before-world-war.html. Accessed 2 May 2022.

Palmer, Alexandra. 'Fashion follows form: patterning a relationship between function and fashion'. *ROM Magazine* Summer 2014. 18–23.

Pears, Matthew, Kola-Palmer, Susanna, and Beretta De Azevedo, Liane. 'The impact of sitting time and physical activity on mental health during COVID-19 lockdown'. *Sports Sciences for Health* 18 (2022) 179–191.

Power O'Donoghue, Nannie. *Ladies on Horseback: Learning, Park-Riding, and Hunting, with Hints Upon Costume, and Numerous Anecdotes.* London: W.H. Allen, 1889.

Pullin, Graham. *Design Meets Disability.* Cambridge: MIT Press, 2009.

Royal Ontario Museum. 'Fashion follows form: designs for sitting'. https://www.rom.on.ca/en/exhibitions-galleries/exhibitions/fashion-follows-form-designs-for-sitting. 2014. Accessed 21 Mar 2022.

Sampson, Ellen. *Worn: Footwear, Attachment and the Affects of Wear.* London: Bloomsbury, 2020.

Sheddon, Diana and Apsley, Violet. *To Whom The Goddess…: Hunting and Riding for Women.* London: Hutchison and Co., 1932.

Steele, Valerie. *The Corset: A Cultural History.* New Haven: Yale University Press, 2003.

Stirling Clarke, J. *The Habit and The Horse: A Treatise on Female Equitation.* London: The Authoress, 1857.

Stuart Menzies, A. C. *Women in the Hunting Field.* London: Vinton, 1913.

Thornton, J. P. *The International System of Ladies' Garment Cutting.* London: The Thornton Institute, 1910 (fifth edition).

CHAPTER 5

The Itches: Embodiment and Distributed Meaning in the Age of Technological Entanglement

Sonia Bernac

The hands want to see, the eyes want to caress
—Johann Wolfgang von Goethe

adhesive nipples, amplifiers, anti-rape condoms, artworks, armour, artificial eyes/limbs/six-packs/skin/teeth/wombs, baby-soothers, binoculars, braces, breast implants/pumps, books, calendars, chastity belts, chest binders, computers, contraception, cutlery, bunny-tail butt plugs, clothes, corsets, dentures, dialysers, drones, drugs, external hard drives, fake eyelashes/nails/tan, formula milk, GPS, guns, gym machines, hearing aids, pacemakers, high heels, incubators, language, corrective/colour-altering/magnifying lenses, machine learning algorithms, microchips, nail extensions, padded underwear, perfume, photography, plasters, robots, senses, sensors, spandex, sperm donors, stoma bags, strap-ons,

S. Bernac (✉)
Royal College of Art, London, UK
e-mail: sonia.bernaciak@network.rca.ac.uk

D. Woolley et al. (eds.), *Wearable Objects and Curative Things*, Palgrave Studies in Fashion and the Body,
https://doi.org/10.1007/978-3-031-40017-9_5

supplements, surgically reconstructed body parts, surrogate mothers, torture machines, vaccinations, vibrators, VR, weightlifting belts, wet-nurses, wigs, wings, wrist bands

5.1 Introduction

This short, arbitrary, and by no means complete list of bodily replacements, corrections, extensions and constrictions signals the diversity of materiality, scale, contexts, and politics of *things* with prosthetic qualities. Certain technologies are easier to accept as belonging to the category of prosthesis than others, and that analytical wrestling itself maps the ontological difficulties, dangers, and opportunities that prosthetics generate. The precision and fairness of that negotiation is of particular importance, as it does not only serve theoretical exercise or accuracy. Rather, it conditions the embodied experience of humans and other sentient beings, often determining who gets included in those categories, whose personhood might be temporarily suspended, and who is thought of as being *one* which has a body. Such political responsibility requires a much more subtle methodological move than creating a concept of prosthetics flexible enough to ensure inclusion of all the bodily replacements, extensions and constrictions. Therefore, the act of mapping the category of prosthetics needs to include empathy as part of its logic, not as something introduced or executed at a level of implementation by 'real life' organisations, such as public health systems, or even more dangerously, by the dynamics of the market.

A prosthesis is considered here as a specific type of technological entanglement rather than a device of some auxiliary function. Critically, this entanglement is not a relationship *between* the biotic body and the broadly understood notion of the machine. In fact, the disruption of this neat conceptual duality (of technology and body) is crucial for understanding the ontological potential of prosthesis. Hence, the vision of prosthetic tension as a singular boundary located *between* the uniformly biotic body and the coherently artificial prosthetic device is replaced in this chapter by complex anatomies of new hybrid-emergent selves.

Another aspect of prosthetic entanglement examined here is the pivotal difference between prosthetic relationships and other types of interdependencies with technology. What follows is an analysis of those particular features of prosthetic attachment: its articulation with corporeal trauma, its distributed nature, and the particular kind of intimacy that it produces. The idea of prosthetic touch will also be revised in the context of digital technologies that do not always require physical articulation, yet remain material. As a consequence, the definition of prosthetic as that which *touches* the body becomes extended by the complication of the very notion of touch.

The category of prosthesis is not merely presented here as an object of theoretical investigation but proposed and tested as a philosophical instrument, one that can be utilised in order to examine ideas of the fragment, the whole, and the boundary. Those questions have become gradually more urgent with the growing global importance of distributed systems and learning algorithms and, more importantly, with the blurring of the boundaries between that which is assuredly robotic-artificial and that which, until recently, was considered essentially biotic-human.

The methodological approach enacted here is a materialist investigation that assumes that meaning cannot exist beyond or outside of matter. This approach brings together analytics based on post-Newtonian physics and complexity theory with a particular emphasis on emergence.

5.2 Methodological Paradoxes: Edges, Essences, and Distributions

Previous historical or genealogical investigations into the notion of prosthetics show that the line between technologies of care and embodied oppression might be ambiguous, or more precisely, that grasping the intensity of prostheses through supposedly oppositional concepts does not account for their hybrid tendencies. This means that prostheses often emerge as a paradoxical device, having a particular predilection for being many things simultaneously. It is a situation rendered impossible by the laws of Newtonian physics, which assumes that two things cannot simultaneously occupy the same space.

In lieu of more effective analysis, this simultaneity is often negotiated by mapping the prosthetic through classically oppositional or antithetical pairs, including but not limited to notions of: lack–excess; illness–recovery (*getting back to normal*); constriction–extension; replacement–augmentation; interiority–exteriority; biotic–synthetic; necessity–vanity; corporeal–psychological (*that which is related to the mind, identity, or consciousness*); functional–aesthetic; reconstructive–enhancing; or real–artificial. However, even if we accept the assumption that the extremes of these binaries are not definite or ultimate, and that prosthetics always negotiate, conflate, or transgress these polarities, those biaxial or even multiaxial systems are still at work. Thus, one is set the impossible task of mapping the meaning of the prosthetic entities somewhere *in-between* or *within* the network of those spectral markers. In this spectral scenario, for example, a device cannot be an object of intense vanity and great necessity at the same time, since these are presented as polar oppositions.

More refined analytical frameworks that still uphold the binary, such as Hegelian dialectics, do allow for certain forms of plurality as a result of the sublation of thesis and antithesis, which together form a synthetic unity, in turn providing the ground of the concept. This mode of understanding enables the articulation of certain paradoxes and contradictions, for example, the fact that many prosthetic technologies can be devices of severe pain or great pleasure without ever reaching the middle ground—that of becoming a neutral tool.[1] A corset, in this analytical framework, can be rightly presented as a form of embodied othering—a mutilating device which constrains the female body and its movement and, simultaneously, a source of joy and pleasure when it is used in a drag performance, for example. This situation of occupying two extremes of meaning at the same time: bodily oppression and freedom of sexual expression, would be analytically inexpressible in the spectral logic of in-betweenness.

Hegelian dialectics becomes less helpful, however, in the articulation of other prosthetic features. As a universal logic, it assumes that meaning would be *true* everywhere at all times regardless of context.[2] This does not explain why certain technologies can be acknowledged as prosthetic only in very particular situations. For example, a glass eye is more easily classified as such if inserted to an empty eye socket, rather than mixed with marbles in a decorative bowl. This contextual flickering undermines the essentialism and universalism of the teleological move.

The shift towards smart devices and the Internet of Things (IoT) complicates the very notion of prosthetics even further, exposing the insufficiency of any binary-based methodologies. With multiple devices at work and users' data perpetually uploaded to external servers, prostheses can no

[1] This is because thesis and antithesis are not contradiction or oppositions. Rather, they are sublated *together* to form the ground of the concept. For example, everything that is pleasure (thesis) and everything that is not-pleasure (antithesis) lead to the formation of *the concept* of pleasure.

[2] This critique of the shortcoming of the dialectical method is indebted to the research group and the lecture series *Entanglement* led and developed by Johnny Golding at the Royal College of Art.

longer be analysed as singular objects with clearly defined, palpable edges. The majority of these prosthetic technologies are algorithmically designed and tested, or remain a part of the perpetually updating software circuit. Here, the human-versus-prosthetic-machine relationship is dismantled and replaced by complex feedback loops and distributed ontologies. This radical shift is not merely the optimisation or advancement of already prosthetic technologies. Growing algorithmisation and the densifying network of the IoT are producing forced dependencies and entanglements that make previously non-prosthetic technological tools touch and articulate with the body in new, far more intimate ways. Touch, and a particularly intimate relationship with a body, become crucial for the understanding of prostheses, differentiating it from other types of technological devices and systems.

There is something ontologically disruptive about prosthesis, in the particular way that it articulates the body, drawing attention to its edges and questioning the barrier of tissues, concepts, and selves. Prostheses touch the skin in a unique fashion, refusing to be merged with it—unlike a transplant—and (ad)dressing bodily traumas more directly and relentlessly than, for example, clothes or jewellery.

The questioning and preoccupation with prosthetics' characteristic edge makes the customary starting points of academic explorations unsuitable as methods. Investigation into prosthetic meanings cannot be initiated through a dictionary definition; analysis of etymological ambiguities; or the common-sense application of a term. The prosthetic always points to the edge of its own meaning, complicating ideas of the whole and the fragment. Therefore, grasping the intensity of prosthetics does not emerge as a problem of definition, but rather as part of a wider onto-epistemological move which necessarily deals with notions of lack, substance, essence, transgression, and, much more importantly, entanglement and emergence.

5.3 Corporeality of Absence: Gaps, Wounds, and Scars

Absence, like all other kinds of apparent nothingness, points to forms of distributed or non-physical materialities. This does not mean that they require a metaphysical move, or that their meaning should only be considered within the constructs of linguistics. Absences, lacks and gaps are not placeholders for what once was and is not any longer, the same way a memory is not just a phantom trace of a *real* event. The often painful presence of absence can become a point, towards which the trajectories of an entity orientate. In that sense, it is not dissimilar to mathematical attractors pulling the trajectories of dynamics systems towards themselves. Ingmar Bergman said that 'if your tooth hurts, your tongue keeps going there. You are always conscious of a wound'. The pull of the wound applies to all forms of compulsive return: tracing the lines of scars with one's fingers; nervous glancing at the gaps that disrupt well-known sequences; getting stuck at parts of one's world concealed by dementia or the recollection of a stubborn memory.

Prosthetics have a particular relationship with a strange form of being that is often described as lack. Understood thus, bodily extensions act as replacements of something that is missing or has been lost, creating a kind of longing. The image of that apparent absence is crucial for the ontology of prosthetics. If that absence is understood as the lack of being, then: 'it is not the lack of this or that, but lack of being whereby the being exists'.[3] In this sense, the Lacanian psychoanalytic move is different to the dialectical image of absence understood as non-being, constituting the antithetical side of sublated synthetic unity. As a consequence, in the dialectical move, the present is analytically impossible to occupy. In the Lacanian sense, lack has a form of paradoxical presence *productive* of desire—it is something rather than a form of void. However, despite its productivity, the Lacanian lack is not fully present.

Therefore, prosthetics can be thought of either as the presence of something where something else is missing, or as something that articulates with a strange form of being that is already there. That ontologically weird entity not only is productive but can also be strategically designed, produced and multiplied. Different forms of absence, lack and loss can be generated by the normative discourse of their time (which can itself be a part of a premeditated political strategy). By that understanding, a prosthetic device corrects faults and inadequacies; moulds the embarrassing excess of flesh or sexuality; patches over illness and wrongness; meets *special* needs; enables looking, feeling, and living *normally*. Unfortunately, the normal or its close relatives—the universal and the standard—are extremely narrow categories, despite their pretences. It is not so much a

[3] Jacques Lacan, *The Ego in Freud's Theory and in the Technique of Psychoanalysis, 1954–1955*, ed. Jacques-Alain Miller, trans. Sylvana Tomaselli, Revised ed. Edition, New York, N.Y: W.W. Norton & Co., 1991.

problem of their equalising nature, particularly unkind to the fringes and particularities, but rather that as much as the Lacanian lack produces desire, this desire can also produce lack. In that model, the universal is not the averaged status quo but rather an aspirational (and never fully achievable) essentialist idea. Paradoxically, the realm of those eternal, immutable forms constantly changes according to the type of philosophical idealism and the political or historical context. It is reflected by the consistently unattainable but rapidly changing beauty standards. What remains fixed are the awkward and shameful bodies stuck in their entropic imperfection, ridden by disease and affected by accidents. If the desire or *telos* give meaning, direction and presence to lack or becoming in universal philosophies, then prosthetic technologies are props enabling malformed bodies to chase the idea of some wholeness, convenience, beauty, and normality. In that sense, they are teleological devices allowing (some)body to be placed on the beneficial dialectical side.

Following that logic, it could be argued that absences, gaps, and inadequacies are *artificially* or *externally* created. If the fully able(d), healthy, strong, young, symmetrical, white body is no longer conceptualised as a universal, neutral idea of the human, then all forms of previously othered, differently bodied beings should, seemingly, return from their ontological exile. However, if absence does not exist as an analytical or material category, one seems to be at risk of ignoring or relativising the trauma of loss that is often connected to prosthetic technologies. The feeling of inadequacy or lack is not just a result of a normative social imperative—a form of, by definition, unattainable desire—but can also be an act of longing for the past self, unaffected by the trauma of illness or an accident. The lived experience of long sickness, a sense of humiliation, alienation, chronic pain, and fear, do not seem to be taken into consideration in transgressive ideas of a body that perpetually expands its biological essence through technological entanglement. The kind of trauma in question here is not an unpleasant memory *of* the past but an ontologically transforming event always located in the present, productive of space and time.[4] Conceptualising prosthetics requires a methodological framework that could account for

[4]A similar argument about temporality of trauma is formulated by Christina Sharpe in *In the Wake: On Blackness And Being*. In Sharpe's work, the emphasis is put on trauma of black bodies captured and analysed through the figure of 'the wake'.

Christina Sharpe, *In the Wake: On Blackness And Being*, Illustrated edition, Durham: Duke University Press, 2016

the parts of the self affected by accidents or wronged by other beings; it necessitates rethinking of bodies, consumed and often alienated by disease, without assuming an idealised essence.

Catherine Malabou talks about the destructive plasticity of the certain kinds of wounds that open up an irreversible cycle of transformation:

> Transformation would no longer be a trick, a strategy or a mask always ready to be lifted to reveal the authentic features of the face. Transformation would betray an existential underground, which, beyond the round of metamorphoses, would enable the subject to become unrecognisable. Unrecognisable less because of a change in appearance than on account of a change in nature, a molting of the inner sculpture.[5]

The destructive plasticity in Malabou's understanding is not simply tantamount to entropy of a system. Rather, it is a force that cannot be inscribed within the creative-destructive opposition, being often violently productive of new, emergent selves. The destructive plasticity of a wound is crucial for understanding prosthetics not as something that replaces a lack, but rather as a technology which articulates *with* a bodily trauma; a trauma that is itself a material *thing*, a present plastic entity.

5.4 Siloying of Senses: Skin, Sensors, and Synaesthesia

Lyotard opens his *Libidinal economy* with a figure of a vivisected body. Its anatomy is disrupted; organs and parts are opened and laid flat so that they form a surface. The body's interiority and exteriority are undermined and questioned; the boundary delineated by the membrane of the skin no longer exists.

> Don't forget to add to the tongue and all the pieces of the vocal apparatus, all the sounds of which they are capable, and moreover, the whole selective network of sounds, that is, the phonological system, for this too belongs to the libidinal 'body', like colours that must be added to retinas, like certain particles to the epidermis, like some particularly favoured smells to the nasal

[5] Catherine Malabou, *The Ontology of the Accident: An Essay on Destructive Plasticity*, Cambridge: Polity Press, 2012.

> cavities, like preferred words and syntaxes to the mouths which utter them and to the hands which write them.[6]

The edge of the body is problematised by the expanded functionalities, affiliations and predilections of its elements. In that sense, a body is neither a sum of the collection of organs nor a well-designed machine, the parts of which are subservient to the meaning of the whole. Most importantly, its meaning does not originate externally, being projected onto organs through the context, neither is a result of some internal (genetic, evolutionary or creationist) essence. Lyotard also criticises the structuralist approach, in which meanings are never fully present and are only graspable through difference, in relation and reference to other elements.

Though the 'organic body' and 'the great ephemeral skin' do not serve as metaphors or concepts, nor can they be applied in a literal manner to understand separate bodies of individuals.[7] Lyotard proposes an ontological move which implies forms of polymorphous circulations, investments and intensities. In that sense, *Libidinal Economy* is a work about always already pluralised matter and meaning. The meaning of a body, or rather embodied meaning, is always material, dynamic, distributed, and prone to mutation. Understood thus, the Lyotardian move allows a rethinking of the relationship between a body, contemporary prosthetic technologies, and trauma. Its philosophical subtlety facilitates the grasping of a shift towards distributed systems, and demonstrates the artificiality of the division between actual and metaphorical prosthetics.

The first analytical step towards dismantling the difference between the actual and metaphorical prosthetics would be to focus on the senses as undermining the boundary delineated by the tissues, organs, words, and concepts. Glasses and hearing aids are easily accepted as belonging to the category of prosthetic technologies, even though their functionality escapes the *mechanical* articulation of their parts, with which they are believed to be associated. If hearing is considered as that belonging to the ears; smell as a function of noses; sight as an optical endeavour; touch enabled by the skin; and taste as that contained by a mouth, then a body is conceptualised as a sum of elements with specialised functionalities. Contemporary technologies, however, bypass the attachments of senses to the body parts, proposing alternative modes of hearing, seeing, touching.

[6] Jean-François Lyotard, *Libidinal Economy*, Reprint edition, Bloomsbury Academic, 2015.
[7] Lyotard, *Libidinal Economy*.

Cochlear implants, for example, are not amplifiers like standard hearing aids; they stimulate the auditory nerve directly, creating an entirely different way of processing sound in people with profound hearing impairments.[8] Similarly, the first prototypes of non-retinal artificial visual prosthetics directly stimulate the cortex of the brain, receiving information from a video camera.[9] The bypassing of organs considered vital for particular forms of sensing points to functional distribution of ways of *grasping*.

There is, however, some methodological literality in the kind of argument that falls into the trap of the new phrenological-like approach. It follows the logic that, for example, a form of sensing can be acknowledged as a form of seeing, if a part of brain usually responsible for optical vision gets activated during some kind of prosthetic stimulation. In that understanding, 'seeing with one's fingers' or 'hearing through one's body' can be only cognitive metaphors, as long as they do not activate the parts of the brain that usually respond to a particular siloed sense.

However, tracing of faces, objects or even entire spaces with one's fingers can lead to the creation of a clear image or shape in one's mind that will possess certain values usually reserved for aesthetics: colour, volume, and depth. Feeling the warmth of the light on one's skin can lead to (re) cognition of a particular hue, even in the absence of eyesight. Brian Massumi in *The Autonomy of Affect* claims that:

> affect is synaesthetic, implying a participation of the senses in each other: the measure of a living thing's potential interactions is its ability to transform the effects of one sensory mode into those of another (tactility and vision being the most obvious but by no means only examples; interoceptive senses, especially proprioception, are crucial). Affects are virtual synaesthetic perspectives anchored in (functionally limited by) the actually existing, particular things that embody them.[10]

[8] Mara Mills, 'Do signals have politics? Inscribing abilities in cochlear implants', *The Oxford handbook of sound studies* (2012): 320-346.

[9] Rodrigo A. Brant Fernandes, Bruno Diniz, Ramiro Ribeiro, and Mark Humayun. 'Artificial vision through neuronal stimulation', *Neuroscience letters* 519, no. 2 (2012): 122–128.

[10] Brian Massumi, 'The Autonomy of Affect', *Cultural Critique*, no. 31 (1995): 83–109. https://doi.org/10.2307/1354446.

The concept of synaesthesia suggests that each specialised sense receives a different kind of informational input. But, those separate channels can often become merged, associated or replaced under certain conditions, when the sensorial impression is formed. This can produce a situation in which a colour can be cold, or there is a particular sound attached to a certain smell in an individual or a collective mind. Synaesthesia offers a form of redemption to the 'impure' ways of sensing without sending them to the realm of metaphor or linguistic phenomena. However, analytically, the idea of senses being occasionally synaesthetically confused or conjoined is based on an assumption that touch, smell, taste, sight, and hearing usually exist in some pure—essential form, like highly specialised sensors designed to detect one particular chemical, range of temperature or type of movement.[11]

5.5 Acephalic Bodies: Heads, Brains, and Smart Devices

Distributed sensing is a very different proposition to the idea of synaesthesia, as it assumes a profoundly decentralised idea of perception of stimulus that does not answer to one primary organ or a section of a brain. This does not imply relativisation of the senses, nor denial of the involvement of highly specialised receptors in obtaining information from the environment. However, it does undermine the idea of human perception understood as a sum of individualised sensorial networks. Prosthetic paradoxes allow a way into thinking about distributed sensing which is a qualitative rather than a quantitative move.

In Stanislaw Lem's short story, *Are You There Mr. Jones?*, the protagonist Harry Jones has a series of accidents. After each of them, the Cybernetics Company offers him prostheses until all of his body, including half of his brain, has been replaced. As a result, Jones falls into debt, being unable to pay for all the replacement parts. The company sues him and requests a return of all the prostheses, but the court rejects their claim because it would be tantamount to killing Jones. Then, the company tricks Jones into replacing the remaining half of his brain, and claims Jones as their property. The court faces an ethical and analytical conundrum: if Jones is quantitively a piece of technology then he cannot be sued;

[11] The thought developed here originated from discussions at the AiDesign Lab: Artificial and Distributed Intelligence, led by Johnny Golding, based at the Royal College of Art.

otherwise, if he is still a human being, he cannot be (legally) claimed as property.[12]

The example of Harry Jones raises the question of technological substitution in a provocative manner, challenging quantitative understandings of human embodiment. If the body is understood as a sum of diverse parts or networks with specialised functions, then loss of hearing, for example, must always remain a form of subtraction from the standardised wholeness of human abilities. However, contemporary prosthesis in particular allows for the re-construction of bodily performance, which often significantly exceeds the average range, durability, speed or lifespan of *natural* bodily circuits or organs. That functional surplus is difficult to conceptualise in the rigid mathematics of the normalised, *essential* body understood as (some)one.

There are certain types of prosthetics that neither replace what once was or should be, nor try to exceed certain bodily functions. Instead, they offer completely new ways of sensing that are crucial for sustaining life functions, particularly in patients whose conditions require precise medical forecasting, such as diabetes, cardiovascular diseases, or epilepsy. This implies that expanding and extending, often associated with prosthesis, does not have to be tantamount to becoming *more*, or going further in the same (outward) direction, as pre-defined by evolutionary patterns.

Distributed sensing disregards the dialectics of biotic-synthetic and focuses on new, emergent entities that are not necessarily restored sums of pre-existing organs and circuits. Moreover, it shifts the point of tension from that located *between* natural body and technological prosthesis, to the complexity of feedback loops. These can be understood in a straightforward physical way: for example, sensors in a prosthetic limb receive information from a body transmitting neural signals, and the robotic actuators act accordingly. This in turn has the potential to change bodily sensations and dictate subsequent actions. In this case, body and prosthesis form a singular circuit. However, most contemporary wearables are not based on closed feedback loops between users and their devices.

In the age of machine learning and perpetually advancing neural networks, the collected data of all users serves as material for pattern recognition. Feedback loops become complicated, layered and transformed. Algorithms learn not only individual bodily patterns, but also multiple collective rhythms belonging to all active and past users of the given

[12] Stanisław Lem, *Przekładaniec*, Agora: 2018.

wearable. The patterns of heartbeat and sleep, daily excitations, weight fluctuations, meal plans, sports activities, and traumas live in this perpetually learning and mutating code. In a certain sense, all the organs; technological devices imbued with sensors and actuators; algorithms; servers; and cables become parts of a bio-synthetic organism, distributed both temporally and spatially.

Mercedes Bunz in the *Internet of Things* describes this strange flow of information—clients' data—through *smart* devices, acknowledging that the smartness of wearables does not imply some Machiavellian intelligence or advancement of singular pieces of technology. Quite the opposite: cheap and often devoid of a firewall, smart devices display high vulnerability to being hacked and used in DoS- and DDoS-type attacks.[13] Their accuracy, effectiveness or usefulness is based on the collective body of users' data, and finding patterns for behavioural prognosis therein.

This image of distribution should not be seen as a network, as that would not fully account for the complexity of the localised connections of distributed sensing. It does not mean simply that those connections are complicated, but rather that the system shows principles of complexity: emergence, non-linearity and undecidability. It is not enough to say that the bodily and the digital algorithms are in a mutual simultaneous interaction, consistent with Newton's Third Law. Human matter lives in the distributed code as much as digital algorithms become entangled with human bodies. This effect can be observed in behavioural influence, when algorithms change the code of daily activities, for example by pushing notifications that warn users against possible bodily traumas or encourage them to change unhealthy actions, such as irregular sleep patterns or lack of movement. It is also a purely physical phenomenon of new neural connections forming, particularly in patients who use smart neuromusculoskeletal prostheses—those which are attached to nerves, muscles and a skeleton simultaneously.[14] Algorithmic prosthetics become distributed in subliminal ways as well, activating a dopamine response in reaction to the

[13] Denial-of-service and distributed-denial-of-service cyberattacks cause disruption to the accessibility of a website that becomes overloaded with requests and, as a consequence, does not respond to legitimate demands; the DDoS attack comes from several different sources.

Mercedes Bunz and Graham Meikle, *The Internet of Things*, Cambridge, UK; Malden, MA, USA: Polity Press, 2017.

[14] Max Ortiz-Catalan, Enzo Mastinu, Paolo Sassu, Oskar Aszmann, and Rickard Brånemark. 'Self-contained neuromusculoskeletal arm prostheses', *New England Journal of Medicine* 382, no. 18 (2020): 1732–1738.

notification sounds of various apps and portable devices. This ontological re-coding and re-distribution in prosthetic interaction seems to be more profound than the principles of mutuality or Newtonian reciprocity.

5.6 Distributed Attachments: Cyborgs, Joints, and Entanglements

The difference between a cyborg and the creature sutured by Doctor Frankenstein seems to lie in distinctive categories of matter being put together. Victor Frankenstein's creation was an amalgamation of corporeal parts that all formerly belonged to human beings. The challenge was to transform dead matter into living. In many ways, Frankenstein's task seemed easier than the current cyborgian one, as it dealt with coherently human and uniformly dead ingredients. Cyborgs, conversely, as assemblages of organic and inorganic (cyborgian) matter, face the difficulty of negotiating between ontologically different codes. The difference between a prosthesis and, for example, a transplant, is that the prosthetic implies an assemblage of the corporeal body and some ontologically different *thing*—often, but not necessarily, abiotic or artificial—that alters the body's functionality. There is a form of tension at the heart of prosthetic emergence; an unsolvable difference that, much like Malabou's plasticity, inevitably transforms the whole system.

The problem of the attachment of one thing to another seemingly only lies at the physical border of entities. The corporeal biotic body is often thought of as displaying a pluralised but united front, neatly delineated by the edge of the skin, and allied with a common telos of some vaguely understood well-being. However, the alliance of organs, tissues and parts is fragile, far from the Renaissance conceptualisation of the human body as a perfect design. Bodies as wholes often lose their integrity: tissues sabotage organs; harmless bacteria or fungi overgrow and become pathological; leftover vestigial structures from the past lead to infections; singular cells multiply uncontrollably and attack the whole system, leading to its failure.

It is easier to conceptualise enemies, selves, technologies or misfortune as clearly separable *things*, equipped with a functional core located at the centre, and diverse parts responsible for various functions. This implies particular logics of knowing, grasping and defence, as well as a specific image of hybridity and entanglement. The methodological consequence of the reductionist assumption that a whole is the sum of its parts, is knowing through taking apart. However, there are many phenomena that reveal the insufficiency of such thinking. Auto-immune and oncological diseases cannot be fully understood through the analysis of singular cells without taking into consideration the dynamics of spreading, circulation and distribution; and acknowledgement that the same structures can display radically different behaviour in different circumstances. Similarly, algorithmic technologies and the growing and densifying network of the IoT cannot be grasped through the analysis of its constituent parts.

If neither the corporeal body, nor the algorithmic technologies which are more and more frequently involved in prosthetics, cannot be understood as closed entities, the notion of attachment changes its shape. It is not so much about disrupting notions of interiority and exteriority—even old-fashioned dentures or glass eyes question the idea of prosthesis as an external add-on. The idea of distribution forces one to think about attachment not as a tension-cohesion *between* a body and a prosthetic thing, but as a form of difference-repetition that becomes part of the code of a new, emergent entity. Entanglement—prosthetic or otherwise—is not, as Karen Barad rightly points out in the *Meeting the Universe Half Way*, a quality of being 'intertwined with another as in the joining of separate entities'.[15] Rather, it is a state of connection that does not include communication, wherein one thing cannot be separated from the whole nor defined independently of another. This does not mean that meaning is relational or that a body becomes defined through prosthetics. Instead, it speaks of the deep intimacy of prosthetic connection and of its productive potential.

This productivity is not about instrumentalist production; an outcome or utility. Heidegger, in his *Question Concerning Technology*, observes that technology is not exclusively a means to an end; it is not a process during which the new things are made, nor the human ability to produce them. He defines the essence of technology as 'by no means anything technological', by which he means that the logic of techne belongs to 'bringing forth' in a form of poiesis: 'the arising of something from out of itself'.[16] The act of 'revealing'—bringing out of concealment—could be seen as part of the Heideggerian phenomenological move, the 'phenomenology

[15] Karen Barad, *Meeting the Universe Halfway: Quantum Physics and the Entanglement of Matter and Meaning*, Illustrated edition, Durham: Duke University Press, 2007.

[16] Martin Heidegger, *The Question Concerning Technology: And Other Essays*, Reissue edition, New York; London Toronto: Harper Perennial, 2013.

of the inconspicuous'. This 'unconcealment' or 'truth revealing' should not be seen as a metaphysical or essentialist move, but as the realisation of a new arrangement out of the possibilities of matter. In that understanding, that which is '*Unscheinbaren*'—translated as 'inconspicuous' *or* 'inapparent'—would have a strange ontological status that cannot be contained in the dialectics of absence-presence. That which is invented, used or discovered is neither summoned from the unrealised world of ideas, nor conceived in the creator's mind. Rather, it is part of a plural move of grasping the out-there and being grasped by it (at the same time), expressed by Heidegger's principle of identity as: A=A.[17] That apparently tautological equation marks a principle of being that is always already in the world; that collapses the neat division of matter between subjects, objects and contexts.[18] Building on the Heideggerian move, Johnny Golding proposes to read A=A as an encounter of embodied exchange, where the ontological base of all being is always already plural. In Golding's work, meaning is perpetually emergent, based on thickening feedback loops, and always requires a form of matter.[19,20]

Prosthetic entanglement is necessarily based on the technological revealing and plurality crucial to its understanding, without which one might resort to the image of intertwined binaries of biotic-mechatronic or human-robotic. Prosthetic bodies are entities with distributed entanglements that run through their emergent codes. In many ways, the question concerning prosthetics is simultaneously a question concerning technology; one which places its emphasis on the aspects of embodiment, intimacy, and emergence.

5.7 Prosthetic Intimacies: Screens, Wings, and Sex Devices

All forms of prosthetics are technological in the expanded Heideggerian sense, but stating that all forms of technology are prosthetic seems to be a rushed conclusion. The question concerning prosthetics implies some

[17] Martin Heidegger, *Identity and Difference*, trans. Joan Stambaugh, 2nd ed. Edition, Chicago: University of Chicago Press, 2002.

[18] Johnny Golding, 'The Courage to Matter', *Data Loam: Sometimes Hard, Usually Soft (the Future of Knowledge Systems)*, 2021. https://doi.org/10.1515/9783110697841.

[19] Golding, 'The Courage to Matter'.

[20] Johnny Golding, 'Friendship' *Edinburgh Companion to Animal Studies*, 1st edition, EUP, 2017.

dark sensuousness or tension that does not seem to refer to the universal qualities of things, but to the form of attachment—touch—formed with the corporeal body. Prosthetic attachment requires a form of matter, but in the age of wireless technologies and sensors it is not controversial to state that connection can take many invisible forms. That is not to say that those ways of pairing are immaterial or metaphorical. A prosthesis is not an objective physical category of concrete device or technology, but rather a specific form of encounter that addresses corporeal trauma. Similarly, that trauma can take many forms and should not be considered as measurable damage or a particular kind of (universally traumatic) event.

Addressing trauma thus does not come with a fixed form of ethics; it does not have to be tantamount to healing, re-pairing, or facilitating. In that sense, a prosthetic can be an oppressive device: nudging, correcting, embarrassing, and shaming the body. That corrective move does not need to have a clear telos. Quite the opposite: the sadism of unrealistic body standards is not a result of the unattainable perfection of the ideal corporeal form, but rather a signal that those ideals themselves are contradictory, paradoxical, and dynamic. However, it needs to be acknowledged that there are some bodies that are particularly subject to those mechanisms of shaming. Black, brown, female and trans bodies, or those whose needs are marked as *special*, become objects of perpetual scrutiny that can operate on the basis of assumed inadequacy—or the opposite: an apparent glorification, often slipping into forms of fetishisation. Prosthetics as corrective-fetishising devices can become tools of an embodied othering or cruelty that, sadly, does not require an analytically correct excuse.

An oppressive prosthetic device can take the form of a tangible object, such as a wig worn to conceal naturally textured hair; padded underwear that imitates voluptuous tissues of breasts or buttocks; or a clip that makes the bridge of a nose more prominent, but it can also take much more subtle routes. Recommendation algorithms can create radicalisation echo-chambers that slowly rewire one's thinking, and, more importantly, feeling and sensing patterns. These entangled preferences, excitations, and annoyances become a part of the circulating recommendation code distributed between people, servers, and devices. It could be argued that these forms of technology do not *touch* the body in a specified way, therefore failing to fulfil the requirement of prosthetics. However, that digital virtuality wrongly gets the status of the not-quite-real, or non-material. Personal devices are one of the most frequently touched objects, and the complicated rhythm of tapping, sliding, clicking, and pressing is entangled with the reactions of the human nervous system. Screens and keyboards are covered with traces of those daily engagements; with the grease, sweat, and dirt of touch.

The corrective rewiring of patterns of behaviour that addresses bodies can be also observed in the forms of their policing, executed through various technologies of surveillance. In that understanding, corporate or governmental data hoarding enables the profiling, seducing, disciplining and punishing of a corporeal body of consumers or citizens, acting as a Panopticon-like prosthetic conscience. This violation of privacy moves with stealth, as the recording, processing, and selling of most private data is performed through forced intimacy with technology; through the introduction and reinforcement of drones, security cameras, wearables, and algorithms attuned to trace the most subtle of human movements.

Johnny Golding claims that any encounter—the space-moment of meaning-making—must necessarily require pluralised attraction and difference.[21] In that sense, the prosthetic encounter is libidinal, which does not necessarily imply forms of sexuality. The intimacy of prosthetic grasping and being grasped is described in David Burrows' and Simon O'Sullivan's *Fictioning: The Myth Functions of Contemporary Art and Philosophy*. Here, they develop the Lacanian notion of *extimacy*—an intimate exteriority that collapses the dichotomy of outside and inside. In their work, the contemporary moment of technological singularity is defined as extimate, characterised by radical mytho-technic processes that do not distinguish between human and machine, but rather weave (together) the lived experiences extended and embodied through intimacy with technology.[22]

The taboo around prosthesis—when understood as a technological extension-transgression of the human essence—is not a new concern. Some of Daedalus' inventions led in turn to some of the best-known mythological miseries. The wax in the prosthetic wings of Icarus melted when he flew too high, getting dangerously close to the sun. Pasiphaë, cursed with a zoophilic passion for a beautiful Cretan bull, asked Daedalus to construct a costume-machine resembling a cow, so a fooled animal would copulate with her. Daedalus' son fell into the sea and drowned. The wife of Minos ended up giving birth to a monstrous hybrid, the Minotaur.

[21] Golding, 'The Courage to Matter'.

[22] David Burrows, and Simon O'Sullivan, *Fictioning: The Myth-Functions of Contemporary Art and Philosophy*, Edinburgh University Press, 2019.

These resounding failures seem to express certain fears around twisting and bending the will of gods or nature with the help of technological instruments.

Those different attitudes to technological intimacies are echoed in positions around artificial intelligence mapped by Hugo de Garis, who predicated a conflict between Terrans, who see a danger to humanity in the expanding forms of algorithmisation of life (representing the more broadly understood biotic); Cosmists, who see *Homo sapiens* as an evolutionary middle man between animals and higher forms of intelligence; and Cyborgs, who intend to exceed the human essence by technological means.[23] All these approaches wrongly assume some form of human or biotic essence that is either: endangered, might happily fulfil its evolutionary duty, or can become outdated. The transgression in Garis' understanding resembles crossing a boundary, adding on, or stretching the essentially unmovable core.

5.8 Automated Ethics: Drones, Response-Abilities, and Military Algorithms

Technological prostheticisation, with algorithmic, distributed decision-making at its base should be perceived as a broader, systemic process. Prosthetic devices and systems emerge as technologies inscribed in the wider process of progressing automation and distribution. If the notion of prosthetics is extended to systemic phenomena, it could be argued that contemporary technology is becoming more and more prosthetic—it creates distributed intimacies, dependencies and entanglements with corporeal human and non-human bodies. A consequence of that process is a gradual suspension of the notion of intention, traditionally always anchored to (human) subjects and their centralised brains. Benjamin Bratton rightly notices that: 'the world is made and re-made not just by political decision, but by its dissolving of decision into automatic and prosthetic systems […] what is most important for the plan is the difficult understanding of how our own physical embodiment and urbanism not only makes use of these automated prostheses, but are also themselves the effects and outcomes of those systems. We are the creature at the end of the tether'.[24]

[23] Hugh De Garis, *The Artilect War: Cosmists Vs. Terrans*, Palm Springs, Calif: Etc Pubns, 2005.

[24] Benjamin Bratton, *The Terraforming*, Strelka Press, 2019.

Prosthetic technologies, or rather, the new prosthetic dimension of distributed technology, necessities philosophical investigations into the types of human data and knowledge that have been consciously or inadvertently circulated in global systems. The question of algorithmisation is not just an issue of the violation of users' data privacy. Despite technological pretences to objectivity, delegation of responsibility or limitation of human factors in systemic decision-making is not tantamount to suspension of ablism, sexism, racism, homophobia, and all other forms of othering. Human-created prosthetic systems are likely then to suffer from the same biases, or to resonate with extant technologies of oppression. In this way, prosthetic technologies as distributed, algorithmic decision-makers face a responsibility to perpetually determine, examine, and judge whose body gets included in the category of human, citizen or sentient being.

Apparently objective systemic decisions, for example, algorithmic bank assessments regarding credit ratings, do not explicitly link race with financial responsibility. However, zip code information is correlated with generations of racial inequalities, non-intentionally affecting the creditworthiness of individuals. In those situations, algorithms, digital or otherwise, become, as Cathy O'Neil calls it: 'Weapons of Math Destruction', using biased data from the past to perpetuate inequality in the future, under pretence of scientific objectivity or bias-blindness.[25]

There seems to be some rightly sensed but often misdiagnosed danger in automated, algorithmic decision and suggestion making. That feeling gives rise to new luddite arguments exhorting people to return to some undefinable, pre-technological or, at least, pre-digital past. It becomes crucial to determine to what extent that algorithmic delegation of the ethical is a new process related to computerisation. Algorithms are often mistakenly perceived as some form of new technology, necessarily associated with the digital age or, more recently, with machine learning and artificial intelligence. In fact, their history goes back to mediaeval 'algorism' which meant, simply, performing calculation on natural numbers. Nowadays it is believed that algorithms should rather be perceived as sets of instructions for solving a problem or accomplishing a task following an established sequential order.[26] Taina Bucher claims that they are 'step-by-

[25] Cathy O'Neil, *Weapons of Math Destruction: How Big Data Increases Inequality and Threatens Democracy,* New York: Crown, 2016.

[26] That echoes Taina Bucher's paraphrase of Donald Knuth in 'If… Then. Algorithmic Power and Politics' Taina Bucher, *If…Then: Algorithmic Power and Politics*, New York: Oxford University Press, 2018.

step guides that prescribe how to obtain a certain goal, given specific parameters'.[27] In that most basic sense, a culinary recipe or a health and safety procedure are forms of an algorithm—an automated code of conduct leading to a particular result.

In Hannah Arendt's proposition of 'banality of evil' formulated in reports on the trial of Adolph Eichmann, the conditions leading to the crisis of ethics and atrocities of Holocaust do not emerge from some innate monstrous tendencies of the perpetrators, the inhuman environment or chaos of war. Instead of focusing on the psychological analysis of one of the main organisers of the Final Solution, she observed that he had often simply followed the conduct of bureaucratic procedures, rather than indulging in some sadistic, evil tendencies.

The Second World War often serves as the main reference point in the analysis of the machinery of exclusion and organised, systemic violence on a large scale. However, numerous military or even humanitarian interventions prove that the procedural mathematics of violence has become an important part of the contemporary economy of war. In *The Least of All Possible Evils* Eyal Weizman analyses the principle of lesser evil that ideologically frames the quantifiable collateral damage used to facilitate or automatise decision-making, especially in case of possible fatalities. The imperative of utility and the illusion of lesser evil sets up (and operates on the basis of) an assumption that the economy of inevitable military conflict follows, at least locally, a zero-sum game, in which balancing acts are possible. Indeed, Weizman quotes Daniel Reisner, former head of the International Law Divisions in the Israeli Army, who speaks of incredible usefulness of numbers and thresholds in setting up equivalences whilst making decisions regarding the deaths of civilians versus soldiers, or weighing up the losses of men, women, and children. The Researchers from Tel Aviv University developed a formula that allows for the calculation of the number of members an army must eliminate from a hostile or resistant organisation in order to suppress it. The formula, taken from systems theory, applies entropic behaviour of molecules in a gaseous state to volatile human actions. The algorithmic automation of a decision in a form of a mathematical formula or a procedure that enables the suspension of the ethical can be contained in one line of text.

[27] Bucher, *If...Then.*

$$Q = 1 - \left(\frac{q \ln q + 1}{q \ln 1 / q} \right)$$

Q= the probability of an organisation collapsing
q= the percentage of members requiring neutralisation[28]

Considering the widespread military use of decision-making algorithms that help to assess risk, losses and targets, and enable the measuring of human lives against each other, the problem with algorithmic ethics is an issue that does not seem to lie in potential failures of not yet perfected code behind, for example, image recognition.[29] The biggest danger posed by prosthetic decision-makers is not the possibility of a digital glitch—such as misrecognition of a target by a drone—but rather, the replacement or suspension of ethics by an algorithmically executed procedure.

International humanitarian law (IHL) therefore seeks to limit or rectify *disproportional* or *excessive* attack of military reaction. The automatisation of difficult ethical decisions becomes reduced to the problem of measurement—the difficulty involved in calculating the probability of destruction and injury—as well as the assessment of risk—the apparent inevitability of so-called *human losses* involved in the proportionality principle.

5.9 Conclusion

Mapping the shifted meaning of prosthetics in the age of algorithms and big data allows for the tracing of vulnerabilities embedded in globally distributed systems and the logics of their implementation. The analysis reveals diverse underlying onto-epistemological assumptions behind the narratives of technological support, facilitation and optimisation, as well as those hidden in more dystopian scenarios of coexistence with the machines.

Prosthesis understood as a particular type of a relationship of a single-agent or a multi-agent body with technology cannot be considered in terms of reciprocity or mutuality of influence. The prosthetic encounter takes a form of entanglement that should not be understood here as two

[28] Eyal Weizman, *The Least of All Possible Evils: Humanitarian Violence from Arendt to Gaza*, Verso, 2012.

[29] Weizman, *The Least of All Possible Evils*.

or more intricately connected and interdependent entities. That entanglement follows a non-Newtonian logic of connection which implies that the elements in question cannot be defined independently of another.

Prosthesis, a body and technology, even in their most extended and non-physical renditions analysed here, remain material and should not be treated as cognitive metaphors or concepts illustrating certain philosophical ideas. Prosthetic bodies are entities with distributed entanglements that run through their emergent codes. In many ways, the question concerning prosthetics is simultaneously a question concerning technology; one which places its emphasis on the aspects of embodiment, intimacy, and emergence.

However, the difference between prosthesis and other types of technological relations with a body is that prosthesis is an instrument that articulates with a form of a corporeal wound. That trauma is understood here not as a gap, lack or inadequacy, but as a material but not necessarily physical *thing*, a plastic entity always located in the present. The prosthetic encounter irreversibly transforms the systems, being, often violently, productive of new, emergent ones and selves.

Prosthetic devices always question, twist, and undermine ideas of the fragment, the whole, and the boundary, enabling ways of sensing and feeling that are not simply an extension of any previously known biotic abilities or their synaesthetic combinations. Distributed prosthetic sensing disregards the dialectics of biotic-synthetic and focuses on new, emergent entities that are not necessarily restored sums of pre-existing organs and circuits. In that sense, prosthesis enables a way into thinking about distributed sensing which is a qualitative rather than a quantitative move. That functional surplus is often difficult to conceptualise in the rigid sum of the normalised, *essential* body understood as (some)one. The idea of distribution forces one to think about attachment, not as a tension-cohesion *between* a body and a prosthetic thing, but as a form of difference-repetition that becomes part of the code of a new, emergent entity. It shifts the point of tension from that located *between* natural body and technological prosthesis, to the complexity of feedback loops.

Addressing trauma does not come with a fixed form of ethics; it does not have to imply healing or re-pairing. Prosthesis can easily slip into a form of oppression—an embodiment of exclusionary bias of its time. With the algorithmic and distributed systems at work that bias or cruelty can become multiplied and circulated within the globally connected networks. Therefore, the prosthetic decision-makers are at risk of emulating historical biases, creating futures that are teleological derivatives of the past. The biggest danger that emerges from this detailed analysis of the ontology and dynamics of prostheticisation is automation of responsibility, where, in the circuit of algorithmic delegation, ethics become decontextualised and suspended.

It could be argued that technological prostheticisation is not threatening to the integrity and independence of humans as individual systems, but rather, that it challenged the conviction that it is possible to talk about intelligence, consciousness, and humanity without seeing it as always distributed. However, this should not encourage relativisation of the radical change in how information is now amassed, stored, circulated, and used as material. As much as humans have always been corporally, culturally, or politically distributed, the algorithmic age has introduced a qualitative change in the way technologies are wired into human existence.

The notion of prosthetics emerges as a philosophical issue; a way into thinking about the response-ability of global network-systems, IoT, sensors, wearables, and other smart devices. More importantly, prosthetics draw attention to the imperative of ethical design: the introduction of care and consent into these new distributed systems on the level of code, without hoping solely for their responsible implementation. The simplest and most naive questions often become the most urgent.[30] A prosthesis as a philosophical device is not a physical apparatus, but a poietic instrument that pertinaciously calls for new answers to questions of what it means to be human in the algorithmic age.[31]

Acknowldegement I would like to thank Eliot Allison, who helped to generate many thoughts behind this chapter.

[30] These are paraphrased words from a poem 'The Century's Decline' from *View With a Grain of Sand* by Wisława Szymborska.

[31] The use of *poesis* here echoes Martin Heidegger's remarks in *The Question Concerning Technology*, where it is understood as an ontological act of revealing. That 'bringing forth' is not, however, assigned to the creative power of the subject who animates-names-innovates but rather 'the bursting open belonging to bringing forth not in itself, but in another'. In that sense, the moment of creation is inextricably linked to belonging together, it is always already distributed. See Martin Heidegger, *The Question Concerning Technology: And Other Essays*.

References

Barad, Karen. *Meeting the Universe Halfway: Quantum Physics and the Entanglement of Matter and Meaning*. Illustrated edition. Durham: Duke University Press, 2007.

Bratton, Benjamin. *The Terraforming*. Strelka Press, 2019.

Bucher, Taina. *If... Then: Algorithmic Power and Politics*. New York: Oxford University Press, 2018.

Bunz, Mercedes, and Meikle, Graham. *The Internet of Things*. Cambridge, UK; Malden, MA, USA: Polity Press, 2017.

Burrows, David, and O'Sullivan, Simon. *Fictioning: The Myth-Functions of Contemporary Art and Philosophy*. Edinburgh University Press, 2019.

De Garis, Hugh. *The Artilect War: Cosmists Vs. Terrans*. Palm Springs, Calif: Etc Pubns, 2005.

Fernandes, Rodrigo A. Brant, Diniz, Bruno, Ribeiro, Ramiro and Humayun, Mark. 'Artificial vision through neuronal stimulation'. *Neuroscience letters* 519, no. 2 (2012): 122–128.

Golding, Johnny. 'The Courage to Matter'. *Data Loam: Sometimes Hard, Usually Soft (the Future of Knowledge Systems)*, 2021. https://doi.org/10.1515/9783110697841.

Golding, Johnny. 'Friendship'. *Edinburgh Companion to Animal Studies*, 1st edition, EUP, 2017.

Heidegger, Martin. *The Question Concerning Technology: And Other Essays*. Reissue edition. New York; London Toronto: Harper Perennial, 2013.

Heidegger, Martin. *Identity and Difference*. Trans. Joan Stambaugh. 2nd ed. Edition. Chicago: University of Chicago Press, 2002.

Lacan, Jacques. *The Ego in Freud's Theory and in the Technique of Psychoanalysis, 1954–1955*. Ed. Jacques-Alain Miller. Trans. Sylvana Tomaselli. Revised ed. Edition, New York, N.Y: W.W. Norton & Co., 1991.

Lem, Stanisław. *Przekładaniec*. Agora: 2018.

Lyotard, Jean-François. *Libidinal Economy*. Reprint edition. Bloomsbury Academic, 2015.

Malabou, Catherine. The Ontology of the Accident: An Essay on Destructive Plasticity. Cambridge: Polity Press, 2012.

Massumi, Brian. 'The Autonomy of Affect'. *Cultural Critique*, no. 31 (1995): 83–109. https://doi.org/10.2307/1354446.

Mills, Mara. 'Do signals have politics? Inscribing abilities in cochlear implants'. *The Oxford handbook of sound studies* (2012): 320–346.

O'Neil, Cathy. *Weapons of Math Destruction: How Big Data Increases Inequality and Threatens Democracy*. New York: Crown, 2016.

Ortiz-Catalan, Max, Mastinu, Enzo, Sassu, Paolo, Aszmann, Oskar, and Brånemark, Rickard. 'Self-contained neuromusculoskeletal arm prostheses'. *New England Journal of Medicine* 382, no. 18 (2020): 1732–1738.

Sharpe, Christina. *In the Wake: On Blackness And Being*. Illustrated edition. Durham: Duke University Press, 2016.

Weizman, Eyal. *The Least of All Possible Evils: Humanitarian Violence from Arendt to Gaza*. Verso, 2012.

COVERING

Ellen Sampson

> *We intuit the meanings of enveloping, draping, covering and clothing as gestures of touching, possessing and protecting (Doy 2002). We intuit the significance of wrapping as a prosthesis of touch, the continued existence of the hand in the absence of the body that offers touch. We intuit the imbrication and interplay between touch and sight. We sense the antithetical dynamic between hiding and revealing, concealment and exhibition.*[1]

Garments hold, cover and contain the body, concealing and revealing through drape, cut and fold. At its most basic, the function of clothing is to cover, to provide an additional boundary between the body and the world. Yet as we know, acts of dressing are not simply responses to bodily need, but instead complex negotiations; both with the cultures and spaces which we navigate, the materials available to use and identities, of the status and allegiances we wish to convey. Covering the body is coded and these codes overlap, intersect and contradict one another as we dress and wrap, and shroud. Enclothed bodies convey identity and contain experience, and in the context of the 'curative', 'protective' and 'palliative' these processes acquire further layers of meaning. Though cloth and clothing are not one and the same, the textile surface is a site on which multiple negotiations, and incorporations are performed and occur. Textiles are simultaneously communicative, protective and intimate; surfaces which

[1] Claire Pajaczkowska, 'On Stuff and Nonsense: The Complexity of Cloth', *TEXTILE*, 3:3 (2005). 223.

touch us and through these tactile interactions become both part of the body schema and separate to it, objects which are to borrow from D.W. Winnicott both 'me and not me'.[2] As textile theorist Claire Pajaczkowska observes 'our ambiguous relationship to textiles that we experience [them] as neither object nor subject, but as the threshold between'.[3]

This second section of the book explores these thresholds; objects which augment the body schema, offering both physical and psychic protection, and through tactile exchange changing the physical composition of our bodily selves. In doing so each chapter touches upon ideas of containment—the experience and (real or imagined) benefits of being wrapped or held. Holding in this context is both metaphorical and material, from the containment of anxiety, to garments imbued with bacteria designed to rebalance the skin microbiome. Though there is a lineage of thinking about containment from the medical humanities[4] and fashion studies,[5] the particular value of containment is most directly explored in psychoanalytic theory where, as R.D. Hinshelwood writes, 'the notion of 'containing' has become a decisive concept for most British forms of analytic psychotherapy'.[6] The physical and psychic act of holding as central to wellbeing, underscores much of the work of twentieth-century psychoanalysts Winnicott,[7] Bion,[8] Bick[9] and Anzieu.[10] For these theorists the experience of being held is central to infant development, allowing a fragile or fragmentary sense of

[2] D. W. Winnicott, 'Transitional Artefacts and Transitional Phenomena—A Study of the First Not-Me Possession', *International Journal of Psycho-Analysis*, 34 (1953) 89–97.

[3] Pajaczkowska, 'On Stuff and Nonsense', 223–229.

[4] See for example Elaine Scarry, *The Body in Pain: The Making and Unmaking of the World*, New York and Oxford: Oxford UP, 1985.

[5] See for example Emma McCracken, 'Fashion and Beauty: Transgression, Utopia, and Containment', *Decoding Women's Magazines*, Palgrave Macmillan, London 1993.

[6] R. D. Hinshelwood, *A Dictionary of Kleinian Thought*, London: Free Association Books, 1989.

[7] For Winnicott, holding in both a physical and psychic sense is essential for the infant's wellbeing: the parent must physically hold the infant in their arms but also hold it in their mind, so that the child is attended to in multiple ways. See D. W. Winnicott, 'Transitional Artefacts and Transitional Phenomena—A Study of the First Not-Me Possession', *International Journal of Psycho-Analysis*, 34 (1953) 89–97.

[8] Wilfred Bion, *Learning from Experience*, London: Heinemann, 1962.

[9] Esther Bick, 'The experience of skin in early object relations', *International Journal of Psychoanalysis*, 49 (1968) 484–86.

[10] Didier, Anzieu, *The Skin-Ego*, trans. N. Segal. London: Routledge, 1985 [2016].

self to be maintained. Whilst for Winnicott this holding is both physical and psychical, being held in the parent's arms and being held in their mind, Anzieu's Skin-ego, 'a containing and unifying wrapping around the Self; as a protective barrier for the psyche'[11] is internal, an interior form holding.[12] Though the objects in this volume cover, envelop and bind in multiple ways, the following chapters all address the containment that textile surfaces afford. The garments and objects explored in this section, 1990s menswear, probiotic bodysuits, and 1930s sun wear, do more than cover: through their real and imagined porousness they mediate the environments we inhabit, functioning as curative, protective or preventative objects.

The use of textile, as a preventive measure to mitigate environmental risk and assuage cultural anxiety, is evident in both Christopher M. Rudeen's 'Securing a Place in the Sun: Clothing, Exposure, and Health' and Andrew Groves' 'Palliative Prototypes or Therapeutic Functionality? Examining C.P. Company's Urban Protection Collection'. Here the porous nature of fashion objects, their capacity to move between the material and symbolic, the fantasy of protection and the risk of damage is bought to the fore. For Rudeen the very permeability of Celanese (a form of rayon) to ultraviolet light, belies the complex layers of protection it afforded. Marketed as fabric which could expand access to the healing power of the sun's rays, Rudeen explores how the marketing and manufacture of Celanese reveal broader cultural anxieties around skin, nudity and race, and in doing so the hegemonic power structures which underscore them. This capacity of cloth to contain, mediate and make visible anxieties around porousness and fragmentation is equally apparent in Andrew Groves' 'Palliative Prototypes or Therapeutic Functionality? Examining C.P. Company's Urban Protection Collection'. Though these garments purport to mitigate real environmental risks, through mask filters and ID cards, Groves explores how they acted as defences to anxieties inherent in the performance of late twentieth-century urban masculinity. Groves' unpacking of millennial urban anxiety and the ways that both designers and wearers deployed fashion objects to counteract it, recalls Anzieu's

[11] Didier, Anzieu, *The Skin-Ego*, trans. N. Segal. London: Routledge, 1985 [2016] 105.

[12] Anizieu makes this distinction himself writing that 'Just as the skin fulfils the function of supporting the skeleton and muscles, the Skin-ego fulfils the function of maintaining the psyche' (106).

writing on the Skin-ego, of a self constantly at risk of fragmentation, which must be held together by a mediating surface so as not to fall apart.[13]

The final chapter in this section, Rosie Broadhead's 'Skin and textile interaction and the future of fashion as therapeutics', draws out a different kind of porousness; the material and living interaction between these surfaces of the body and the surfaces of the garments we wear. Taking perhaps the most directly curative approach in the volume, this design-led chapter explores the ways that garments might be used to promote a healthy skin microbiome, through nurturing the plethora of bacteria which live on and in the body. In exploring how a more holistic understanding of the body self comprising not only of human flesh but of multiple living organisms can aid development of 'curative' things, Broadhead returns us to the two-sided relationship between body and cloth and the processes of giving and taking, meeting and exchange which underscore these interactions. Thus, just as Merleau-Ponty[14] writes of touching and being touched, the experience of being covered is not passive or one sided but a continual meeting and exchange between the me and not me. The curative, preventative or protective qualities of Broadhead's prototypes and of the other garments in this section, present a particular understanding of the body schema of a bodily and psychic self which is constituted and held together by multiple surfaces other than its own: an uncontainable porous body both intermingled with and vulnerable to the atmospheres and affects of the world it inhabits.

References

Anzieu, Didier, 1985 [2016]. *The Skin-Ego*, trans. N. Segal, London: Routledge.

Bick, Esther, 1968, 'The experience of skin in early object relations', *International Journal of Psychoanalysis*, 49, 484–86.

Bion, Wilfred 1962, *Learning from Experience*. London: Heinemann.

Hinshelwood, R. D., 1989, *A Dictionary of Kleinian Thought*. London: Free Association Books.

Merleau-Ponty, M., 1968. *The visible and the Invisible*. Evanston, Illinois: Northwestern University Press.

[13] Anzieu, *The Skin-Ego*, 105.

[14] Maurice Merleau-Ponty, *The visible and the Invisible*. Evanston, Illinois: Northwestern University Press, 1968.

Pajaczkowska, Claire, 2005. On Stuff and Nonsense: The Complexity of Cloth, TEXTILE, 3:3, 223.

Winnicott, D. W., 1953, 'Transitional Artefacts and Transitional Phenomena—A Study of the First Not-Me Possession', *International Journal of Psycho-Analysis*, 34, 89–97.

CHAPTER 6

Securing a Place in the Sun: Clothing, Exposure, and Health

Christopher M. Rudeen

6.1 Introduction

'Your place in the sun'. That is what a roundup of products published by the journal *Britannia and Eve* in 1939 promised its readers. Above a picture of footprints in the sand were several scenarios one might face when outdoors trying to achieve that elusive perfect tan: 'If You Can Take It', 'If You Want to Go Half Way', 'If You Get Caught'. There were products for each case, guiding the reader through these possibilities. For those who wanted to look tan without tanning, for instance, '*Helena Rubinstein's Rose Tan* make-up has been specifically designed for wearing with the mauvy blues, lime, clear blues and pinks, that we like for sports clothes this summer'. While on the beach, '*Leichner* has a liquid body make-up that

C. M. Rudeen (✉)
Harvard University, Cambridge, MA, USA
e-mail: cmrudeen@g.harvard.edu

D. Woolley et al. (eds.), *Wearable Objects and Curative Things*, Palgrave Studies in Fashion and the Body,
https://doi.org/10.1007/978-3-031-40017-9_6

stays put even in the sea...It won't come off on your swimsuit or light dresses and will prevent sunburn when you lie out on the beach'.[1]

How does one make sense of this dizzying array of products required to achieve one's 'place in the sun'? Why would someone want this place at all? This chapter investigates the intersection of fashion and health in early-twentieth-century Great Britain using the case of Celanese, one such product that, ten years prior, also promised readers a place in the sun. Celanese was a fabric that was permeable to ultraviolet light, thereby allowing its wearer to feel the sun on their skin while remaining fully clothed. Those behind the product hoped to expand access to the healing power of the sun's rays to improve the well-being of the British people. In so doing, it also sought to treat specific anxieties of belonging to the white British elite.

Celanese is a form of artificial silk, generally called rayon, made up of cellulose acetate. Before it was a fiber, cellulose acetate was used as part of a varnish to strengthen airplanes during the first World War. The British government invited Henry and Camille Dreyfus, the Swiss brothers who had developed the chemical solution, to move to Great Britain and help the government in its war efforts. After the fighting ceased, the two men looked for other outlets for their synthetic process, setting their sights on artificial silk. Thus, Celanese was born.[2] The brothers' next challenge was to distinguish the fabric from the more commonly known viscose rayon. While substantial research was conducted on matters of dyeing and production, marketers used their own tools to try to sell the products. It is in these advertisements that we can see the position of Celanese—and the white middle class—in Great Britain in the early twentieth century.

This subject has received scattered attention in the history of medicine and fashion studies literature. Authors have turned to sunshine as part of ongoing relationships between the environment and health. Daniel Freund in particular has chronicled the changing views of the sun in the American context, where he argued that different groups sought to commodify nature in the face of new fears about modern society.[3] In a related vein, Simon Carter has argued that in the early twentieth century, 'the social

[1] 'Your Place in the Sun', *Britannia and Eve* 19, no. 2 (August 1939): 39.

[2] Robert K. Fourness, 'The Development of Disperse Dyes for Acetate Fibres', *Coloration Technology* 90, no. 1 (1974): 15.

[3] Daniel Freund, *American Sunshine: Diseases of Darkness and the Quest for Natural Light* (Chicago: The University of Chicago Press, 2012).

and material figuration of the body in sunlight changed dramatically'.[4] Carter's sociological analysis focuses on the emergence of what he calls the 'helio-human', an assemblage of people, light, and technology informed by the ideal of the 'healthy body'. In this context, Carter briefly discusses tourism, bathing suits, and sun cream.[5] The present chapter seeks to expand on this intriguing idea. In addition, various organizations promoting this fight against 'diseases of darkness', most notably the Sunlight Society, have been studied in New Zealand and in the context of wider reform groups in Britain in the interwar period, including those focused on dress.[6] Finally, artificial silk, as will be explored in more detail below, has mostly been associated with health problems, especially of factory workers.[7] Sunlight, as many of these authors indicate, tends to ignore boundaries, and so this present work is necessarily interdisciplinary, drawing on these various literatures to understand a single case study that has largely escaped historical attention.

This chapter proceeds in five parts. The first discusses the Sun Bathing Society, whose frustration with laws banning semi-nudity in public parks illustrated a broader problem to be overcome by proponents of the sun's rays. The solution to this issue of modesty, the second section argues, was found in material goods that expanded access to the sun. Sun lamps, vitamins, and new types of glass brought the sun into the home, while Celanese allowed tanning even when fully clothed. The third section focuses on Celanese as a material. In contrast to wool or cotton, the artificiality of the cellulose acetate made it a blank slate for advertisers, who focused on its functionality and versatility. The fourth and fifth sections look at the specific visions of class and race, respectively, imagined by the fabric's marketers. The well-being one received from the sun was, in part, the ability to emulate the upper classes. Tanned skin also illustrated how whiteness was fragile and constructed by technologies such as Celanese

[4] See Simon Carter, *Rise and Shine: Sunlight, Technology and Health* (Oxford: Berg, 2017), 5.

[5] Carter, *Rise and Shine*, See especially Chapter 8.

[6] Nadia Gush, 'The Beauty of Health: Cora Wilding and the Sunlight League', *New Zealand Journal of History* 43, no. 1 (2009): 1–17; Barbara Burman and Melissa Leventon, 'The Men's Dress Reform Party 1929–37', *Costume*, no. 21 (1987): 75–87; and Joanna Bourke, 'The Great Male Renunciation: Men's Dress Reform in Inter-War Britain', *Journal of Design History* 9, no. 1 (1996): 23–33.

[7] On the relationship between fashion and ill health, see Alison Matthews David, *Fashion Victims: The Dangers of Dress Past and Present* (London: Bloomsbury Visual Arts, 2015).

that allowed ownership of nature. In sum, I argue, Celanese was a curative thing that helped alleviate anxieties around exposure and identity.

6.2 Everything Under the Sun

In the early twentieth century, attention turned to sunlight as part of social reform. Notable in this regard is the Sun Bathing Society. Formed in 1930 in London, the group boasted members such as Julian Huxley, a biologist and eugenicist and the brother of writer Aldous Huxley; J. C. Flügel, a psychologist and psychoanalyst who had just published a monograph on the 'psychology of clothes'; and Elizabeth Sloan Chesser, a physician and medical journalist who wrote widely on issues of women and children. Its ranks also included A. C. Jordan, a prominent member of related health organizations such as the New Health Society and the Men's Dress Reform Society.[8]

Writing to the editor of *The Times* of London in 1932, the group expressed two major components of their mission. First, the society emphasized the growing support in the medical community for the power of the sun. 'It is becoming increasingly manifest to the observant that this nation is rapidly awakening to the fact that so-called "sun bathing," or to be more correct "active air bathing," is extremely beneficial to the health and happiness of the indoor worker', the group argued. What is more, the sun could do what medical technology could not. 'We have constantly before us', they wrote, 'the evidence of high medical authorities that, in spite of the development of medical science, the health of people in general and school-children in particular does not materially improve'.[9] The authors continued, however, that 'these authorities...are satisfied that it would be definitely improved if more light and fresh air were allowed to act directly on the skins of indoor workers and school-children'.[10] These groups were the focus of many reformers of the time, as they stood in for the future of the nation.

Second, the group bemoaned standards of public decency that prevented people from directly experiencing the sun on their skin. Discussing

[8] As fashion historian Barbara Burman has argued, these groups were part of a loose cluster of progressive movements in the interwar period heavily influenced by eugenics. See Barbara Burman, 'Better and Brighter Clothes: The Men's Dress Reform Party, 1929–1940', *Journal of Design History* 8, no. 4 (1995): 275–290.

[9] 'Sun Bathing: Benefits of Light and Air', *Times* (London, England), March 18, 1932, 10.

[10] 'Sun Bathing: Benefits of Light and Air', 10.

the value of the sun, the letter noted 'that the discarding of all but a minimum of clothing for outdoor exercises and certain sports materially adds to their enjoyment'.[11] As part of their work, the society had set up a sunbathing center in Regent's Park, a project that had been featured in medical journals such as the *Lancet*.[12] Looking back on that project, members of the Sun Bathing Society noted that over 150 individuals attended, clad, 'in spite of the weather, [in] less than a bathing costume'.[13] Similar attempts to found sites for 'air bathing' had not met with the same success. 'Many other groups have been formed to practise air bathing, but have found it necessary to secrete themselves in the woods round London in order to avoid the attention of the public, the Press, their friends, and their neighbors'.[14] The group continued by lamenting that 'This need for secrecy is an iniquitous state of affairs! Semi-nudity can be viewed on the stage by paying for it, but cannot, it seems, be indulged in for health and well-being in the open air, until for lack of it one is ill enough to go to a hospital or a home for crippled children!'[15] If sunbathing were to become widespread practice, some even suggested, hospitals could become obsolete.[16]

This problem of modesty became a key sticking point for professionals hoping to expand the practice of sunbathing. Articles published in the *Times* recounted instances of men brought before the court after attempting to sunbathe in public places. In a case from 1927, a 44-year-old schoolmaster was charged after appearing in a park 'on an overcoat on the grass by the western end of the Serpentine-road in clothing consisting only of shorts'.[17] The Magistrate stated that while 'It might be a very desirable thing for one to lie in one's garden or room, out of sight, practising what was termed sunbathing, to get the full benefit of the violet rays…to expose the upper part of one's body, the torso, was indecent. It was likely to shock persons of ordinary susceptibilities'.[18] A similar case from 1933 found a young clerk charged with personal exposure after

[11] 'Sun Bathing: Benefits of Light and Air'.

[12] See 'Sun-Bathing in a London Park', *Lancet* 216, no. 5600 (December 27, 1930): 1409–1410.

[13] 'Sun Bathing: Benefits of Light and Air'.

[14] 'Sun Bathing: Benefits of Light and Air'.

[15] 'Sun Bathing: Benefits of Light and Air'.

[16] 'Sun-Bathing for Children: New Centre in Regent's Park', *Times*, August 19, 1930, 7.

[17] 'Sun Bathing: Benefits of Light and Air'.

[18] 'Magistrate on Sun-Bathing in Public', *Times*, August 6, 1927, 12.

sunbathing at the Welsh Harp Recreation Ground. The judge, in binding him over, similarly emphasized 'that no attack was being made on sunbathing, which was an admirable thing if decently conducted'. However, 'what was not to be allowed was for a man willfully to expose himself in a public place'.[19] These cases emphasized both an increasing acknowledgment of the value of sunbathing and strong legal precedent against exposing skin in public.

A key issue at stake in these debates was the propriety of the 'manly chest'. In 1932, an individual named A. P. Herbert wrote to the editor of the *Times* with an entreaty. 'Sir', the letter began, 'someone in authority—and what authority could be better than you?—should give the nation a definite ruling on the troublesome question of masculine swimming-wear'. The author noted that while some borough councils had 'boldly announced' that only a 'slip' was required for swimming or sunbathing, others required the 'university costume' and 'beach inspectors and policeman use stern language to the bather if a single shoulder be exposed to the sun'. The author mused on the question, 'Is the male chest indecent or not?' and settled upon the answer that 'some clever tailor, hosier, or haberdasher realized that he could charge more money for a long bathing-dress than he could for a short one'. He thereby called for abolishing this 'nonsense' rule, which was 'one of the many small things which makes our country ridiculous, incomprehensible, and undesirable to the foreigner'.[20]

Almost exactly one year later, an article on the situation in France was published in the *Times*. It was reported that the mayor of Moliets-et-Maa had forbidden undress on the beaches, 'considering that improper costumes cannot be tolerated on the beach during the holiday season, and considering, further, that persons hardly clothed, on the pretext of taking a sun cure, disport themselves in the sight of their fellow-men, and, especially, of children'. The author ended the account by quipping, 'As for morality, the French will at least be unable any longer to point the finger of scorn at long-suffering English municipalities'.[21]

The formation of the Sun Bathing Society, as well as debates in newspapers over questions of nudity, help to explain the particular marketing of Celanese fabric. At a time when many worried about how best to extend

[19] 'Sun-Bather Bound Over', *Times*, October 19, 1933, 4.

[20] A. P. Herbert, 'The Manly Chest; Aesthetics of the Beach; Costume and Convention', *Times*, July 28, 1932, 13.

[21] Herbert, 'The Manly Chest', 11.

the health-giving properties of the sun to more groups, technology offered a solution backed by the imprimatur of modernity.

6.3 Selling the Sun

Many people alighted on a means to 'materially improve' the health of populations via the sun, I argue, in *material* ways—in objects that used technology to circumvent the problem of modesty. Take, for instance, the case of one disgruntled reader of the *Times* in the winter of 1924. While it was 'all very well for your Correspondent to praise the holiday cruises which enable those who can afford them—a mere handful—to enjoy the sun in the winter', the writer sought a more approachable solution: 'What I want, and have long wanted', the letter continued, 'is some means of bottling up the warmth of summer for use in the winter'. The writer turned his attention to scientists, asking, 'Cannot science, whose triumphs are dinned into our ears often enough, give us something more immediate and better than this?'[22] Many scientists and salesmen did have something to say in this matter. By the late 1920s there was an array of products being marketed for that very purpose, so much so that the *Times* published a special 'number' on 'Sunshine and Health' in 1928 filled with advertisements and articles introducing the reader to the consumer marketplace available to people in search of the sun.

A reader who picked up the edition on 'Sunshine and Health' would have been confronted with a flood of information on the 'new science' of sunlight as a healing agent. They could have read its articles to learn about 'ultra-violet radiation and its measurement', the 'cure of rickets', or the curiously named 'sunshine milk'. They could have turned to the section on health resorts to see for themselves the different communities around the world catering to those looking for the sun's rays. What is perhaps most striking in the din of words and images, however, is the wealth of products advertised to get access to the supposed benefits of the sun.[23]

The special issue offered its readers many means of accessing sunlight, whether in food, through glass, or from special lamps. The reader who had been hunting for a bottle of sunshine, for instance, could find on the back cover an advertisement for glass bottles filled with Radiostol, 'the scientific substitute for sunshine', sold by the British Drug Houses, Limited. 'Vita'

[22] A. Shadwell, 'Bottling the Sun', *Times*, November 23, 1924, 10.
[23] 'A New Science', *Times*, May 22, 1928, x.

Glass promised 'health through your windows' by 'bringing indoors the natural health-giving rays of ultra-violet light that ordinary window glass shuts out entirely'.[24] And a variety of special lamps promised 'artificial sunlight' for home use.

It is among these advertisements that one finds half a page devoted to Celanese (Fig. 6.1). Whereas other products were developed to overcome questions of modesty by bringing the sun into the home, British Celanese Limited told consumers they could 'live in [their] own Lido', another name for the type of exotic beaches advertised in the same pages. This compromise between traveling to far-off health spas and indirectly accessing sunlight in private thereby offered a unique material solution to the problem of the manly chest and its potential indecency in the public realm.

The advert declares that, with Celanese, one can 'Secure a place in the sun this summer'. The rays of a simply drawn sun punctuate this message, and below it is a beach scene with a noticeable amount of fabric and covered skin. 'Everyone knows that sunshine gives a sense of well-being', the copy began, but 'only within the last decade has the reason for this been proved and applied. The secret is the action of the sun's ultra-violet rays on the skin'. Echoing the concerns of the Sun Bathing Society, the advertisement goes on to note that 'When the strength of the sun coaxes women to wear their filmiest garments and urges men to light-weight white attire, an extra fitness results because the ultra-violet rays are given easier access. But to harness the sun rays as a definite treatment for many of the ills of our age, these wonderful rays must be applied directly to the skin'. Those traveling to beaches could get access to rays by 'dispens[ing] with heavy, ray-resistant clothing'. Those who could not, however, had Celanese, which offered not 'the slightest barrier' to the sun's rays. 'It is a fact', the advertisement noted, 'that one can be fully clothed in "Celanese," wearing several layers of the material, and yet be in a state of Lido-like receptivity to ultra-violet rays'. Put another way, 'Under all conditions "Celanese" is a staunch ally of the sun in promoting health'. The advertisement included a note that indicated a 'distinguished Harley Street specialist' had recommended Celanese fabric and endorsed the claims of the copy.[25]

[24] British Drug Houses Limited, 'Radiostol: The Scientific Substitute for Sunshine', advertisement, *Times*, May 22, 1928, xl; Pilkington Brothers Ltd., '"Vita" Glass', advertisement, *Times*, May 22, 1928, xxxviii.

[25] British Celanese, Ltd., 'Secure a Place in the Sun This Summer', advertisement, *Times*, May 22, 1928, xxxv.

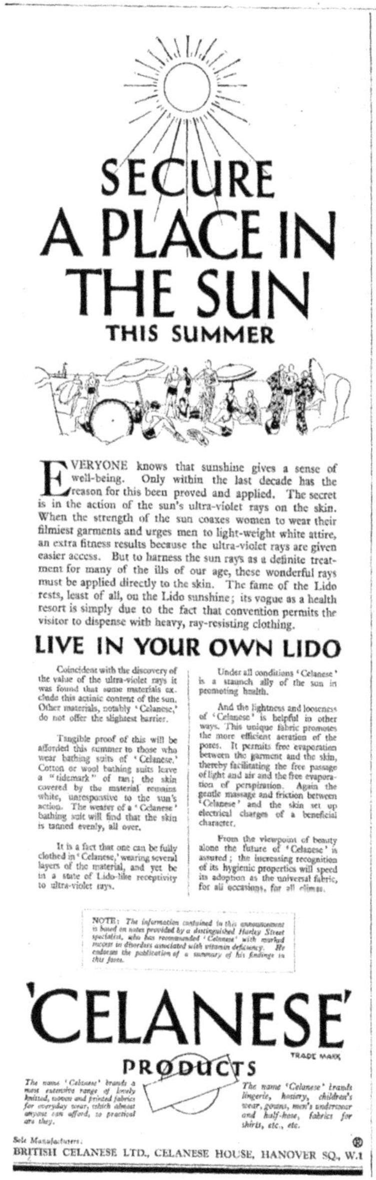

Fig. 6.1 An advertisement for Celanese products from a May 22, 1928, issue of the *Times* in London

This diverse and sizeable marketplace illustrates the profound anxiety of British society about 'diseases of darkness'. The functional and social properties of materials such as Celanese allowed certain individuals a chance to 'secure a place in the sun'. However, the fabric also indexed broader concerns of race, class, and exposure in early twentieth-century Britain.

6.4 Material Improvements

There was much confusion in the early twentieth century about rayon and how to explain it to the consumer. An article in the *Journal of Retailing* from 1931 defined rayon as follows: 'Rayon is the generic name of filaments made from various solutions of modified cellulose by pressing or drawing the cellulose solution through an orifice and solidifying it in the form of a filament, or filaments, by means of some precipitating medium'. While the major types of rayon then in production—viscose, nitro cellulose, and cuprammonium—all used pure cellulose, Celanese was manufactured using a compound of cellulose and acetic acid.[26]

Celanese intended to capitalize on this difference yet hoped to retain the familiarity of the term rayon. The article noted that acetate yarns had different properties than those of pure cellulose. Most notably, they reacted differently to dyeing and held less water, qualities that were to be emphasized to the consumer. As the author put it, 'The diversity of weave, finish, soft luster, richness, and originality of color and design give fabrics made of these yarns an especial style value'. While still appropriately called rayon, the consumer had to be sure to alert the drycleaner that the cloth was 'acetate', since it reacted differently to heat and organic solvents than other forms of synthetic silk.[27]

In 1925, *The Economist* published an article on 'The Artificial Silk Industry' in one of its monthly supplements, arguing that the development, production, and management of rayon were inextricably tied to Great Britain.[28] In that same year, the British Parliament debated a revenue duty on silk—both natural and artificial—as part of a new finance act,

[26] Isabel B. Wingate, 'Acetate Rayon', *Journal of Retailing* 6, no. 4 (January 1931): 119–121.

[27] Wingate, 'Acetate Rayon'.

[28] 'The Artificial Silk Industry', *The Economist Monthly Supplement*, no. 31 (December 26, 1925): 47.

which indicated its growing importance for the financial status of the country.[29] Silk was an especially popular fabric in the booming 1920s, and there was great enthusiasm as to the future of the trade.[30] On the business side, British companies wanted to be clear about the provenance of the material.

The *Economist* article noted that the world production of artificial silk was close to two hundred million pounds in 1925, just shy of double the amount produced two years prior. While the great bulk of this material was derived from the viscose process, the correspondent indicated that other methods—including the cellulose acetate process used by British Celanese Limited—were in fact higher in quality but had yet to experience the same commercial success. In addition, the field as a whole was dependent not upon seasonal harvests but was instead 'at the mercy of fashion's whims'. As such, the production of artificial silk 'required an almost unique combination of chemical and technical textile brains working in close harmony with the commercial or sales side of the business'.[31] This report thus explains not only the particular focus of Great Britain on this type of fiber, but also the resources expended in attempting to market Celanese. In the mid-1920s, Great Britain was importing more silk than any other type of fabric, in large part due to limited internal production (as indicated by low export figures), and so artificial silk represented a great potential source of revenue, especially if manufacturers could determine the best way to sell it to the British public.[32] For those companies that produced Celanese, finding a way to unseat the dominance of viscose rayon in this market necessitated an stronger reliance on the sales and marketing.

[29] Parliament of the United Kingdom, 'Finance Act, 1925', 15 & 16 Geo. 5, Ch. 36, June 30, 1925, https://www.legislation.gov.uk/ukpga/1925/36/pdfs/ukpga_19250036_en.pdf. See also 'Silk [Customs),' Commons Hansard 183 (May 11, 1925), 1476–1587, https://hansard.parliament.uk/Commons/1925-05-11/debates/a5a77e07-a72d-4dc1-9e22-0a84284a85d1/SilkCustoms).

[30] In the case of the United States, historian Nelson Klose noted that the 1920s saw increasing imports of silk as 'laborers indulged in the luxury of silk shirts'. While the depression decreased demand, 'public resentment of Japanese aggression' helped artificial silk regain some of this market. By midcentury, artificial silk had taken over for its natural counterpart. See Nelson Klose, 'Sericulture in the United States', *Agricultural History* 37, no. 4 (1963): 233.

[31] 'The Artificial Silk Industry', 47.

[32] See 'Commercial Reports', *The Economist* C, no. 4260 (April 18, 1925): 784–785.

Marketing synthetic fabrics required creativity, and often new markets were created for the products to avoid competition with established natural fibers. This was especially the case for Celanese, which had to find its niche in the booming artificial silk trade. Fashion historian Regina Lee Blaszczyk has argued, for instance, that DuPont found its greatest success in marketing new fabrics in men's sportswear. While businessmen were 'cotton snobs, turning up their noses at nylon, polyester or acrylic dress shirts', they were more willing to experiment in weekend wear and sports tops.[33] In the case of Celanese, entering the bathing suit market similarly allowed the hope of inroads against established fabrics. Customers, especially those hoping to sunbathe without ending up in court, were more likely to try new styles, which added to the sense of exclusivity.

Part of the problem was the prevailing design of the bathing costume, which offered space for companies to experiment. Fashionable bathing suits at the time emphasized, as much as possible, exposing skin to the sun. This was often done through an open, low-cut, or V-shaped 'sun-back'.[34] However, as the Celanese advertisement noted, materials that excluded the 'actinic content' of the sun's rays still left parts of the body unsusceptible. 'Cotton or wool bathing suits leave a "tidemark" of tan', it noted, and 'the skin covered by the material remains white, unresponsive to the sun's action'. On the other hand, 'the wearer of a "Celanese" bathing suit will find that the skin is tanned evenly, all over'.[35] Referencing the standard 'natural' fibers by name, Celanese was offered as an alternative.

Medical professionals reported on the detrimental effects that could result from untanned skin. For instance, a New York doctor published on a case of pityriasis rosea in the journal *Archives of Dermatology and Syphilology*. The patient, a man named M. R., had 'acquired a deep tan on the body during the summer of 1937'. In January of the following year, he experienced an eruption of pinkish lesions. These were located 'exactly on the area covered by the bathing trunks'. The article used the case to conclude that 'in a person whose body has been tanned by exposure to the

[33] Regina Lee Blaszczyk, 'Ernest Dichter and the Peacock Revolution: Motivation Research, the Menswear Market and the DuPont Company', in *Ernest Dichter and Motivation Research: New Perspectives on the Making of Post-War Consumer Culture*, ed. Stefan Schwarzkopf and Rainer Gries (New York: Palgrave Macmillan, 2010), 131.

[34] For contemporary accounts of summer fashions, see 'Summer Fashions: Bathing Costumes and Wraps', *Times*, June 26, 1931, 17, and 'London Fashions: For Sun and Sea,' *Times*, June 22, 1934, 17.

[35] British Celanese, advertisement, xxxv.

sun an eruption of pityriasis rosea may avoid the tanned areas'.[36] Beyond simply benefitting from the sun's rays, skin excluded from healthful tanning was thus classed as a health risk.

In practice, however, rayon was often associated instead with illness, especially for those producing the fabric. While its proponents argued that cellulose acetate was superior to pure cellulose fibers, both types of rayon were implicated in scandals over their negative health effects. Paul David Blanc's book *Fake Silk* details the dangers of viscose rayon in particular, which harmed workers and released toxic chemicals into the manufacturing plants' surrounds.[37] Cellulose acetate was also embroiled in controversy. An article in the *British Medical Journal* reported the case of a child who presented with acute poisoning after being treated with cellulose acetate solution on her knee.[38] This article inspired several responses objecting to the particulars of the case. Writers emphasized that cellulose acetate was a solid that did not have fumes, and that it was 'non-poisonous, very stable, odorless, and non-inflammable'. The authors did note, however, that the solvents used to make cellulose acetate had toxic properties.[39] Fumes were also implicated in the deaths of a handful of factory workers at the plants of British Celanese.[40]

In this context, then, emphasizing novel health benefits for the wearers of the fabric served two purposes. It created a new market for the fiber while simultaneously stressing the relationship between Celanese and well-being in the public mind. The advertisement in question includes even more functional benefits of the fabric besides its permeability to the sun. 'This unique fabric promotes the more efficient aeration of the pores. It permits free evaporation between the garment and the skin, thereby facilitating the free passage of light and air and the free evaporation of perspiration. Again the gentle massage and friction between "Celanese"

[36] Maurice J. Costello, 'Pityriasis Rosea Sparing Tanned Areas of The Skin (Bathing Trunk Distribution)', *Archives of Dermatology and Syphilology* 38, no. 1 (1938): 75–76.

[37] Paul David Blanc, *Fake Silk: The Lethal History of Viscose Rayon* (New Haven: Yale University Press, 2016).

[38] Godfrey Carter, 'Acute Poisoning by Fumes from Cellulose Acetate', *British Medical Journal* 2, no. 3324 (1924): 456.

[39] See, for instance, Sidney A. Welch, 'Cellulose Acetate', *British Medical Journal* 2, no. 3327 (October 4, 1924), 644; and M. T. Callimachi, 'Cellulose Acetate', *British Medical Journal* 2, no. 3327 (October 4, 1924), 644.

[40] 'British Celanese Worker's Death: Story of Fumes', *Manchester Guardian*, February 15, 1934, 12.

and the skin set up electrical charges of a beneficial character'.[41] This deluge of medical information created new associations for the reader, marketing the fabric as a tool for maintaining one's health.

Celanese also fit into the broader goals of the so-called rational dress movement of the late nineteenth and early twentieth centuries, which stressed simplicity and lightness of clothing as an aid to physical health.[42] The advertisement asserted that 'from the viewpoint of beauty alone the future of "Celanese" is assured', but that 'increasing recognition of its hygienic properties will speed its adoption as the universal fabric, for all occasions, for all climes'.[43] Ken Montague has investigated the visual culture of the dress reform movement, where he argues that the appeals to 'naturalness' in the shape of the body sought to stabilize forms of difference at a time of rapid change.[44] As will be discussed in the following sections, Celanese was thereby implicated in broader attempts to delineate boundaries of class and race. While it aimed to universalize access to aspects of the upper classes, namely their ability to travel and tan, the devaluing of white skin was hard to square with logics of white supremacy.

6.5 Celanese and the Social Body

As indicated by the letter writer from 1924 mentioned above, access to the sun was highly dependent upon one's class status—some individuals could afford to travel on cruises or to the beaches of far-off health resorts, while others were left hoping for affordable, bottled sunshine. The well-being promised by the makers of Celanese, then, hinged partially on emulation of the upper classes and their privileged access to ultraviolet rays.

This was explicitly discussed in a study on consumer attitudes toward Celanese fabrics conducted three decades later across the Atlantic. Ernest Dichter, an Austrian immigrant to the United States, founded his Institute

[41] British Celanese, advertisement, xxxv.

[42] On the dress reform movement in the nineteenth century, see the classic text by Stella Mary Newton, *Health, Art & Reason: Dress Reformers of the 19th Century* (London: John Murray, 1974). On its extension into the twentieth century, see Barbara Burman and Melissa Leventon, 'The Men's Dress Reform Party, 1929–1937' and Joanna Bourke, 'The Great Male Renunciation'. For some of the connections between these movements, see Michael Carter, 'J.C. Flügel and the Nude Future', *Fashion Theory* 7, no. 1 (2003): 79–101.

[43] Ibid.

[44] Ken Montague, 'The Aesthetics of Hygiene: Aesthetic Dress, Modernity, and the Body as Sign', *Journal of Design History* 7, no. 2 (1994): 91–112.

for Motivational Research to help companies gather information on the behavior of their customers. Motivational Research was premised on the idea that the tools of psychology and psychoanalysis could uncover unconscious feelings people had toward products, which could guide future advertising to increase sales. Dichter's institute performed such studies for hundreds of companies in a variety of industries, including many on clothing and personal appearance.[45]

In early 1957, the institute sent a proposal to the American Celanese Corporation for a study on customers' views of the company and its products. The first suggested area of research entailed 'the psychology of women's apparel and the expressive power of Celanese'.[46] In much of his writing, Dichter emphasized that objects were engaged in dynamic relationships with their owners—objects had 'souls', which could be uncovered through projective testing and depth interviews.[47] Dichter found that 'women, of course, regard clothes as not only instruments that enable them to demonstrate the contours of their bodies but also as the means of satisfying definite basic emotional and psychological needs'.[48] In delineating potential avenues of this research, the proposal highlighted the connection between Celanese and status. 'A dress, according to the lesson of several of our previous studies, is the badge of a woman's social standing. Or, at least, it is seen that way *psychologically*, by many women'. More specifically, Dichter argued that clothing was a means by which women sought to psychologically climb the social ladder. 'Many women', the proposal continued, 'are "clothes snobs." Their emotional demand is for clothes that do not appeal so much to their sense of beauty as to their deep-seated need to appear to belong in a high social class'. Wealthy women, on the other hand, want to be sure 'that the clothes they wear will not be seen on every "Joan, Jane, and Jennie"'.[49]

[45] See Ronald Fullerton, 'Ernest Dichter: The Motivational Researcher', in *Ernest Dichter and Motivation Research: New Perspectives on the Making of Post-War Consumer Culture*, ed. Stefan Schwarzkopf and Rainer Gries (New York: Palgrave Macmillan, 2010), 58–72.

[46] 'A creative problem analysis and suggested areas of research for a motivational research study affecting the advertising and merchandising areas of the Celanese Corporation', January 1957, 849A, Box 33, Ernest Dichter papers (Accession 2407), Hagley Museum and Library, Wilmington, Delaware.

[47] Ernest Dichter, *The Strategy of Desire* (New Brunswick, N.J.: Transaction Publishers, 1960), 86.

[48] 'A motivational research study affecting the advertising and merchandising areas of the Celanese Corporation', 7.

[49] 'A motivational research study', 11–12.

It is not clear that this research was ever performed. Dichter's papers include a follow-up letter with amendments to the proposal from late January after a meeting between Institute researchers and representatives of the Celanese Corporation, but there is no final report.[50] However, the proposal is still helpful in analyzing the advertisement for Celanese and the class aspirations stitched into the fabric. The first few pages of the *Times* supplement on sunshine and health are littered with advertisements for health spas around the world, which make clear their status as places for the upper classes. Under adverts for French spas, for instance, was a list of hotels under the heading 'The Palaces of the "Elite"'.[51] The advertisement for the Lido in Venice is subtler, featuring a drawing of a woman lying on the sand under the tagline, 'La Plage des Bronzes Vivants'. The copy reads, 'bronzing on the silvery, pleasantly hot sands, with a lazy, appreciative eye for the sunburst of color of the Pyjama Parade—no wonder they call it "La Plage du soleil et des pyjamas"'.[52] The names of precious metals and the invocation of leisure signal that this is a place for only a select few. This is literally underscored by the advertisement below it. 'Resorts, spas, & hotels wishing to attract the most desirable class of visitors', it stated, 'should reserve space in the Special ADVERTISEMENT TRAVEL COLUMNS of "The Times"—"The World's Leading Medium for Travel Advertising"'.[53] This placed the Lido unequivocally as a rarefied institution with an exclusive clientele.

In the section on health resorts, the Milan correspondent for the *Times* provided a short piece on the Lido in Venice. This article likewise emphasized the exclusivity of the resort. Echoing the advertisements earlier in the issue, the correspondent wrote about the variety of 'charming' accommodations, including 'several rich new palaces'. In no uncertain terms, the writer concluded that the Lido 'has become the most aristocratic, the most beautiful, and the most fashionable bathing resort in Italy'.[54] The name of this particular resort, the Lido, would later become synonymous with beaches and pools all over England, standing in for aspirational access

[50] 'Proposed motivational research for Celanese Corporation', January 22, 1957, 849.1A, Box 33, Ernest Dichter papers (Accession 2407), Hagley Museum and Library, Wilmington, Delaware.

[51] 'The Palaces of the "Elite"', advertisement, *Times*, May 22, 1928, iii.

[52] Lido Venice, advertisement, *Times*, May 22, 1928, iv.

[53] The *Times* Travel Department, advertisement, *Times*, May 22, 1928, iv.

[54] 'The Lido', *Times*, May 22, 1928, xxv.

to exclusive sites in which to experience the sun's rays.[55] Just as this naming was a way to democratize the Italian spa, the Celanese fabric sought to let every consumer 'live in your own Lido'. This was an invitation to become a living bronze statue, all without the expenses of travel. The goal was to 'secure a place in the sun this summer', but, more generally, the idea was to secure one's status as 'a member of the most desirable class'.

As the court cases around exposure indicated, access was a big part of the issue. Nudity was tolerated 'in one's garden or room, out of sight'. When the body was 'exposed', however, was when the trouble began. Just as only some members of British society had the means to travel to health spas, only a small portion could access private space in which to sunbathe without exposure. Underlying the Celanese advertisement, then, as well as debates around semi-nudity on the stage, was a critique about class exclusion. Built into these concerns, though still distinct, was commentary on race and national belonging, a subject to which I now turn.

6.6 Light and Color

Throughout the promotional material for the Lido described above, the vibrant colors of the spa are highlighted. The piece on the resort in the *Times* ends, for instance,

> The tents and cabins that stretch out for two or three kilometres along the smiling sea-shore are brightly and variously decorated; and in the full blaze of the sun out of a proverbially Italian sky the bizarre jangle of colors from the tents and the striking bathing costumes and cloaks of the fashionable multitude that drawl out the long hours on the sun-warmed sand compose a landscape unrivaled in Europe for its impression of warmth and sun-worshipping gaiety.[56]

Indeed, color was a key part of sun worship. The right color was believed to do wonders to one's well-being. In an article in the *Times* reporting on a meeting of the British Medical Association in Plymouth in July of 1938, the value of sunbathing was discussed by Dr. W. R. G. Atkins. While light therapy was primarily successful in treating diseases such as

[55] For more on Lidos, which referred to either beaches or, increasingly, to open-air swimming pools, see Janet Smith, *Liquid Assets: The Lidos and Open-Air Swimming Pools of Britain* (London: English Heritage, 2005).

[56] Ibid.

rickets, lupus, and tuberculosis, 'on the healthy population the mental effect of bright daylight was so cheering that one was compelled to regard it as of significance for the body also, especially when it was a very variable stimulus'. The article continued, 'No one could see the splendid general tone of the skin of those who took even short regular sun-baths on the sea front in Plymouth without realizing that an unsunned skin was unnatural and might consequently be expected to fail when extreme calls were made on its heat-regulating powers'.[57] Aesthetics and health were tied squarely to color, spelling out a warning for those who looked 'unnatural' to the privileged observer.

Other medical studies substantiated this belief. In a paper delivered before the Royal Institute of Public Health in 1925, Henry Gauvin and C. R. McRae reported on their use of 'phototherapy'. The authors reflected that 'In an institution where light treatment is seriously and systematically practiced one is struck not only by the appearance of robust health and improved physique exhibited by the large majority of patients treated, but also by the vivacity, happiness and general alertness of the patients'.[58] To test this perception, mental testing was conducted in two institutions: special schools in London for children suffering from a variety of physical ailments and a hospital in Alton for those with 'surgical' tuberculosis. The researchers found a noticeable difference in 'mental ratio', the measure of children's mental age divided by their chronological age. They proposed four hypotheses for this difference, discussed in turn: differences in heredity, educational facilities, the seriousness of 'physical defects', and treatment. While they found no noticeable differences between the two groups in the parents' occupations (their proxy for heredity) and found the average rates of class attendance to be, in fact, much lower in Alton due to many children's bedridden state, the researchers suggested that 'it seems certain that the improvement brought about in the body-pole of the organism by exposure to sunlight and artificial light is accompanied by a corresponding improvement in the efficiency of the mind-pole'. The authors noted that 'while the bodily improvement recorded and the raised metabolism noted as the result of exposure to sun, sea bathing and open

[57] 'Mental Factors in Illness; A Gap in Medical Teaching; Value of Sun-Bathing', *Times*, July 22, 1938, 11.

[58] Henry Gauvin and C. R. McRae, 'The Effect of Heliotherapy and Artificial Light Treatment on the Mentality of Patients' *Journal of State Medicine* 33, no. 12 (December 1, 1925): 551–562. This study was reported in the popular press as well. See 'Light as Brain Food: Effect on Patients' Mentality', *Times*, May 29, 1925, 5.

air would of itself be likely to have an indirectly beneficial effect on mental activity', this was not likely to fully account for the differences in mental activity observed. Instead, the researchers pointed to studies where light was used to treat rickets to argue that light fortifies tissues such as the blood and thus might do the same for the brain.[59] In making these claims, Gauvin and McRae indicated not only that there was an indirect effect of light on mental health but also that they believed its effect to be so great that physical processes had to be at work as well.

This claim is striking when compared to discourses of 'civilization' and the racial science of intelligence testing from this same period. If access to the sun led to increases in mental activity in this case, why would those who had supposedly evolved to have darker skin not have gained similar advantages? Instead of conferring mental advantage, melanin was pathologized in medical literature.[60] Writing in the *British Medical Journal*, H. J. Fleure argued that 'the character of the skin and hair...seems to be in some degree an indicator of the general constitution, and especially of the mechanism of heat regulation. And these differences of constitution seem to connect themselves, not only with adaptability to certain climates, but also with resistance to various diseases'. Looking at the 'variations of colour in inter-tropical Africa', Fleure included a handful of hypotheses, including 'That regions with specially lowly societies, refugees of ancient types, societies on poor soil, apart from forest, tend to be specially dark', and 'the better lands usually have lighter coloured peoples'.[61] Levels of civilization, he believed, could be read on the skin.[62] In this case, darker skin conferred health benefits but decidedly did not improve mental aptitude.

[59] Gauvin and McRae, 'Artificial Light Treatment on the Mentality of Patients', 556–560.

[60] For a specific example, see 'Melanin', *Lancet* 236, no. 6100 (July 1940): 109–110. On the history of skin lightening, see Shirley Anne Tate, 'Skin Lightening: Contempt, Hatred, Fear', in *Black Women's Bodies and the Nation: Race, Gender, and Culture* (Hampshire: Palgrave Macmillan, 2015), 146–163.

[61] H. J. Fleure, 'Racial Characters of Skin in Relation to Health', *British Medical Journal* 2 (November 20, 1926): 953–955.

[62] Historian Tony Kushner takes Fleure, a progressive man who never fully abandoned racial categories, to be paradigmatic of race thinking in Britain at this time. See Tony Kushner, 'H. J. Fleure: a paradigm for inter-war race thinking in Britain', *Patterns of Prejudice* 42, no. 2 (2008): 151–166.

This was largely a question of nationhood as it intersected with race.[63] To take one example, reporting on the 1919 race riots in Cardiff and Liverpool emphasized the inability of nonwhite peoples to be incorporated into the nation. As one article put it, 'The heritage of Grecian and Roman thought, with twenty centuries of Christianity imposed upon it, has given us ideals and standards which the coloured races cannot share nor understand. So we cannot admit them to share our citizenship'. The article noted that British citizens tended to ignore 'race distinction', largely because many ignored the presence of nonwhite peoples in the metropole until events such as these riots made their presence all too clear.[64]

The ambiguous racial implications in scientific studies on sunbathing can be explained, however, by situating Britain as a colonial power interested in managing its empire. The above article continued,

> One of the secrets of good British colonisation among coloured races has been the instinctive recognition of this fact by the British man, as soon as he goes abroad to help to administer a coloured colony. He does not mix with the natives, though he governs them justly and mercifully as a rule. (European Peoples who do not 'draw the colour line' so strictly do not succeed so well.)[65]

One way to 'draw the colour line' was through clothing. Medical men of this time were often preoccupied with how to keep white men safe in the colonies, particularly when it came to the sun. It was in these contexts that the frailty of white skin really came to light, leading to what historian Warwick Anderson called 'pigment envy' in the case of United States occupation of the Philippines.[66] This reduced any comparative advantage to the level of chemicals, divorced from bodies and especially from minds. The invocation of medicine and the purposeful use of technology to

[63] On this point, see Tony Kushner, *We Europeans? Mass-Observation, 'Race' and British Identity in the Twentieth Century* (Burlington, VT: Ashgate, 2004).

[64] 'The Negro Riots: A Lesson for England', *Morning Post* (London, England), June 13, 1919.

[65] 'The Negro Riots'. For more on these riots, see Michael Rowe, 'Sex, 'race' and riot in Liverpool, 1919', *Immigrants & Minorities* 19, no. 2 (July 2000): 53–70.

[66] Warwick Anderson, *Colonial Pathologies: American Tropical Medicine, Race, and Hygiene in the Philippines* (Durham: Duke University Press, 2006), 83–84.

achieve what evolution had done was then used to obscure this weakness and 'reify' race and white supremacy in the process.[67]

Writing about tropical clothing, physician Louis Sambon wrote in 1907 that 'the most striking and important difference between the inhabitants of the temperate zone and the native of tropical regions is *colour*'. Over a lifetime, the skin of 'the white man' may become 'somewhat tanned, but otherwise there is no change in the colour of his skin'. It is only 'in the course of generations', he argued, that such changes could be effected. From his observations, Sambon experimented with the 'skin of dark-coloured races' and concluded that 'the white man in the Tropics should wear black, red, or orange clothing'. The practice of wearing white, 'adopted in imitation of native custom', ignored 'the all-important fact that the native is already fully protected by a natural armour of pigment'.[68] Commenting on Sambon's findings, another writer emphasized that 'by imitating nature...the white man can hope to overcome this defect in his cutaneous covering, and Dr. Sambon has shown us with scientific precision how this can be successfully accomplished'.[69] In short, Sambon's work objectified darker skin into a 'natural armour'. Emphasizing its hardiness, Sambon thereby participated in broader eugenic discourses around 'endangered whiteness'.[70]

Sambon, who was born in Italy and practiced in Britain, is known for having developed a fabric to regulate the relationship between the skin and the sun. Notably, however, his 'Solaro' material sought to inhibit the same 'actinic' rays that Celanese touted, keeping them from reaching the body at all. This fabric was even tested on thousands of American soldiers in the Philippines, who were given orange-red underwear by the United States Army Board in the hopes it would reduce disease and increase fitness.[71] Sambon is the subject of work by historian Ryan Johnson, who

[67] Troy Duster, 'Race and Reification in Science', *Science* 307, no. 5712 (2005): 1050–1051.

[68] Louis W. Sambon, 'Tropical Clothing', *The Journal of Tropical Medicine and Hygiene* 10, no. 4 (February 15, 1907): 67–68. Emphasis added.

[69] J. C. [James Cantlie], 'Tropical Clothing', *The Journal of Tropical Medicine and Hygiene* 10, no. 4 (February 15, 1907): 71. Emphasis added.

[70] Laura Briggs, 'The Race of Hysteria: 'Overcivilization' and the 'Savage' Woman in Late Nineteenth-Century Obstetrics and Gynecology', *American Quarterly* 52, no. 2 (June 2000): 250.

[71] James M. Phalen, 'An Experiment with Orange-Red Underwear', *The Philippine Journal of Science* 5, no. 6 (December 1910): 525–46. See also 'Orange-Red Clothing: No Improvement', *Journal of the American Medical Association* 54, no. 22 (May 28, 1910): 1793.

investigates the intertwining of tropical medicine and imperial power at the turn of the twentieth century. Johnson locates Solaro, for instance, as part of 'a vast commodity culture that upheld climatic etiologies in practice'. Solaro's failure to improve the health of soldiers, in this context, indicates the complex transition to a microbial understanding of disease.[72]

Comparing Solaro to Celanese, however, indicates not only changing ideas around the health effects of sunlight in the 1920s but also the role of the colonies in the construction of racial categories. Following the work of Ann Laura Stoler on the colonial origins of Michel Foucault's theories of sexuality, we might say that clothing likewise illustrates how colonies functioned as 'laboratories of modernity' in which European culture was first tested.[73] In the colonial setting, Solaro attempted to maintain whiteness both literally and figuratively. Its failure, then, can be read as part of a growing difficulty to use physical measures alone to create racial categories.[74] In the metropole, Celanese emphasized instead how pale skin was unhealthy and unbecoming, a sign of the ill or the lower classes. The clothing was sold based on ties to a fledgling science of heliotherapy, which stood in for a more complex understanding of race as including other factors related to civilization, namely technology and medicine. The use of intelligence tests in understanding the action of the sun's rays, then, is emblematic of these strands of race-making coming together in the early twentieth century. Both tans and orange-red clothing were temporary, and it was in the achievement of 'imitating nature' that white supremacy was built. White skin's 'defect', that is, was only skin deep.

6.7 Conclusion

In the early twentieth century, sunbathing swelled in popularity in England as doctors and reformers touted the health benefits of ultraviolet rays. These groups ran into trouble, however, when it came to the question of how much skin one should show. Companies marketed a variety of consumer products to deliver the sun's benefits while preserving modesty,

[72] Ryan Johnson, 'European Cloth and "Tropical" Skin: Clothing Material and British Ideas of Health and Hygiene in Tropical Climates', *Bulletin of the History of Medicine* 83, no. 3 (Fall 2009): 530–560.

[73] Ann Laura Stoler, *Race and the Education of Desire: Foucault's* History of Sexuality *and the Colonial Order of Things* (Durham: Duke University Press, 1995), 15.

[74] George W. Stocking Jr., 'The Turn-of-the-Century Concept of Race', *Modernism/modernity* 1, no. 1 (1994): 4–16.

including personal sunlamps and vitamin D supplements. One such product was Celanese fabric, an artificial silk that promised to help its wearer 'secure a place in the sun' without indecency. Celanese fabric was therefore an answer to moralists' concerns around exposure and reformers' hopes to dispense with heavy clothing that obstructed the skin. Clothes made from cellulose acetate were marketed to increase one's well-being—through the action of the sun upon the skin, as well as through emulation of the upper classes and their ability to travel to lidos and health spas. As I have argued, Celanese products thus promoted a specific type of healing that ameliorated anxieties relating to class, race, and other aspects of identity.

This history has lots to tell us about our world today. In 2000, a show premiered on Channel 4 called *A Place in the Sun*. The program follows British couples hoping to buy property, usually in a sunny locale on the continent. In the past two decades, the show has expanded to include a wealth of spin-offs and an online 'overseas property portal' all designed to help 'house-hunters find their dream holiday home in the sun'.[75] The show's immense popularity builds on the story detailed in this chapter—nearly a century after British Celanese advertised their fabric with that language, the British people are still looking for ways to secure their 'place in the sun'.

There is therefore a long history of marketplaces geared around access to the sun. For those who cannot afford to travel or purchase homes in Spain or Greece, there are a wealth of products bringing the sun home to the British people. Celanese fabric and real estate television shows are just some of many things that capitalize on cultural anxiety around environment, disease, and aesthetics. As this chapter has argued, underneath these claims are broader concerns about the nation, especially around questions of belonging. Consumer goods can democratize institutions to some degree, but it is important to remember the often-disregarded consequences of curative things and the new barriers they can create. Securing a place in the sun by necessity casts a shadow.

[75] The program's full website can be found at https://www.aplaceinthesun.com, and its Channel 4 page is https://www.channel4.com/programmes/a-place-in-the-sun Accessed September 1, 2022.

References

Anderson, Warwick. *Colonial Pathologies: American Tropical Medicine, Race, and Hygiene in the Philippines*. Durham: Duke University Press, 2006.

'The Artificial Silk Industry'. *The Economist Monthly Supplement*, no. 31 (December 26, 1925): 47.

Blanc, Paul David. *Fake Silk: The Lethal History of Viscose Rayon*. New Haven: Yale University Press, 2016.

Blaszczyk, Regina Lee. 'Ernest Dichter and the Peacock Revolution: Motivation Research, the Menswear Market and the DuPont Company'. In *Ernest Dichter and Motivation Research: New Perspectives on the Making of Post-War Consumer Culture*, edited by Stefan Schwarzkopf and Rainer Gries, 126–139. New York: Palgrave Macmillan, 2010.

Briggs, Laura. 'The Race of Hysteria: "Overcivilization" and the "Savage" Woman in Late Nineteenth-Century Obstetrics and Gynecology'. *American Quarterly* 52, no. 2 (June 2000): 246–273.

'British Celanese Worker's Death: Story of Fumes'. *Manchester Guardian*, February 15, 1934, 12.

Burman, Barbara. 'Better and Brighter Clothes: The Men's Dress Reform Party, 1929–1940'. *Journal of Design History* 8, no. 4 (1995): 275–290.

Burman, Barbara and Melissa Leventon, 'The Men's Dress Reform Party 1929–37'. *Costume* 21 (1987): 75–87.

Bourke, Joanna. 'The Great Male Renunciation: Men's Dress Reform in Inter-War Britain'. *Journal of Design History* 9, no. 1 (1996): 23–33.

Callimachi, M. T. 'Cellulose Acetate'. *British Medical Journal* 2, no. 3327 (October 4, 1924): 644.

C., J. [Cantlie, James], 'Tropical Clothing'. *The Journal of Tropical Medicine and Hygiene* 10, no. 4 (February 15, 1907): 71.

Carter, Godfrey. 'Acute Poisoning by Fumes from Cellulose Acetate'. *British Medical Journal* 2, no. 3324 (1924): 456.

Carter, Michael. 'J.C. Flügel and the Nude Future'. *Fashion Theory* 7, no. 1 (2003): 79–101.

Carter, Simon. *Rise and Shine: Sunlight, Technology and Health*. Oxford: Berg, 2007.

'Commercial Reports'. *The Economist* C, no. 4260 (April 18, 1925): 784–785.

Costello, Maurice J. 'Pityriasis Rosea Sparing Tanned Areas of The Skin (Bathing Trunk Distribution)'. *Archives of Dermatology and Syphilology* 38, no. 1 (1938): 75–76.

Dichter, Ernest. *The Strategy of Desire*. New Brunswick, N.J.: Transaction Publishers, 1960.

Duster, Troy. 'Race and Reification in Science'. *Science* 307, no. 5712 (2005): 1050–1051.

Fleure, H. J. 'Racial Characters of Skin in Relation to Health'. *British Medical Journal* 2 (November 20, 1926): 953–955.

Fourness, Robert K. 'The Development of Disperse Dyes for Acetate Fibres'. *Coloration Technology* 90, no. 1 (1974): 15–21.

Freund, Daniel. *American Sunshine: Diseases of Darkness and the Quest for Natural Light.* Chicago: The University of Chicago Press, 2012.

Fullerton, Ronald. 'Ernest Dichter: The Motivational Researcher'. In *Ernest Dichter and Motivation Research: New Perspectives on the Making of Post-War Consumer Culture*, edited by Stefan Schwarzkopf and Rainer Gries, 58–72. New York: Palgrave Macmillan, 2010.

Gauvin, Henry and C. R. McRae, 'The Effect of Heliotherapy and Artificial Light Treatment on the Mentality of Patients'. *Journal of State Medicine* 33, no. 12 (December 1, 1925): 551–562.

Gush, Nadia. 'The Beauty of Health: Cora Wilding and the Sunlight League'. *New Zealand Journal of History* 43, no. 1 (2009): 1–17.

Herbert, A. P. 'The Manly Chest; Aesthetics of the Beach; Costume and Convention'. *Times* (London, England), July 28, 1932, 13.

Institute for Motivational Research. 'A creative problem analysis and suggested areas of research for a motivational research study affecting the advertising and merchandising areas of the Celanese Corporation'. January 1957, 849A, Box 33, Ernest Dichter papers (Accession 2407), Hagley Museum and Library, Wilmington, Delaware.

Institute for Motivational Research. 'Proposed motivational research for Celanese Corporation'. January 22, 1957, 849.1A, Box 33, Ernest Dichter papers (Accession 2407), Hagley Museum and Library, Wilmington, Delaware.

Ryan Johnson, 'European Cloth and "Tropical" Skin: Clothing Material and British Ideas of Health and Hygiene in Tropical Climates'. *Bulletin of the History of Medicine* 83, no. 3 (Fall 2009): 530–560.

Klose, Nelson. 'Sericulture in the United States'. *Agricultural History* 37, no. 4 (1963): 225–234.

Kushner, Tony. *We Europeans? Mass-Observation, 'Race' and British Identity in the Twentieth Century.* Burlington, VT: Ashgate, 2004.

Kushner, Tony. 'H. J. Fleure: a paradigm for inter-war race thinking in Britain'. *Patterns of Prejudice* 42, no. 2 (2008): 151–166.

'Light as Brain Food: Effect on Patients' Mentality'. *Times* (London, England), May 29, 1925, 5.

'London Fashions: For Sun and Sea'. *Times* (London, England), June 22, 1934, 17.

'Magistrate on Sun-Bathing in Public'. *Times* (London, England), August 6, 1927, 12.

'The Manly Chest: French Mayor's Warning to Sun-Bathers'. *Times* (London, England), July 27, 1933, 11.

Matthews David, Alison. *Fashion Victims: The Dangers of Dress Past and Present*. London: Bloomsbury Visual Arts, 2015.
'Melanin.' *Lancet* 236, no. 6100 (July 1940): 109–110.
'Mental Factors in Illness; A Gap in Medical Teaching; Value of Sun-Bathing'. *Times* (London, England), July 22, 1938, 11.
Montague, Ken. 'The Aesthetics of Hygiene: Aesthetic Dress, Modernity, and the Body as Sign'. *Journal of Design History* 7, no. 2 (1994): 91–112.
'The Negro Riots: A Lesson for England'. *Morning Post* (London, England), June 13, 1919.
'A New Science'. *Times* (London, England), May 22, 1928, x.
Newton, Stella Mary. *Health, Art & Reason: Dress Reformers of the 19th Century*. London: John Murray, 1974.
'Orange-Red Clothing: No Improvement'. *Journal of the American Medical Association* 54, no. 22 (May 28, 1910): 1793.
Phalen, James M. 'An Experiment with Orange-Red Underwear'. *The Philippine Journal of Science* 5, no. 6 (December 1910): 525–546.
Rowe, Michael. 'Sex, 'race' and riot in Liverpool, 1919'. *Immigrants & Minorities* 19, no. 2 (July 2000): 53–70.
Sambon, Louis W. 'Tropical Clothing'. *The Journal of Tropical Medicine and Hygiene* 10, no. 4 (February 15, 1907): 67–68.
Smith, Janet. *Liquid Assets: The Lidos and Open-Air Swimming Pools of Britain*. London: English Heritage, 2005.
Stocking Jr., George W. 'The Turn-of-the-Century Concept of Race'. *Modernism/modernity* 1, no. 1 (1994): 4–16.
Stoler, Ann Laura. *Race and the Education of Desire: Foucault's* History of Sexuality *and the Colonial Order of Things*. Durham: Duke University Press, 1995.
'Summer Fashions: Bathing Costumes and Wraps'. *Times* (London, England), June 26, 1931, 17.
'Sun Bathing: Benefits of Light and Air'. *Times* (London, England), March 18, 1932, 10.
'Sun-Bather Bound Over'. *Times* (London, England), October 19, 1933, 4.
'Sun-Bathing for Children: New Centre in Regent's Park'. *Times* (London, England), August 19, 1930, 7.
'Sun-Bathing in a London Park'. *Lancet* 216, no. 5600 (December 27, 1930): 1409–1410.
Shadwell, A. 'Bottling the Sun'. *Times* (London, England), November 23, 1924, 10.
Tate, Shirley Anne. 'Skin Lightening: Contempt, Hatred, Fear'. In *Black Women's Bodies and the Nation: Race, Gender, and Culture*, 146–163. Hampshire: Palgrave Macmillan, 2015.

Welch, Sidney A. 'Cellulose Acetate'. *British Medical Journal* 2, no. 3327 (October 4, 1924), 644.

Wingate, Isabel B. 'Acetate Rayon'. *Journal of Retailing* 6, no. 4 (January 1931): 119–121.

'Your Place in the Sun'. *Britannia and Eve* 19, no. 2 (August 1939): 39.

CHAPTER 7

Palliative Prototypes or Therapeutic Functionality? Examining C.P. Company's Urban Protection Range

Andrew Groves

Human trauma—the body damaged and degraded, the mind uneasy, anxious and disturbed—was a reoccurring motif in art and fashion at the end of the twentieth century, with designers including Alexander McQueen, Hussein Chalayan and Comme des Garçons mobilising a dystopian aesthetic of decay and deathliness.[1] At the same time, a more optimistic—indeed, utopian—response to the imagined challenges of the impending

[1] On trauma and art, see Hal Foster, 'Obscene, Abject, Traumatic', *October* 78 (1996): 106–24. On fashion, see Caroline Evans. *Fashion at the Edge: Spectacle, Modernity and Deathliness.* New Haven and London: Yale University Press, 2003, and Rebecca Arnold. *Fashion, Desire and Anxiety* (London and New York: I.B. Tauris, 2001.

A. Groves (✉)
University of Westminster, London, UK
e-mail: grovesa@westminster.ac.uk

D. Woolley et al. (eds.), *Wearable Objects and Curative Things*, Palgrave Studies in Fashion and the Body,
https://doi.org/10.1007/978-3-031-40017-9_7

twenty-first century was proposed by designer Moreno Ferrari, whose Urban Protection menswear range for C.P. Company embedded augmented technology within hybrid garments, creating multifunctional barriers intended to protect the wearer against the harms of the contemporary urban environment. Produced at a moment of collective cultural anxiety, these distinct approaches suggested fashion's anticipation of the future as both dystopian threat and utopian promise.[2]

This chapter examines the Urban Protection range through a thematic analysis of ten objects from the collection, emphasising the complexity of Ferrari's proposition. The Urban Protection range was initially interpreted as embodying a utopian vision of the future in which wearable technology would augment the human body to withstand the challenges of the modern metropolis. However, the passing of time has repositioned these garments. While the inherent obsolescence of technology means that the garments' original functionalities have today been rendered ineffective, Ferrari's metaphysical framework, which employed a variety of semiotic strategies, has enabled the garments to transcend their material limitations. Accordingly, this chapter reads these garments as a rejection of the technology that they ostensibly embraced, and locates them in the context of a long tradition of artists and designers with a quasi-spiritual desire to start again from zero.

This chapter situates the Urban Protection range in relation to this volume's concept of 'curative things', paying particular attention to two frameworks: the palliative and the therapeutic. The term 'palliative' typically denotes a medical situation where there is no prospect of cure, and where treatment is therefore aimed at relieving symptoms and offering comfort.[3] The etymology of palliative, from the Latin verb *palliare*, meaning to cloak, cover or conceal, provides a conceptual connection to the Urban Protection line, which consisted primarily of outerwear that cloaked, covered and protected the body.[4] This chapter argues that the

[2] On culture and anxiety at the end of the twentieth century, see Renata Salecl's *On Anxiety* (2004) and Timothy Bewes' *Reification* (2002).

[3] On the changing use of 'palliative' in medical journals from the mid-nineteenth century onwards, see Taubert M, Fielding H, Mathews E, *et al.* 2013, 'An exploration of the word 'palliative' in the 19th century: searching the BMJ archives for clues', *BMJ Supportive & Palliative Care* 3: 26-30.

[4] Lori Wiener et al., 2015. 'Threading the Cloak: Palliative Care Education for Care Providers of Adolescents and Young Adults with Cancer,' *Clinical Oncology in Adolescents and Young Adults* 5: 1–18

garments in the Urban Protection range were initially understood as essentially palliative in intent, intended to soothe the somatic symptoms triggered in the wearer by the implicitly unhealthy urban environment. However, closer attention to Ferrari's semantic framing of these garments reveals that the garments were able to serve a psycho-therapeutic function, engaging the wearer on a metaphysical and spiritual, as well as merely physical, level.[5]

7.1 Antecedents to the Urban Protection Range

In 1909, the Italian poet F. T. Marinetti published the 'Founding and Manifesto of Futurism' in several newspapers, including on the front page of *Le Figaro*.[6] The manifesto championed aggression, speed, poetry, automobiles, and the modern industrial city, and lauded man's technological triumph over nature. Central to their artistic practise and dissemination of their revolutionary ideas was the creation of written clothing through the printed word. In 1914, Giacomo Balla, a key proponent of the Futurist movement, published The Futurist Manifesto of Men's Clothing.[7] It stated:

> We want Futurist clothes to be comfortable and practical:
> Dynamic
> Aggressive
> Shocking
> Energetic
> Violent
> Flying (i.e. giving the idea of flying, rising and running)
> Peppy
> Joyful
> Illuminating (in order to have light even in the rain)
> Phosphorescent
> Lit by electric lamps.

[5] Deriving from the Greek *therapeutikos*, meaning to attend or to treat, the therapeutic is an elastic concept that sits somewhere between the palliative and the curative (a complex term unpacked in the introduction to this book).

[6] Christine Poggi, 2009, *Inventing Futurism: The Art and Politics of Artificial Optimism*. Princeton N.J.: Princeton University Press, 1.

[7] Giacomo Balla, *Le Vêtement Masculin Futuriste: Manifeste*, Milan: Direction du mouvement futuriste (IS), 1914.

This litany of physical, emotional and technological characteristics associated with Futurist clothing can be understood as a direct precursor to Ferrari's approach. As Clark points out, 'the Futurists were not dress designers but painters, sculptors and poets. Dress to them was only one more active canvas upon which to work rhetorically'.[8]

In 1919, nearly 80 years before the Urban Protection range was created, the Italian Futurist Ernesto Michahelles, under the alias Thayaht, designed the TuTa, or what we now refer to as the boiler suit. Thayaht, who later worked for Madeleine Vionnet, saw the fusion of fashion and art as an opportunity to imagine utopian clothing and, in doing so, posed the question, could fashion begin again from zero?[9] Thayaht's revolutionary aim of creating a rational and utopian garment, that was functional, democratic, and transcended the restrictions of fashion, can be seen as a direct forerunner of the Urban Protection range. Thayaht disseminated the TuTa through the reproduction of images and its pattern in the Florentine newspaper *La Nazione* in July 1920, as well as through the distribution of a short film, postcards, and a brochure he had produced to promote the TuTa.[10] It is this dissemination, not primarily as a physical garment, but as what Barthes calls 'written clothing' and 'image clothing', that enabled the TuTa to undergo a transformation from functional garment to spectacle.[11] As Loscialpo argues, the TuTa symbolised a break with the past, a transition to a 'new' period, a pragmatic solution capable of bridging the 'real' and the 'ideal'.[12] Five years after the TuTa's emergence, Gerard Heard, the British writer and philosopher, was predicting the convergence of man, machine, and dress:

> But, if living beside a car has already had such effect, how much greater modification may be expected when the association becomes more intimate, and the man is seldom visible outside the machine, when it is his clothing?

[8] Judith Clark, 'Looking Forward Historical Futurism', in *Radical Fashion*, ed. Claire Wilcox, Victoria & Albert Publications, 2001, 14

[9] Djurdja Bartlett, *FashionEast: The Spectre That Haunted Socialism*, Cambridge, Mass: MIT Press, 2010, 1.

[10] Flavia Loscialpo, 'Utopian Clothing: The Futurist and Constructivist Proposals in the Early 1920s', *Clothing Cultures* 1 (1 October 2014): 229, https://doi.org/10.1386/cc.1.3.225_1.

[11] Roland Barthes, *The Fashion System*, trans. Matthew Ward and Richard Howard, London: Cape, 1985, 235.

[12] Loscialpo, 'Utopian Clothing.'

> If like a snail possessed, we learn to carry a rushing house everywhere with us, it will be our costume and habit.[13]

As Wilson notes, dress had always played a central part in literary utopias.[14] For Thomas More, who coined the term, Utopia was a place where people wore plain clothes and fashion never changes.[15] Throughout the twentieth century, fashion designers returned to the concept of utopian dress, most notably in the 1960s, when, fuelled by the space race, designers began to present collections that appeared to suggest an egalitarian vision of dress in the twenty-first century. Among them were Pierre Cardin, André Courrèges, Paco Rabanne, and Hardy Amies, who also designed the costumes for Stanley Kubrick's 1968 film *2001: A Space Odyssey*. The use of uniformity of dress to suggest an idealised utopia was central to how these designers portrayed this predicted future. As Quinn observes: 'These visions of the future suggested fashion would eventually evolve away from the system that had existed for centuries towards a single, functional style of clothing'.[16]

Cardin's futuristic space-age Cosmocorps collection, shown in Paris in 1967, included womenswear outfits with abstract cut-outs as a decorative motif; however, such ornamental features were absent from the menswear presented. Instead, the designs emphasised the functional elements of the men's outfits such as zippers, belts, and pockets. Cardin's aesthetic echoed Thayaht's in this regard, proposing menswear stripped down to its most utilitarian and functional components. The American designer Rudi Gernreich further pared back clothing, augmenting what remained with innovative technology to propose a utopian, genderless future. By the 1970s, Gernreich foresaw a future of functional clothing in which: 'Jewelry will exist only as a quality—that is, to hold something up or together, like a belt, of for information, like a combination wristwatch, weather indicator, compass and radio'.[17] As Palomo-Lovinski noted 'Gernreich envisioned an era in which designers would become technicians, "Once a designer can spray on clothing or transmigrate fabrics to the body, new

[13] Gerald Heard, *Narcissus an Anatomy of Clothes* (London: Kegan Paul, Trench, Trubner & Co Ltd, 1924.

[14] Elizabeth Wilson, 2003, *Adorned in Dreams: Fashion and Modernity*, Rev. and updated ed. London: I. B. Tauris, 220.

[15] Thomas More, 1901, *Utopia*. London: Cassell, 56

[16] Bradley Quinn, 2002, *Techno Fashion* Oxford: Berg Publishers, 6.

[17] Rudi Gernreich, 9 January 1970, 'Fashion for the '70s', *LIFE*.

things will happen"'.[18] In the 1970s, these visions of the future were still utopian, treating clothing as indicative of a benign, calming, and peaceful technological future. In contrast, the cultural discourse of the 1990s displays a marked anxiety about the coming of the new millennium.

7.2 The Anxious Future

Writers such as Renata Saleci and Timothy Bewes identified the 1990s as a 'new age of anxiety', linking this to apparently unresolvable threats such as terrorist attacks and new illnesses, as well as to rapidly changing ideas about identity and subject-hood, and to the social and cultural anxieties of late capitalism.[19] The end of the twentieth century prompted numerous apocalyptic predictions included the second coming of Jesus Christ, the Tribulation, the Rapture, and the beginning of the war of Armageddon, whilst increased reliance on technology led to the fear that with the arrival of the year 2000, computing infrastructures for industries ranging from banking to aviation would fail, with catastrophic consequences.[20]

For fashion designers working in the 1990s, the end of the twentieth century represented a significant source of anxiety for other reasons. The temporal nature of fashion meant that they were faced with the challenge of designing for a future that was both rapidly approaching and had already occurred: the fashion futurology of designers such as Cardin, Courrèges and Gernreich had already staked a claim on this future, forcing contemporary designers to adopt a different approach. As the artist Ad Reinhardt observed: 'The present is the future of the past, not the past of the future.'[21] This paradox presented new challenges, as by consciously destroying the past, fashion reaffirms its existence.[22]

[18] Noel Palomo-Lovinski, *The World's Most Influential Fashion Designers: Hidden Connections and Lasting Legacies of Fashion's Iconic Creators*, 1st edition New York, N.Y: B E S Pub Co, 2010, 126.

[19] (On Anxiety, 2004 and Reification, 2002).

[20] Michele A Schottenbauer et al., (1 January 2004) 'Computers, Anxiety, and Gender: An Analysis of Reactions to the Y2K Computer Problem', *Computers in Human Behavior* 20, no. 1: 67, https://doi.org/10.1016/S0747-5632(03)00044-X.

[21] Ad Reinhardt. 'Twelve Rules for a New Academy', *Art News* 56, no. 3 (1957) 37–38.

[22] Caroline Evans and Alessandra Vaccari, eds., *Time in Fashion: Industrial, Antilinear and Uchronic Temporalities*, London: Bloomsbury Visual Arts, 2020, 119.

In response to this collective anxiety, fashion designers became fixated on the temporal nature of fashion, transitioning from fashion as a form of industrial capitalism designed solely to sell clothes to fashion as a form of cognitive capitalism in which their practise utilised 'the body as a site for the deployment of discourses'.[23] Some designers, including Alexander McQueen, Olivier Theyskens, and Comme des Garçons chose to locate their response to this anxiety within the decaying, diseased, or deceased body: for McQueen in particular, this was often combined with a latent sexuality.[24] These designers reaffirmed Benjamin's observation that fashion initiates a 'dialectical exchange between woman and ware—between carnal pleasure and the corpse.'[25]

For other designers, such as Hussein Chalayan, Simon Thorogood, and Moreno Ferrari, their response was to see the body as a site for augmentation, transformation, and metamorphosis via its interface with technology. Both positions can be interpreted as a reaction against the increasingly commodified environment in which designers were expected to operate at the turn of the twentieth century. The establishment of the luxury fashion conglomerate Moët Hennessy Louis Vuitton (LVMH) in 1987 and the retail conglomerate Pinault-Printemps-Redoute (PPR) in 1994, meant the designer's role became both elevated and expendable, with couture houses employing and dismissing creative directors at an accelerating rate. A new generation of designers began to question their role within this corporate system and started to subvert the parameters in which their practice was situated by using the mechanisms and artefacts of the fashion system to explore ideas that resisted commodification and challenged the fashion industry's value system. Julian Roberts launched the label Nothing Nothing in 1998 by sending press and buyers invitations to a non-existent show; Alexander McQueen presented models wrapped in cling film; and Martin Margiela displayed garments sprayed with mould that grew across their surfaces. While Barthes once described fashion as a 'vengeful present' that sacrifices the signs of the previous year, these designers were

[23] Valerie Steele, 'Letter from the Editor', *Fashion Theory* 1, no. 1 (1997) 1–2, https://doi.org/10.2752/136270497779754589.

[24] Arnold, *Fashion, Desire and Anxiety*, 85.

[25] Walter Benjamin, *The Arcades Project*, ed. Howard Eiland and Kevin MacLaughlin, First Harvard University Press paperback edition Cambridge, Mass. and London: The Belknap Press of Harvard University Press, 2002, 62.

determined to collapse fashion's temporal structure further by sabotaging their work at the time of its creation.[26]

All of these acts (the collection which does not exist, the garment that exists only once, and the clothes that are already decaying) can be interpreted as a continuation of the Futurists' utopian aspirations to determine whether fashion could start again from zero.[27] At the same time as these designers were trying to reset fashion's clock, others were also attempting to reframe our perception of time itself. Established in 1996, The Long Now Foundation sought to promote slower, better thinking, proposing the construction of the Clock of the Long Now, which would keep time for 10,000 years, ticking only once a year.[28] This desire to think beyond the short term was simultaneously taking place within multinational corporations such as Philips which had identified fashion as an effective vehicle for integrating its emerging technology to make it more palatable to consumers. Their 1996 *Vision of the Future* exhibition in Eindhoven posed the question: 'How would life be in 2005?' The project explored new product and service concepts across multiple 'domains' of life—personal, domestic, public, and mobile.[29] Their proposals included multimedia clothing with embedded radio chips and drawstring collars equipped with earpieces.[30] Philips launched their Wearables project in 1997 in response to the event, which resulted in a collaboration with Levi's Industrial Clothing Division and the commercial release of four wearables in 2000.[31] Though the accompanying book identified the compression of time and an ever-increasing rate of living as critical issues to address, the project itself only gazed ten years into the future. Looking too far ahead can cause us to ponder a time when we are either no longer alive or, worse, have become obsolete. As Arnold noted: 'Perhaps the greatest anxiety has been that the encroachment of technology will cause loss of self, that machines will take over the work and leisure activities of humans, and identity will

[26] Barthes, *The Fashion System*, 288.

[27] Bartlett, *FashionEast: The Spectre That Haunted Socialism*, 1.

[28] Tim Radford, 'The Time of Our Lives', *The Guardian*, 12 June 1999, 43

[29] Stefano Marzano, *Vision of the Future*, Fourth Edition, Philips, 1998.

[30] Miller Freeman, 'Future Perfect – Philips Vision of The Future,' *Electronics Times*, 20 June 1996.

[31] Joseph Gleasure, 'An Expanded History of Levi's ICD+ & Philips' Wearable Electronics Program – Shell Zine,' *Shell Zine* (blog), accessed 10 February 2022, https://shellzine.net/levis-icd/.

be lost through such interaction.'[32] Joe Hunter and Adam Thorpe, who founded Vexed Generation in 1995, were among the first designers to react against the growing intrusion of this technology into everyday life. In response to the increased use of surveillance on the streets in London they created a series of garments designed to conceal the wearer from closed-circuit television cameras (CCTV). While in Tokyo, Kosuke Tsumura created Final Home, a jacket designed as a wearable shelter, with pockets that could be filled with newspaper for insulation and then donated to a homeless shelter after it had been used.[33] While at Samsonite, Milan-based designer Neil Barrett was researching wearable technology and developing garments that had pop-up reading lamps and built-in cell phone earpieces.[34]

7.3 C.P. Company and Moreno Ferrari

In 1971, designer Massimo Osti established the Italian menswear label C.P. Company.[35] During its first 25 years, it primarily produced menswear from natural fibres such as linen, cotton, leather, and wool. Even though the brand's ideal man might not actually live in the countryside, they wore clothing that reflected romanticised notions of nature and its materials. In 1997, following Massimo Osti's departure, Moreno Ferrari was appointed creative director of C.P. Company. Ferrari immediately repositioned the brand, abandoning its material connection to nature in favour of an exploration of the urban man-made environment. His designs were unified by the use of an industrial nylon, Dynafil TS-70, in the construction of nearly all of the Urban Protection collection. This industrial material was discovered by Ferrari while researching the capabilities of safety workwear to protect the wearer from polluted environments. It provided a barrier that was resistant to abrasion, tearing, oil, and water. Ferrari rejected the notion that natural fabrics were intrinsically superior, opting instead for the fabric of the industrial worker, echoing More's vision of dress in Utopia, '...why should a fine thread be thought better than a coarse one?'[36] In its

[32] Arnold, *Fashion, Desire and Anxiety*, 27.

[33] Andrew Bolton, *The Supermodern Wardrobe*, 1st edition, London: V&A Publications, 2002, 48.

[34] Natasha Singer, 'The Suit That Makes You Feel as Good as Prozac', *The New York Times*, 11 June 2000. Sec 6, 72

[35] Daniela Facchinato, 2012, *Ideas from Massimo Osti*, 01 edition, Bologna: Damiani.

[36] More, *Utopia*.

materiality, Ferrari's work exemplified Benjamin's assertion that: 'Fashion stands in opposition to the organic. It couples the living body to the inorganic world.'[37] Speaking in 2019 about his radical repositioning of the C.P. Company aesthetic Ferrari said:

> I was intrigued by the notion of people migrating from the countryside to the city. There was already an idea of a smart city, an idea of pollution, and an idea of how your body could act as a shield. I was interested in ways of reducing rather than producing, in ways of condensing everything that can be done around a piece of clothing into a body, and in ways of making the item functional in a meaningful way for the person wearing it.[38]

In this regard, Ferrari's approach is aligned with Loschek's assertion that the body's appearance is always the constructed body; that it is not a representation of nature, but of culture.[39] Talking about his approach to design, Ferrari said: 'There are so many things one can do with a body and an object that becomes inseparably attached to it as a sort of artificial extension!'[40] His creation of the Urban Protection range, which incorporated complex, mostly concealed technology into each garment, could be considered a form of prosthetics, a method of augmenting, extending, and enhancing the body and its functions.

Informed by Balla's *Futurist Manifesto of Men's Clothing* and emulating Thayaht's TuTa, Ferrari proposed a series of rational garments that explored the relationship between man and his environment. These included a jacket that detected pollutants in the air and alerted users via a light-emitting diode (LED) screen; a parka with an inbuilt anti-smog filtration mask; a trench coat enhanced with hidden electronics that played soothing music; and a jacket with an integrated personal safety device that emitted a loud, piercing scream. However, while the physical garments had inbuilt functionalities that appeared to address specific physical and environmental challenges, Ferrari, like Thayaht and Balla before him, was more interested in the creation and dissemination of his ideas as written

[37] Benjamin, *The Arcades Project*, 8.

[38] Jonathan Faiers, 'In Conversation – Lorenzo Osti and Moreno Ferrari' (Ambika P3, London, 31 October 2019).

[39] Ingrid Loschek, *When Clothes Become Fashion: Design and Innovation Systems*, English ed. Oxford and New York: Berg, 2009, 169.

[40] Cristina Morozzi, *Carlo Rivetti: C.P. Company – Stone Island* Milano: Automobilia, 2001, 84–85.

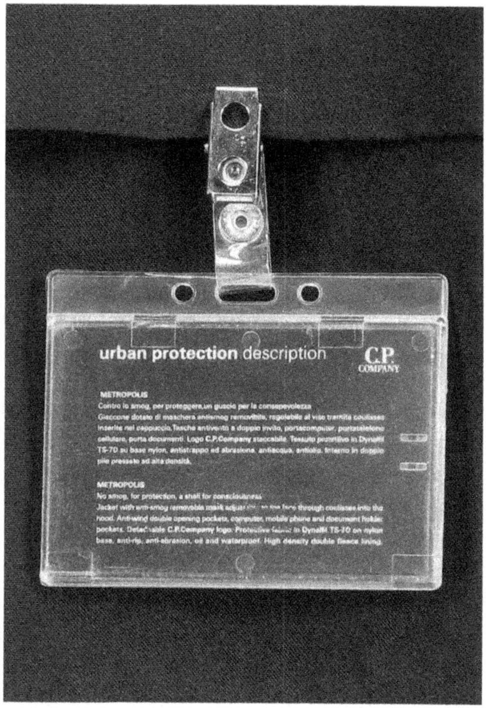

Fig. 7.1 Attached to the various Urban Protection jackets is an identification card holder. Photograph ©Andrew Groves

clothing. He employed a variety of semiotic strategies to create both 'vestimentary clothing' and 'written clothing', with the latter serving as a signifier for the former (Fig. 7.1).[41]

Ferrari developed a linguistic taxonomy for the Urban Protection range, giving the garments evocative names such as Metropolis, Atlas, Munch, Life, and Amaca. Attached to each garment within the Urban Protection range was a clear plastic clip-on holder containing an identification card detailing the garment title, materiality, and technical properties. The accompanying text also alluded to ancient concepts of protection by including a phrase that spoke to the garment's more abstract qualities:

> No noise, for inner life, a new womb to listen to silence-
> Freedom of thought, poetry for the soul
> Between sky and earth man's consciousness

[41] Barthes, *The Fashion System*, 25.

These cards are critical to understanding Ferrari's intent with the Urban Protection range. They appropriate the conventions of the art gallery label (listing the title, maker, and medium) to frame our understanding of these objects as abstractions of their ostensibly functional purpose. In doing so Ferrari, like Thayaht before him, produced a poetic mutation, as his work shifted from function to spectacle.[42] This linguistic structure established a system for viewing Ferrari's artistic output as a continuous body of work that transcended the temporal constraints of the seasonal fashion system.

7.4 Object-Based Analysis of the Urban Protection Range

In contrast to the normal practise in the fashion industry, where designers frequently change direction each season, the overarching concept of the Urban Protection range remained consistent from 1997 to 2001. The continuity of material, colour, and process across multiple seasons was a rejection of the fashion system's temporal structure, which demands constant seasonal change. Ferrari refused to employ any of the conventional design techniques typically used by fashion to signify seasonal change. This resistance rendered the garment's surface devoid of print, embellishment, or texture, echoing the TuTa's modernist, unadorned aesthetic. By rejecting the desire to engage with the materiality of the garment's surface, he further abstracted each item to its conceptual narrative. Indeed, his use of materials seemed to align his work to More's Utopia, which envisaged clothing to all be monochrome and cut to the same silhouette.[43] Yet these are not the utopian garments predicted in the 1960s by designers such as Cardin, Courrèges, and Paco Rabanne for the new century. Ferrari was far too close to the dawn of the twenty-first century to regard it as some distant utopia. Neither was his work part of the dystopian vision of the future created by other designers in the 1990s such as Alexander McQueen, Martin Margiela, and Rick Owens. Instead Ferrari positioned his work outside the norms of the fashion system, where the passage of time could not be measured by the shifting seasonal changes inherent to men's attire. It could, therefore, be viewed as existing in a heterotopia, a termed coined by Michel Foucault to describe a distorted utopia that can

[42] Barthes, *The Fashion System*, 235.
[43] Wilson, *Adorned in Dreams*, 220.

exist within the world, reflecting, yet distorting other spaces.[44] Lefebvre defined heterotopia as 'the other space and the space of the other'.[45] While for Dehaene and De Cauter it characterised 'the tension between place and non-place'.[46] Marc Auge's exploration of the non-place in his 1995 book *Non-Places: Introduction to an Anthropology of Supermodernity* influenced Ferrari's approach to the Urban Protection range.[47] Curator Andrew Bolton noted that their functionality aligned with the transitional spaces of the airport, highway, and subway,[48] while Ferrari described these non-places as, 'anonymous spaces which annul our soul; a soul which we all pretend to forget about, but which can suddenly re-emerge to remind us who we are and what we really need' (Fig. 7.2).[49]

In their materiality and design, the objects produced for the Urban Protection range intentionally resist a surface reading. The similarity of these objects' external appearance necessitates the inclusion of detailed descriptions as part of this approach. The following section investigates the Urban Protection range through an object-based analysis, grouping them according to the themes of sound, air, and motion. Several of Ferrari's contemporaries in fine art explored similar motifs in their work, which provide an additional framework for understanding his output.

7.5 Air

The first three garments examined in this chapter are concerned with air and its relationship to health: the air of the polluted city; the air used in flotation devices to keep us alive; or the possibility that the air may contain lethal contaminants that could cause us serious harm.

In 1997, the Metropolis jacket became the very first garment to be released from C.P. Company as part of the Urban Protection range.[50] The

[44] Michel Foucault, 'Texts/Contexts: Of Other Spaces', in *Grasping the World*, ed. Donald Preziosi and Claire Farago, 1st ed. Routledge, 2019, 371–79, https://doi.org/10.4324/9780429399671-24.

[45] Henri Lefebvre, *La révolution urbaine*. Paris: Gallimard, 1970, 172.

[46] Michiel Dehaene and Lieven de Cauter, eds., *Heterotopia and the City: Public Space in a Postcivil Society* London and New York: Routledge, 2008, 5.

[47] Marc Auge, *Non-Places: Introduction to an Anthropology of Supermodernity*, trans. John Howe. London; New York: Verso Books, 1995.

[48] Bolton, *The Supermodern Wardrobe*, 66.

[49] Morozzi, *Carlo Rivetti*, 84.

[50] C.P. Company, 'Urban Protection Metropolis Jacket' (1999), Westminster Menswear Archive, University of Westminster, https://ukdps.uwestminster-edit.tmp.accesstomemory.org/2016-181-1.

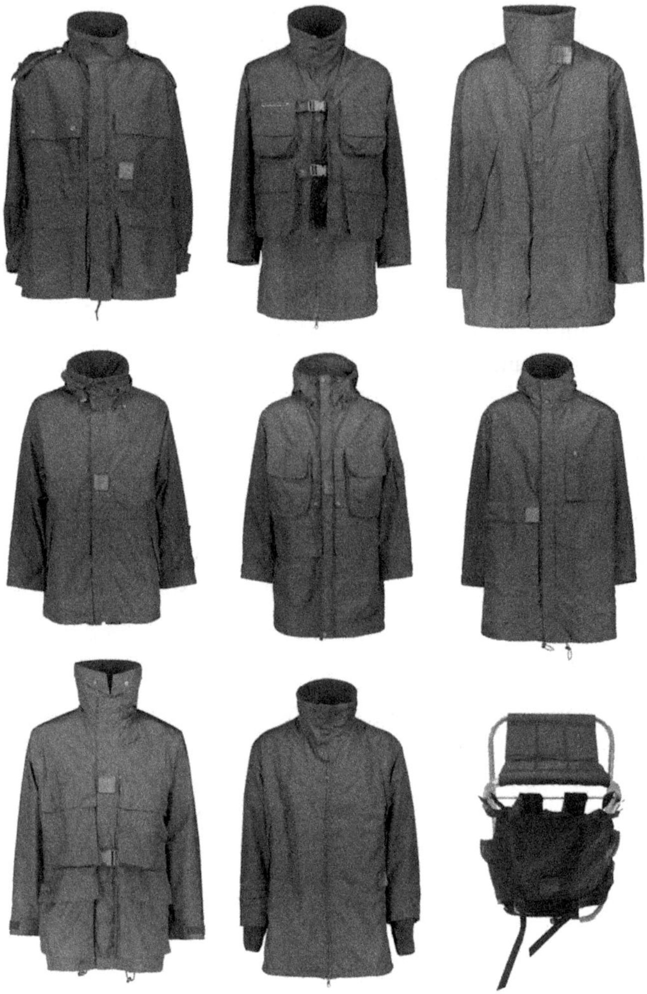

Fig. 7.2 Garments from the Urban Protection range. Top Row: Metropolis, LED, and Atlas. Second row: R.E.M., Life, and YO. Third row: Munch, Move, and Rest. Photograph ©Andrew Groves

black nylon jacket was constructed from Dynafil TS-70 and was lined with a high-density double fleece lining. Its material made it almost indistinguishable from a security guard's jacket. The attached plastic clip-on identification holder further reinforced this interpretation. The ID card for the Metropolis contained the phrase, 'No smog, for protection, a shell for consciousness'. The jacket was advertised as having pockets large enough to accommodate 'computers, mobile phones, and documents' and featured a detachable anti-smog mask that attached to the hood and covered the lower half of the wearer's face. However, the jacket's hip-length cut indicated that it was not designed for cyclists, as might be presumed, but for men moving through an urban environment. Ferrari explained, 'I made the Metropolis jacket to say that C.P. Company has to acknowledge the dystopic city as well'.[51] As a statement of intent, with its use of synthetic textiles and deliberate emphasis on the difficulties of living in polluted cities, it was diametrically opposed to C.P. Company's former 'heritage' aesthetic; Ferrari was starting again from zero (Fig. 7.3).

In 2001, five years after the launch of the Metropolis jacket, the LED jacket was released.[52] Although the LED jacket is slightly longer than the Metropolis, it was also constructed from Dynafil TS-70 and had a similar layout, with four large front pockets and a high-density double fleece lining. It differed in that the upper-right chest pocket contained a Figaro Sensors gas detector made in the United States of America. This was equipped with a microcomputer and a filter and sensor for the detection of methane, propane, Freon, and other gases in the air. Externally visible through a slit on the top of the pocket flap, a long, thin LED display changed from green to red to indicate the wearer's exposure to airborne contaminants. When asked by *The New York Times* who their customer was, a C.P. Company representative stated: 'The gentleman who understands this is beyond normal outerwear. He could be an artist, he could be someone visual. Our customer isn't necessarily looking for basic products. He's looking for exclusivity'.[53]

[51] Lodovico Pignatti Moreno, ed., 2021, *C.P. Company 971-021. An Informal History of Italian Sportswear* Milan: Tristate International SA: 414.

[52] C.P. Company, 'Urban Protection LED Jacket' (2001), Westminster Menswear Archive, University of Westminster.

[53] Sara Ivry, 'News Watch: Apparel; Rain or Shine, a Coat That Checks Air Quality', The New York Times. 31 January 2002, Sec G, 3.

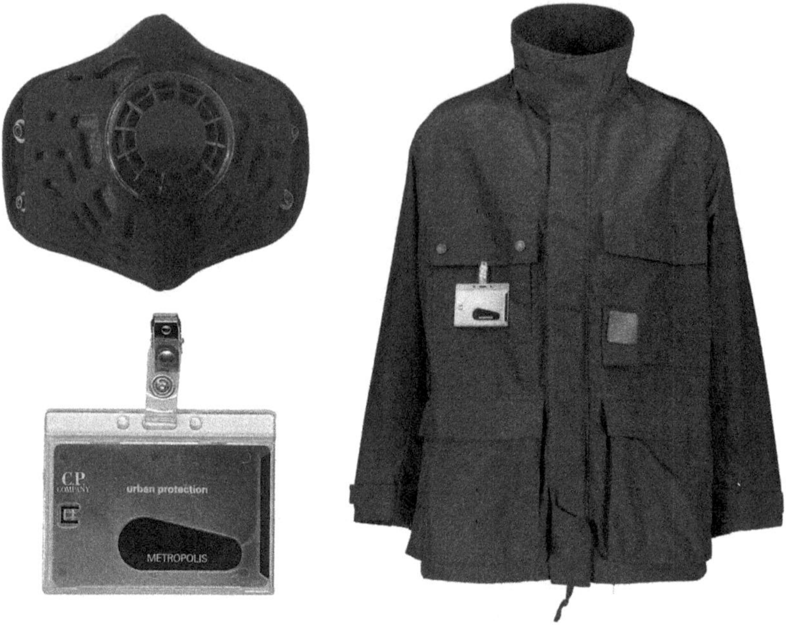

Fig. 7.3 The Metropolis jacket came with a smog mask and an identification card holder which contained the phrase, 'No smog, for protection, a shell for consciousness'. Photograph ©Andrew Groves

Released in 1999, the Atlas jacket was also constructed from Dynafil TS-70 and featured a long tunnel neck collar which housed a large inflatable PVC pillow that could be removed and worn around the neck for support while travelling.[54] The jacket was advertised using the phrase, 'From an ancient myth a support to man's thoughts'. In Greek mythology, Atlas was punished by Zeus and sentenced to forever carry the weight of the sky on his shoulders. Atlas assisted Hercules during the Twelve Labours of Hercules by retrieving apples while Hercules carried the sky. However, Hercules tricked Atlas into switching places on the pretext of

[54] C.P. Company, 'Urban Protection Atlas Jacket' (1999), Westminster Menswear Archive, University of Westminster, https://access.westminster.arkivum.net/2018-86.

acquiring pillows for his shoulders. In doing so, Atlas resumed his punishment carrying the sky.[55]

The American artist Jeff Koons explored similar themes by employing air as a metaphor for support, preservation, and protection in his first solo show *Equilibrium* in 1985. For Koons air was symbolic of the delicate equilibrium between life and death: 'Every time you take a breath, it's like a symbol of life, and every time you exhale, it's a symbol of death.'[56] In his exhibition Koons presented a series of inflatable objects, including an aqualung, snorkel vest and a lifeboat.[57] Each was originally designed to function as a piece of lifesaving equipment but had now been recast in bronze. The alchemy of their new materiality facilitated their transformation from functional design objects to high-status sculpture; Koons saw the recasting of objects in bronze not as transformed but as having been 'recodified'.[58] However, their function had been transformed: they had become symbolic, and their original purpose had become not only obsolete, but lethal. Further by employing the material of ancient statuary, they allude to the object's ability, whether worn or not, to outlive its owner. Their materiality equates to durability, so that we learn to see them not merely as relics from the past, but also as artefacts whose inherently unchangeable character will persist long into the future.[59] Like Jeff Koons' *Aqualung*, at first glance Moreno's garments also appear to offer salvation; however, upon closer inspection, their distinctive approach to materiality reveals that they, too, will outlast us, thereby mocking human fallibility.

7.6 Sound

The following four items are thematically linked to sound as a conduit between inner self and outside world. Like the Metropolis jacket, LED jacket and Atlas jacket, these were all constructed from Dynafil TS-70 and

[55] Robin Hard and H. J. Rose, *The Routledge Handbook of Greek Mythology: Based on H.J. Rose's 'Handbook of Greek Mythology'* London and New York: Routledge, 2004, 271.

[56] Jeff Koons, *Jeff Koons, Versailles*. (Paris: X. Barral, 2008), 111.

[57] Jeff Koons, *Aqualung*, 1985, Bronze, 68.6 x 44.5 x 44.5 cm, 1985.; Jeff Koons, *Snorkel Vest*, 1985, Bronze, 53.3 x 45.7 x 15.2 cm, 1985.Jeff Koons, *Lifeboat*, 1985, Bronze, 30.5 x 203.2 x 152.4 cm.

[58] Michael Archer, 2011, *Jeff Koons: One Ball Total Equilibrium Tank*, London: Afterall Books, 88.

[59] Archer, 13–14.

lined with a high-density double fleece. The R.E.M. came equipped with a Sony ICD-30 Voice Recorder which was concealed within an external mesh pocket on the bottom of the left sleeve.[60] This positioning allowed the user to operate the voice recorder without removing it from the jacket. The device functioned as a note taker by recording the user's voice as they spoke into it. It utilised two separate note files, each of which could store up to 16 minutes of audio in long player mode across 99 notes.[61] The R.E.M. jacket included an identification card with the inscription 'Freedom of thought, poetry for the soul' (Fig. 7.4).

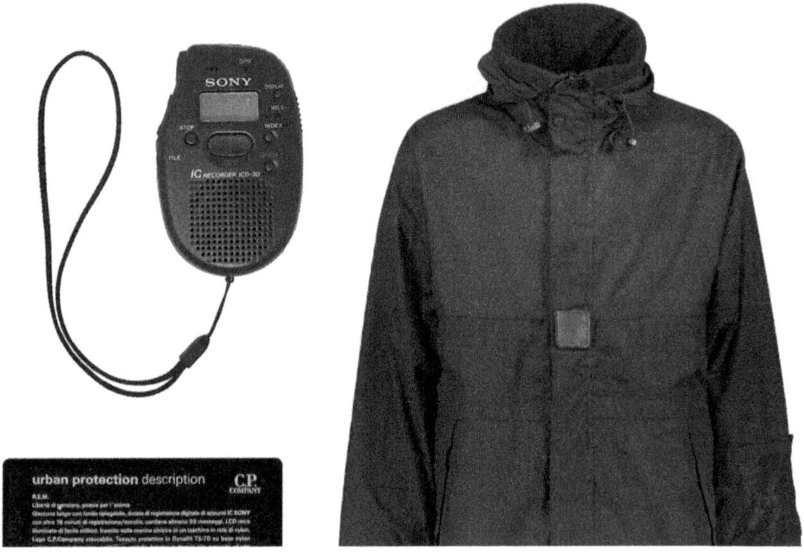

Fig. 7.4 The R.E.M. jacket included a Sony notetaker and an identification card holder with the phrase 'Freedom of thought, poetry for the soul'. Photograph ©Andrew Groves

[60] C.P. Company, 'Urban Protection R.E.M. Jacket' (1999), Westminster Menswear Archive, University of Westminster.

[61] 'ICD-30 Voice Record Instructions' (Sony, 2000).

The Life parka featured four large front pockets and an oversize backpack-style pocket on the rear.[62] It came equipped with a pair of foldable Bilsom 715 noise-proof earmuffs that could be worn over or inside the hood through loops. Founded in 1968, Bilsom are a Swedish company that manufactures personal protective equipment for sound management. Rather than being used to listen to music, as one might assume, these earmuffs were designed to completely isolate the wearer from the sound of the outside world. The parka's accompanying identification card declared, 'No noise, for inner life, a new womb to listen to silence.'

The YO coat featured a large pocket on the upper right and an oversize pocket on the lower front.[63] It included an integrated Sony DE705 ESP2 Discman, which was housed within an internal mesh pocket. The Sony Discman was, at the time, the most advanced portable music player available. The jacket's identity card stated, 'Music as will for growth of inner consciousness.'

Finally, the Munch jacket featured an integrated personal safety device that could be activated by pulling a cord located inside a specially constructed internal pocket.[64] Once pulled, the coat emitted an intensely loud noise like a high-pitched scream, hence the jacket's name. The attached identification card read, 'No panic, a cry as a bridge for a better future.' As McCracken observes, within a consumerist society the acquisition of objects can 'serve as bridges to displaced meanings'.[65] The term 'bridge' is critical to understanding this coat and the rest of the Urban Protection series, as it connects us to Auge's non-place and Foucault's heterotopia. Situated on a bridge on the outskirts of Oslo and the Oslo Fjord, is the location that Munch depicted in *The Scream*.[66] Painted in 1893, this

[62] C.P. Company, 'Urban Protection Life Jacket' (1999), Westminster Menswear Archive, University of Westminster, https://access.westminster.arkivum.net/2019-37.

[63] C.P. Company, 'Urban Protection YO Jacket' (1999), Westminster Menswear Archive, University of Westminster, https://access.westminster.arkivum.net/2016-255-1.

[64] C.P. Company, 'Urban Protection Munch Jacket' (2000), Westminster Menswear Archive, University of Westminster.

[65] Grant David McCracken, *Culture and Consumption New Approaches to the Symbolic Character of Consumer Goods and Activities* Bloomington, Indiana: Indiana University Press, 1990, 113.

[66] Edvard Munch, *The Scream of Nature*, 1893, Oil, tempera, pastel and crayon on cardboard, 1893.

bridge could be viewed as one of the earliest examples of Auge's transitional non-places.[67] In the background of the painting is the city of Oslo, and nearby a slaughterhouse and the mental asylum where Edvard Munch's sister Laura, had been hospitalised; as noted by one of Munch's biographers, 'the screams of the animals being slaughtered in combination with the screams of the insane were reported to be a terrible thing to hear'.[68] By explicitly referring back to an artwork created over a century ago, Ferrari created a bridge between the silent screams on the outskirts of Oslo and those within the non-places of late modernity.

7.7 Motion

The concluding thematic section examines three transformative objects for the Urban Protection series: Move, Rest, and Amaca. Uniquely, Move referred to two garments worn in a specific configuration, rather than to a single garment.[69] The bottom coat, called Glove when worn on its own, featured vertical anti-wind pockets, and extended internal cuffs with fleece half-mittens. On top of this coat, a multipocketed waistcoat could be worn, which housed an aluminium foldable scooter designed for travel through the urban environment. These were made by Micro Mobility Systems Ltd, which had begun selling scooters in Japan in 1999. In this configuration the ensemble was referred to as Move, and the accompanying identification card read 'Movement, protection, comfort on the road'.

Rest was one of the few accessories included in the Urban Protection line.[70] It was a folding aluminium frame chair with an attached multipocketed rucksack with padded straps, and a detachable C.P. Company logo. It was inspired by military rucksacks with integrated field stools that could be transformed into a small folding seat, allowing the wearer to rest momentarily on their travels. Its dual functionality, whether as a backpack with a built-in stool or as a stool with a built-in rucksack, suggests both mobility and immobility.

[67] Marc Auge, *Non-Places: Introduction to an Anthropology of Supermodernity*, trans. John Howe London; New York: Verso Books, 1995.

[68] Sue Prideaux, *Edvard Munch: Behind the Scream* New Haven and London: Yale University Press, 2005, 151.

[69] C.P. Company, 'Urban Protection Move Jacket' (2000), Westminster Menswear Archive, University of Westminster.

[70] C.P. Company, 'Urban Protection Rest Backpack' (2000), Westminster Menswear Archive, University of Westminster.

Amaca, which translates as 'hammock' in Italian, is one of the most conceptual designs in the C.P. Company's Urban Protection series.[71] This extremely long coat could be transformed into a hammock by adjusting the thick nylon tapes at the top and bottom to allow for suspension. In this configuration, it bears a striking resemblance to a shroud or a body bag; thus, it could be interpreted as a final resting place for the body inside, now motionless and inert. When asked about the inspiration for his hammock design, Ferrari stated, 'I liked the idea of taking that bucolic otium and re-contextualising it within a city, which by nature and culture is resistant to this more fluid harmony of time.'[72]

There are parallels here with the work of British artist Lucy Orta. Beginning in the early 1990s, Orta began investigating how clothing functions as a negotiated space between body and world, using the visual language of boilersuits, survival wear, rescue stretchers, and modular tents. Sculptural works such as *Refuge Wear—Mobile Survival Sac with Transformable Rucksack* explored how the transitional spaces offered by these garments can serve as sites for withdrawal and exclusion, and act as a physical and emotional barrier.[73] Speaking about her work, Orta observed: 'Since to inhabit a space means to consider it part of one's body, clothes are fully entitled to become architectural dwellings, temporary shelters affording protection against cold and storms in the stopping-places on the long journey of our existence.'[74] Quinn observed Orta's use of clothing in her artworks: 'By moving beyond their ability to provide protection, she amplifies their inherent power to communicate, negotiate social bonds and unite members of a community.'[75] He notes: 'Orta's designs relate the story of the tension between movement and stillness, between the visible and the invisible.'[76]

[71] C.P. Company, 'Urban Protection Amaca Cape' (2000), Westminster Menswear Archive, University of Westminster.

[72] Morozzi, *Carlo Rivetti*, 87.

[73] Lucy Orta, *Refuge Wear – Mobile Survival Sac with Transformable Rucksack*, 1996, Microporous polyester, PU coated polyamide, silkscreen print, transformable rucksack, zips, 210 x 90 cm, 1996.

[74] Maria Cristina Tommasini. 'Body Architectures, Survival Clothes', *Domus*, March, 2000, 74.

[75] Andrew Patrizio, Bradley Quinn, and Margaret Miller, *Lucy Orta – Body Architecture*, ed. Courtenay Smith and Lucy Orta, 1st edition: München: Silke Schreiber, 2003.

[76] Patrizio, Quinn, and Miller, *Lucy Orta – Body Architecture*.

If the final garments in the Urban Protection collections are symbolic of death, then Ferrari's subsequent Transformables range from 2000, with its transparent, ethereal garments, some of which are designed to float into the sky, suggest a spiritual ascension. All the garments within the Transformables collection were translucent and could convert into various objects, including a tent, an inflatable chair, and a kite. Bolton argues that these garments transcend numerous functionalities to ultimately become non-functional conceptual garments;[77] for Moreno the Transformables were a continuation of the Urban Protection range into ever more poetic, ephemeral and experimental forms'.[78]

7.8 The Future Past

In 2019 the Westminster Menswear Archive staged Invisible Men, the United Kingdom's largest exhibition dedicated to menswear.[79] Divided into 12 thematic sections, the exhibition featured two sections devoted entirely to black clothing. The first, Black Jackets, examined tailoring's pervasiveness as a defining feature of twentieth-century menswear. It featured 13 seemingly identical black jackets created between 1928 and 2010; upon closer inspection, however, each garment revealed its own unique characteristics. This section was mirrored by 13 black garments from the Urban Protection collection, the first time the range had been seen together in 20 years. The passage of time allowed Ferrari's future vision to be reassessed as the future past. The once-new technology they contained has become obsolete. Yet (like the materiality of Koon's statuary) the garments themselves have remained impervious to the passing of time (the Dynafil TS-70 resisting all marks, tears, or stains), underlining the temporal permeance of Ferrari's work. In constructing allegorical 'vestimentary clothing' and 'written clothing', Ferrari enabled these objects to transcend fashion's fleeting nature and to address spiritual and metaphysical themes. As Benjamin noted: 'Only a thoughtless observer can deny that correspondences come into play between the world of modem technology and the archaic symbol-world of mythology. Of course, initially the

[77] Bolton, *The Supermodern Wardrobe*, 19.

[78] Moreno, *C.P. Company 971-021. An Informal History of Italian Sportswear*. 424

[79] Andrew Groves and Danielle Sprecher, *Invisible Men: An Anthology from the Westminster Menswear Archive*, London: Westminster Menswear Archive, 2019.

technologically new seems nothing more than that. But in the very next childhood memory, its traits are already altered.'[80]

7.9 Conclusion

Produced at a moment of cultural and temporal anxiety, the Urban Protection range was initially interpreted as embracing a utopian vision of the future in which the augmentation of the human body with wearable technology would offer a 'curative' remedy to the ills of a toxic urban environment. The augmentation of garments by Ferrari with smog masks, pollution monitors, ear protectors, and personal alarms superficially positioned these 'curative' objects as palliative prototypes for managing (but not curing) the bodily symptoms created by an unhealthy metropolis. The garments' original palliative intentions have been rendered ineffective due to the inherent obsolescence of technology, but Ferrari's philosophical approach has enabled the garments to transcend these initial limitations. It is in their metaphysical representation that they offered therapeutic functionality. Ferrari's work consciously employed Barthes' semiotic methodology for fashion analysis. In *The Fashion System*, Barthes examined the semiotics of fashion and its construction through the vestimentary code of the real garment and its representation in photography and writing. These two other structures, the 'image-clothing', and the 'written-clothing', serve as signifiers for our construction of fashion.[81] Ferrari's garments were purposefully alike in their vestimentary code; they were the same colour, were made of the same material, and had a similar silhouette, with their design language emulating that of the ordinary functional security jacket. However, Ferrari constructed mythical 'written clothing' imbued with therapeutic functionality through the identification cards attached to each garment. Ferrari thus creates both 'vestimentary clothing' and 'written clothing', with the latter serving as the signifier for the former. The transformation from function to spectacle, even when the spectacle disguises itself as a function, allows a poetic metamorphosis to occur.[82]

Over the past two decades, the shift away from wearable technology and towards the development of internal technology, some of which can

[80] Benjamin, *The Arcades Project*, 461.

[81] Barthes, *The Fashion System*, 3–9.

[82] Barthes, *The Fashion System*, 235.

both transmit and receive data, has resulted in the emergence of approximately 200 different medical implants that are currently in use.[83] As a result, there is no longer a need for wearable technology to capitalise on the desirability of fashion to facilitate its adoption to augment the human body. Instead, it once again exploits anxieties about health and well-being to facilitate its assimilation into our bodies. As we enter the transhuman era and nanotechnology is implanted, ingested, or permeates our bodies, clothing no longer functions as a barrier between the internal self and the external world. Therefore, if our threats come from within, our clothing can no longer protect us; it can only serve as a symbolic talisman, impotent to ward off harm or danger. As Baudrillard warned:

> The point when prostheses are introduced at a deeper level, when they are so completely internalized that they infiltrate the anonymous and the micro molecular core of the body, when they impose themselves upon the body itself as the body's 'original' model, burning out all subsequent symbolic circuits in such a way that every body is now nothing but an invariant reproduction of the prosthesis: this point means the end of the body, the end of its history, the end of its vicissitudes. It means that the individual is now nothing but a cancerous metastasis of his basic formula.[84]

Today, under the shadow of COVID-19, we enter a time when our bodies will become increasingly politicised, regulated, and contested. As concerns about the intrusive and pervasive role of technology in this context intensify, these artefacts from the Urban Protection range enable us to reflect on the palliative and therapeutic use of design and technology and the blurring of boundaries between the physical and the spiritual.

References

Archer, Michael. *Jeff Koons: One Ball Total Equilibrium Tank*. London: Afterall Books, 2011.

Arnold, Rebecca. *Fashion, Desire and Anxiety*. London and New York: I.B. Tauris, 2001.

[83] Ghislaine Boddington, 'The Internet of Bodies—Alive, Connected and Collective: The Virtual Physical Future of Our Bodies and Our Senses', AI & SOCIETY, 38, 5 (2023) 1897–1913 https://doi.org/10.1007/s00146-020-01137-1.

[84] Jean Baudrillard, The Transparency of Evil: Essays on Extreme Phenomena, trans. James Benedict and J. S. Baddeley, London; New York: Verso Books, 1993, 119.

Arnold, Rebecca. 'The Brutalized Body'. *Fashion Theory,* 3 no. 4 (November 1999): 487–501.

Auge, Marc. *Non-Places: Introduction to an Anthropology of Supermodernity.* Translated by John Howe. London; New York: Verso Books, 1995.

Balla, Giacomo. *Le Vêtement Masculin Futuriste: Manifeste.* Milan: Direction du mouvement futuriste (IS), 1914.

Barthes, Roland. *The Fashion System.* Translated by Matthew Ward and Richard Howard. London: Cape, 1985.

Bartlett, Djurdja. *FashionEast: The Spectre That Haunted Socialism.* Cambridge, Mass: MIT Press, 2010.

Baudrillard, Jean. *The Transparency of Evil: Essays on Extreme Phenomena.* Translated by James Benedict and J. S. Baddeley. London; New York: Verso Books, 1993.

Benjamin, Walter. *The Arcades Project.* Edited by Howard Eiland and Kevin MacLaughlin. First Harvard University Press paperback edition. Cambridge, Mass. and London: The Belknap Press of Harvard University Press, 2002.

Ghislaine Boddington, 'The Internet of Bodies—Alive, Connected and Collective: The Virtual Physical Future of Our Bodies and Our Senses', AI & SOCIETY, 38, 5 (2023) 1897–1913

Bolton, Andrew. *The Supermodern Wardrobe.* 1st edition. London: V&A Publications, 2002.

Clark, Judith. 'Looking Forward Historical Futurism'. In *Radical Fashion*, edited by Claire Wilcox. London: Victoria & Albert Publications, 2001.

C.P. Company. 'Urban Protection Amaca Cape', 2000a. Westminster Menswear Archive, University of Westminster. https://ukdps.uwestminster-edit.tmp.accesstomemory.org/2018-48-2

C.P. Company. 'Urban Protection Atlas Jacket', 1999a. Westminster Menswear Archive, University of Westminster. https://ukdps.uwestminster-edit.tmp.accesstomemory.org/2018-86

C.P. Company. 'Urban Protection LED Jacket', 2001. Westminster Menswear Archive, University of Westminster. https://ukdps.uwestminster-edit.tmp.accesstomemory.org/2016-093

C.P. Company. 'Urban Protection Life Jacket', 1999b. Westminster Menswear Archive, University of Westminster. https://ukdps.uwestminster-edit.tmp.accesstomemory.org/2019-37

C.P. Company. 'Urban Protection Metropolis Jacket', 1999c. Westminster Menswear Archive, University of Westminster. https://ukdps.uwestminster-edit.tmp.accesstomemory.org/2016-181-1

C.P. Company. 'Urban Protection Move Jacket', 2000b. Westminster Menswear Archive, University of Westminster. https://ukdps.uwestminster-edit.tmp.accesstomemory.org/2017-242

C.P. Company. 'Urban Protection Munch Jacket', 2000c. Westminster Menswear Archive, University of Westminster. https://ukdps.uwestminster-edit.tmp.accesstomemory.org/2017-241-1

C.P. Company. 'Urban Protection R.E.M. Jacket', 1999. Westminster Menswear Archive, University of Westminster. https://ukdps.uwestminster-edit.tmp.accesstomemory.org/2016-298-1

C.P. Company. 'Urban Protection Rest Backpack', 2000d. Westminster Menswear Archive, University of Westminster. https://ukdps.uwestminster-edit.tmp.accesstomemory.org/misc-17

C.P. Company. 'Urban Protection YO Jacket', 1999d. Westminster Menswear Archive, University of Westminster. https://ukdps.uwestminster-edit.tmp.accesstomemory.org/2016-255-1

Dehaene, Michiel, and Lieven de Cauter, eds. *Heterotopia and the City: Public Space in a Postcivil Society*. London and New York: Routledge, 2008.

Evans, Caroline. *Fashion at the Edge: Spectacle, Modernity and Deathliness*. New Haven and London: Yale University Press, 2003.

Evans, Caroline, and Alessandra Vaccari, eds. *Time in Fashion: Industrial, Antilinear and Uchronic Temporalities*. London: Bloomsbury Visual Arts, 2020.

Facchinato, Daniela. *Ideas from Massimo Osti*. 01 edition. Bologna: Damiani, 2012.

Faiers, Jonathan. 'In Conversation – Lorenzo Osti and Moreno Ferrari'. Ambika P3, London, 31 October 2019.

Foucault, Michel. 'Texts/Contexts: Of Other Spaces'. In *Grasping the World*, edited by Donald Preziosi and Claire Farago, 1st ed., 371–79. Routledge, 2019.

Freeman, Miller. 'Future Perfect – Philips Vision of The Future'. *Electronics TImes*, 20 June 1996.

Gernreich, Rudi. 'Fashion for the '70s'. *LIFE*, 9 January 1970.

Gleasure, Joseph. 'An Expanded History of Levi's ICD+ & Philips' Wearable Electronics Program – Shell Zine.' *Shell Zine* (blog). Accessed 10 February 2022. https://shellzine.net/levis-icd/

Groves, Andrew, and Danielle Sprecher. *Invisible Men: An Anthology from the Westminster Menswear Archive*. London: Westminster Menswear Archive, 2019.

Hard, Robin, and H. J. Rose. *The Routledge Handbook of Greek Mythology: Based on H.J. Rose's 'Handbook of Greek Mythology.'* London and New York: Routledge, 2004.

Heard, Gerald. *Narcissus an Anatomy of Clothes*. London: Kegan Paul, Trench, Trubner & Co Ltd, 1924.

Heidegger, Martin, John Macquarrie, and Edward Robinson. *Being and Time*. Malden, Mass.: Blackwell publ, 2007.

Horwitz, Allan V., and Jerome C. Wakefield. *All We Have to Fear: Psychiatry's Transformation of Natural Anxieties Into Mental Disorders*. New York: Oxford University Press, 2012.

'ICD-30 Voice Record Instructions'. Sony, 2000.

Sara Ivry, 'News Watch: Apparel; Rain or Shine, a Coat That Checks Air Quality', The New York Times. 31 January 2002, Sec G, 3.

Kierkegaard, Soren, and Alastair Hannay. *The Concept of Anxiety: A Simple Psychologically Oriented Deliberation in View of the Dogmatic Problem of Hereditary Sin*. New York: Liveright, 2014.

Koons, Jeff. *Aqualung*. 1985a. Bronze, 68.6 x 44.5 x 44.5 cm.

Koons, Jeff. *Jeff Koons, Versailles*. Paris: X. Barral, 2008.

Koons, Jeff. *Lifeboat*. 1985b. Bronze, 30.5 x 203.2 x 152.4 cm.

Koons, Jeff. *Snorkel Vest*. 1985c. Bronze, 53.3 x 45.7 x 15.2 cm.

Lefebvre, Henri. *La révolution urbaine*. [Paris]: Gallimard, 1970.

Loschek, Ingrid. *When Clothes Become Fashion: Design and Innovation Systems*. English ed. Oxford and New York: Berg, 2009.

Loscialpo, Flavia. 'Utopian Clothing: The Futurist and Constructivist Proposals in the Early 1920s'. *Clothing Cultures* 1 (1 October 2014).

Marzano, Stefano. *Vision of the Future*. Fourth Edition. Philips, 1998.

McCracken, Grant David. *Culture and Consumption New Approaches to the Symbolic Character of Consumer Goods and Activities*. Bloomington, Indiana: Indiana University Press, 1990.

More, Thomas. *Utopia*. London: Cassell, 1901.

Moreno, Lodovico Pignatti, ed. *C.P. Company 971-021. An Informal History of Italian Sportswear*. Milan: Tristate International SA, 2021.

Morgan, Stuart, and Frances Morris. *Rites of Passage: Art for the End of the Century*. London: Tate Gallery Publications, 1995.

Morozzi, Cristina. *Carlo Rivetti: C.P. Company – Stone Island*. Milano: Automobilia, 2001.

Munch, Edvard. *The Scream of Nature*. 1893. Oil, tempera, pastel and crayon on cardboard.

Orta, Lucy. *Refuge Wear – Mobile Survival Sac with Transformable Rucksack*. 1996. Microporous polyester, PU coated polyamide, silkscreen print, transformable rucksack, zips, 210 x 90 cm.

Palomo-Lovinski, Noel. *The World's Most Influential Fashion Designers: Hidden Connections and Lasting Legacies of Fashion's Iconic Creators*. 1st edition. New York, N.Y: B E S Pub Co, 2010.

Patrizio, Andrew, Bradley Quinn, and Margaret Miller. *Lucy Orta – Body Architecture*. Edited by Courtenay Smith and Lucy Orta. 1st edition. München: Silke Schreiber, 2003.

Poggi, Christine. *Inventing Futurism: The Art and Politics of Artificial Optimism*. Princeton N.J.: Princeton University Press, 2009.

Prideaux, Sue. *Edvard Munch: Behind the Scream*. New Haven and London: Yale University Press, 2005.

Quinn, Bradley. *Techno Fashion*. Oxford: Berg Publishers, 2002.

Radford, Tim. 'The Time of Our Lives.' *The Guardian*. 12 June 1999.

Reinhardt, Ad. 'Twelve Rules for a New Academy.' *Art News* 56, no. 3 (1957): 37–38.

Schottenbauer, Michele A, Benjamin F Rodriguez, Carol R Glass, and Diane B Arnkoff. 'Computers, Anxiety, and Gender: An Analysis of Reactions to the Y2K Computer Problem.' *Computers in Human Behavior* 20, no. 1 (1 January 2004): 67–83.

Singer, Natasha. 'The Suit That Makes You Feel as Good as Prozac.' *The New York Times*, 11 June 2000.

Steele, Valerie. 'Letter from the Editor.' *Fashion Theory* 1, no. 1 (1 February 1997): 1–2.

Sterbak, Jane. *Vanitas: Flesh Dress for an Albino Anorectic.* 1987. Mannequin, flank steak, salt, thread, color photograph on paper, 62-1/4 x 16-1/2 x 11-7/8 inches.

Tommasini, Maria Cristina. 'Body Architectures, Survival Clothes.' *Domus*, March 2000.

Walker, Christopher. 'Israelis on Alert for Millennium Suicide Invasion.' *The Times*. 22 October 1998.

Wiener, Lori, Meaghann Shaw Weaver, Cynthia J Bell, and Ursula M Sansom-Daly. 'Threading the Cloak: Palliative Care Education for Care Providers of Adolescents and Young Adults with Cancer.' *Clinical Oncology in Adolescents and Young Adults* 5 (9 January 2015): 1–18.

Wilson, Elizabeth. *Adorned in Dreams: Fashion and Modernity*. Rev. and Updated ed. London: I. B. Tauris, 2003.

CHAPTER 8

Skin and Textile Interaction and the Future of Fashion as Therapeutics

Rosie Broadhead

8.1 Introduction

Skin is the largest organ of the human body and the principal site of interaction with the external environment, with the most immediate environment being the clothes we wear. Textiles are an integral part of our lives, from our shirts to our bedsheets and all the materials in between. The relationship between the body, skin and clothing has been widely explored by literary authors, historians and fashion theorists. Beyond their use to regulate our temperature, Virginia Woolf observed that clothes have the ability to change our view of the world and the world's view of us.[1] Claire Pajaczkowska remarks that clothing is the most tactile when it comes to the meaning of surface; while clothing faces the gaze of the viewer, its

[1] S. Thanhauser, *Worn: A People's History of Clothing*, Pantheon, 2022, xvi.

R. Broadhead (✉)
Ghent University, Ghent, Belgium

D. Woolley et al. (eds.), *Wearable Objects and Curative Things*, Palgrave Studies in Fashion and the Body,
https://doi.org/10.1007/978-3-031-40017-9_8

constant contact with the skin means it will remain proximate.[2] Textiles are regularly, if not constantly, in contact with our skin; this surface is a unique ecosystem that can affect individual skin microbiomes.[3]

As a fashion designer and researcher working in the field of bio-design, I focus on what it means to develop therapeutic clothing and nurture our bodies through textile contact. What if the clothes we wear could be tailored to meet our body's needs? For me, this means working with healthy microbes and skin care experts to develop biomaterials and skin microbiome-friendly clothing. The understanding that living organisms are transferred between these surfaces provides us with new insights into the relationship between clothing and skin.[4] This multispecies 'inter and intra action' between humans and non-humans is what Donna Haraway describes as an 'extended synthesis' where transdisciplinary science and arts practices become entwined to form ecologies, technologies, and performances.[5] By exploring the current and future possibilities of these therapeutic materials, it becomes possible to view clothing and the body as one entity. This chapter explores the current research and future developments in the field of skin and textiles microbiomes. Focusing on the skin's constant exposure to clothing in which the exchange of substances living and non-living can influence our body. I conclude that the skin and textile interaction has an impact on human skin biology and may provide a direct way to manipulate the performance of clothing for our future health and well-being.

8.2 The Skin Microbiome

To understand the potential therapeutic applications of clothing we first must understand the skin and body. The skin's surface area is a complex and semipermeable membrane interacting with the immune system, inner

[2] Claire Pajaczkowska, 'On Stuff and Nonsense: The Complexity of Cloth', *TEXTILE*, 3:3, 2005, 223.

[3] C. Callewaert, et al. 'Characterization of Staphylococcus and Corynebacterium Clusters in the Human Axillary Region'. *PLoS ONE*, vol. 8 2013, e70538 Preprint at https://doi.org/10.1371/journal.pone.0070538; N. Dayan, *Skin Microbiome Handbook: From Basic Research to Product Development*, John Wiley & Sons, 2020.

[4] C. Jacques, et al., Effect of skin metabolism on dermal delivery of testosterone: qualitative assessment using a new short-term skin model, *Skin Pharmacol.* Physiol. 27, 2014, 188.

[5] Donna J. Haraway, *Staying with the Trouble: Making Kin in the Chthulucene*, 2016, 29.

body as well as outer environment. The ability of water to permeate the skin's surface can be considered one of the most crucial skin functions that make human life possible.[6] This porous surface is a highly efficient self-repairing barrier designed to maintain the health of the body and protect it from the external environment.[7] The skin gives protection against chemical, physical and biological hazards such as UV radiation and pathogens or insects, respectively. Yet, the different protective functions of the skin are often linked or even co-regulated.[8] The regulatory role of the skin includes moisture release, dehydration prevention, blood pressure regulation and body temperature control.[9] The skin has an indispensable function working hard to allow substances to pass through to protect and preserve the body's equilibrium.

The skin is home to microorganisms that live and feed on its surface.[10] These billions of microorganisms, including bacteria, fungi, and micro-eukaryotes, form the ecosystem called the skin microbiome.[11] It is known that these organisms are more numerous in comparison to the body's own cells: there are approximately 30 trillion body cells in comparison to 39 to 100 trillion microorganisms.[12]

Interdisciplinary artist, Sonja Baumel's work has been documenting the microbial layer that is present as a second surface on our bodies. Analysing where the environment begins and ends, Baumel suggests the skin is not the edge of the human body, yet its surface is expanding into this invisible layer of microbial relations. In her work 'Expanded Self' she explores the skin and its potential by visualising the invisible surface of the human

[6] G. K. Menon & M. Duggan, 'Strategies for improving the skin barrier by cosmetic skin care treatments', *Skin delivery systems: Transdermals, dermatologicals, and cosmetic actives*, Blackwell Publishing, Ames, 2006, 25–42.

[7] A. Williams, 'Transdermal and topical drug delivery from theory to clinical practice', *Pharmaceutical Press*, 2003.

[8] M. Lyman, 'The Remarkable Life of the Skin: An Intimate Journey Across Our Largest Organ', *Atlantic Monthly Press*, 2007; P. M. Elias, 'The skin barrier as an innate immune element', *Semin, Immunopathol.* 29, 2007, 3–14.

[9] N. G. Jablonski, *Skin: A Natural History*, University of California Press, 2006, 1–11.

[10] Jablonski, *Skin: A Natural History*, 164–66.

[11] N. N. Schommer & R. L. Gallo, 'Structure and function of the human skin microbiome', *Trends Microbiol*, 21; 2013, 660–668; A. L. Byrd, Y. Belkaid & J. A. Segre, 'The human skin microbiome'. *Nat. Rev. Microbiol*, 16, 2018, 143–155.

[12] R. Broadhead, L. Craeye, & C. Callewaert, 'The Future of Functional Clothing for an Improved Skin and Textile Microbiome Relationship', *Microorganisms* 9, 2021.

body. Through the support of the bacteriologist Erich Schopf, Baumel creates a human-size agar petri dish to grow the bacteria that inhabit her body. The artwork explores the ongoing evolving perception of what bodies are made of, highlighting the invisible microbial infrastructure that lives in synergy with our own cells.[13]

This leads us to question where these external organisms start and the human cells end, and if this living ecosystem on our skin has become part of the body's natural ecology. Scott Gilbert, argues that the body has never been an individual, suggesting that if the majority of the cells in the body are microbes, then what part is in fact human? When we are born, we primarily receive our symbionts and microbiota from our mother through the birth canal. The microbiome of a newborn is also supplemented by living organisms from the mother's skin, breast milk and local environment.[14] This symbiosis between organism and host or 'holobiont' is a new way of conceptualising the self: 'In theory, the organism is an Individual whose component parts cooperate for the betterment of the whole. But the parts that cooperate can be other organisms living with it'.[15] In this way, there cannot be biological individuality if the majority of our cells are microbial and if we co-metabolise with these microbes then we are not physically individual either. As humans, it's therefore impossible to isolate the body, the genome, and the immune system but it should be acknowledged rather as a complex ecosystem.[16] Biologist and cultural theorist Donna Haraway writes: *'Every living thing has emerged and persevered (or not) bathed and swaddled in bacteria'*.[17] Haraway suggests it is our responsibility for shaping these relationships of multispecies interaction for the future of economies, ecologies, and species living and dying together.

[13] S. Bäumel et al., 'Fifty Percent Human – how art brings us in touch with our microbial cohabitants', *Microb. Biotechnol.*, 11, 2018, 571–574.

[14] S. F. A Gilbert, 'Holobiont birth narrative: the epigenetic transmission of the human microbiome', *Front. Genet.* 5, 2014, 282.

[15] Scott Gilbert, 'The NEW Body Politic: How Knowledge of Our Bodies Can Affect the Wisdom of Our Policies', *Jefferson Journal of Science and Culture*, *1*(4), 2014, 11.

[16] A. L. Tsing, N. Bubandt, E. Gan & H. A. Swanson, *Arts of Living on a Damaged Planet: Ghosts and Monsters of the Anthropocene*, University of Minnesota Press, 71–83, 2017.

[17] Haraway, *Staying with the Trouble.*

8.3 Skin Health and Bio-Design

Optimal skin health depends on the probiotic bacteria or microbes that live on our bodies. Cosmetic products and fabric finishes on clothing can contain toxic chemicals, which disrupt the diversity of bacteria living on our skin. Competition between different bacteria constitutes the body's first line of defence against disease and viruses.[18] For example, some microbes native to the skin are known to exert an immunoregulatory effect, and the skin microbiome plays a part in controlling skin inflammation.[19] Recent papers indicate certain strains of Lactobacillus can reverse symptoms of osteoporosis.[20] It's becoming clear that microbes are critical to bodily function. Different body sites on the skin with their own microbial composition[21] can provide us with a view of how to move towards cross-species entanglement in clothing.[22]

Studies show that the chemical and microbial diversity on our bodies and textiles can change according to the composition, finish and even the fit of a garment. Research into the shared surface between the skin and textiles is a growing field, giving the relationship between clothing and identity a new and more literal meaning. Our clothing is becoming its own biological interface, influencing and being influenced by its wearer. Scientists are now studying clothing's effects on the body, as the garments next to our skin may be closely linked to our health.

In the last few years, there has been a new focus on bio-fabricated material using living organisms within the fashion industry.[23] Bio-design and synthetic biology have meant we can start to use the self-repairing and

[18] Byrd, Belkaid, & Segre, 'The human skin microbiome'.

[19] S. Naik, et al., 'Compartmentalized control of skin immunity by resident commensals', *Science* 337, 2012, 1115–1119; Y. Lai, et al., 'Commensal bacteria regulate Toll-like receptor3-dependentinflammationafterskininjury', *Nat.Med.*,15,2009,1377–1382;B.D.Pessemier et al., 'Gut–Skin Axis: Current Knowledge of the Interrelationship between Microbial Dysbiosis and Skin Conditions', *Microorganisms*, vol. 9 353, 2021, Preprint at https://doi.org/10.3390/microorganisms9020353.

[20] R. A. Britton et al., 'ProbioticL. reuteriTreatment Prevents Bone Loss in a Menopausal Ovariectomized Mouse Model', *Journal of Cellular Physiology*, vol. 229, 2014, 1822–1830 Preprint at https://doi.org/10.1002/jcp.24636.

[21] Callewaert, et al., 'Characterization'.

[22] Karen Barad, *Meeting the Universe Halfway: Quantum Physics and the Entanglement of Matter and Meaning*, Duke University Press, 2007, 220–222.

[23] J. Groll et al., 'Biofabrication: reappraising the definition of an evolving field', *Biofabrication* 8, 2016, 013001.

healing properties found in nature through digital code in the form of DNA. Artist and researcher Daisy Ginsburg suggests synthetic biology could begin to repair this industrialised landscape which threatens our planet through human-powered biology.[24] This technology has provided some clues as to the future direction of performance wear and its interaction with the second skin. Biotechnological and engineering methods will help to expand the functions, properties and potential of textiles surfaces along major frontiers.[25] Examples of materials which utilise living organisms in their manufacture include bacteria, yeast, algae, and mycelium.[26] In living system fabrication, the organism is either harvested and formed into a textile or it grows and becomes the material structure itself, such as mycelium.[27] In all instances, the organisms are terminated before further processing of the material. This differs from 'Microbiome Smart Textile', which relies on the microbial count and enzymatic action on the textiles. In this case, the health and ecology of the skin surface become part of the textile performance. For example, mycelium comprises a sense-transmitting network of ultra-fine threads that enable mushrooms to absorb nutrients.[28] This naturally abundant material is what is being used to produce a range of materials, including mycelium 'leather' which is starting to emerge commercially. In this case, billions of cells grow to form an interconnected 3D network which is then processed with chemicals and hot treatments to make a durable leather-like material.[29] Equally, Mycelium spores and their components also have protective and healing properties for the body.[30] A recent study explored the therapeutic properties of Ganoderma mushrooms, used as a traditional medicine around the world,

[24] D. H. Ginsburg, Synthetic Competition, *Antitrust and Regulation in the EU and US* 2009, Preprint at https://doi.org/10.4337/9781848447394.00006.

[25] Jablonski, *Skin: A Natural History.*

[26] Groll et al., 'Biofabrication'.

[27] 'Understanding "Bio" Material Innovations: a primer for the fashion industry', 2020, https://fashionforgood.com/wp-content/uploads/2020/12/Understanding-Bio-Material-Innovations-Report.pdf Accessed 15 October 2022.

[28] P. Stamets, *Mycelium Running: How Mushrooms Can Help Save the World*, Ten Speed Press, 2011.

[29] J. Raman, D.-S. Kim, H.-S. Kim, D.-S. Oh & H.-J Shin, 'Mycofabrication of Mycelium-Based Leather from Brown-Rot Fungi', *Journal of Fungi* vol. 8 317, 2022, Preprint at https://doi.org/10.3390/jof8030317.

[30] S.-Y. Lin, S.-C. Chien, S.-Y. Wang & J.-L. Mau, 'Nonvolatile Taste Components and Antioxidant Properties of Fruiting Body and Mycelium with High Ergothioneine Content from the Culinary-Medicinal Golden Oyster Mushroom Pleurotus citrinopileatus (Agaricomycetes)', *International Journal of Medicinal Mushrooms* vol. 18, 2016, 689–698 Preprint at https://doi.org/10.1615/intjmedmushrooms.v18.i8.50.

for repairing radiation damage to the body. The findings of this study suggested the polysaccharide derived from *G. lucidum* possessed DNA repair-enhancing properties, which could be a novel future approach to protecting against radiation exposure.[31]

The incorporation of new properties to improve the biological function of natural materials can be achieved at the molecular level.[32] Synthetically produced materials for the body apply biomedical knowledge to wearable applications.[33] These multispecies surfaces work together in unexpected collaborations and combinations.[34] Bacterial and fungal species are known for their ability to decompose organic matter through their enzymatic actions.[35] Thus, probiotic bacteria are being explored as an alternative to toxic biocides and antimicrobials. Probiotics are defined as 'living micro-organisms that provide a positive health effect for the host'.[36] However, if probiotics are used in a product, it is important to ensure that the bacteria stay alive on the substrate as the viability of the bacteria affects the product efficiency.[37] The majority of probiotic investigations in textiles have explored the use of spore-forming *Bacillus* spp to reduce odour on (textile) surfaces.[38] This process of applying live microorganisms to fibres results in natural, non-toxic health benefits to consumers and the environment.[39] However, despite their wide use in industry, *Bacillus* spp is not a

[31] N. N. Schommer & R. L. Gallo, 'Structure and function of the human skin microbiome', *Trends Microbiol.* 21, 2013, 660–668.

[32] Ginsburg, 'Synthetic Competition'.

[33] B. Robertson, J. Johansson & T. Curstedt, 'Synthetic surfactants to treat neonatal lung disease', *Molecular Medicine Today* vol. 6, 2000, 119–124 Preprint at https://doi.org/10.1016/s1357-4310(99)01656-1.

[34] Haraway, *Staying with the Trouble.*

[35] K. Shrimali & E. Dedhia, 'Microencapsulation for textile finishing', *IOSR Journal of Polymer and Textile Engineering* 2, 2015, 1–4.

[36] S. Rokka & P. Rantamäki, 'Protecting probiotic bacteria by microencapsulation: challenges for industrial applications', *Eur. Food Res. Technol.*, 231, 2010, 1–12.

[37] Rokka, 'Protecting probiotic'.

[38] E. Caselli et al., 'Reducing healthcare-associated infections incidence by a probiotic-based sanitation system: A multicentre, prospective, intervention study', *PLOS ONE,* vol. 13 2018, e0199616 Preprint at https://doi.org/10.1371/journal.pone.0199616.

[39] P. Chow & Ciupa, 'Impregnated Odour Control Products and Methods of Making the Same', *Composites,* U.S. Patent No. 2018/0228164, 16.

dominant species on the skin,[40] yet there are many strains of probiotic bacteria that benefit the body and already reside on its surface.[41]

8.4 Skin II—Probiotic Clothing

As a designer I'm fascinated that humans have no anatomical individuality: about half the cells in our bodies contain a human genome and the rest are microbial. The understanding that we live in a symbiotic relationship with microbes changes the way we think about the individual and has changed the way I approach design. My research on Probiotic Clothing embodies the necessity for the co-habitation of human and non-human cells and how the entanglement of these ecologies can work for our benefit. We know our skin's biome is shaped by our environment, and what we choose to wear can have a direct impact on the body. Through my cross-disciplinary practise of fashion design and scientific research I focus on what it means to heal our bodies through the clothes we wear. This means working with healthy microbes and skin care experts to develop biomaterials and skin microbiome-friendly clothing.

Textiles and clothing can form a barrier between the body and the environment and increase the ability of the body to function in a variety of settings. Our relationship with textiles and the body has developed considerably since 1856 when William Henry Perkin, quite unintentionally invented the first synthetic textile dye, mauveine.[42] This became the beginning of a new era of synthetic chemistry and the creation of a new library of materials. The textile industry still uses large amounts of synthetic chemicals throughout the production chain. Weatherproof and water-resistant clothing, although functional and desirable, can contain some of the most harmful chemicals to the human frame.[43] Yet, the permeable

[40] T. C. Scharschmidt & M. A. Fischbach, 'What Lives On Our Skin: Ecology, Genomics and Therapeutic Opportunities Of the Skin Microbiome', *Drug Discov. Today Dis. Mech.*, 2013, 10.

[41] K.-L. Niehaus, 'Viability and Efficacy of Probiotics Printed on a Textile Material', Högskolan i Borås, Akademin för Textil, Borås, Sweden, 201.

[42] A. D. Ginsberg, et al. *Synthetic Aesthetics: Investigating Synthetic Biology's Designs on Nature*. MIT Press, 2017 4–11.

[43] D. D. Smet, D. De Smet, D. Weydts & M. Vanneste, 'Environmentally friendly fabric finishes', *Sustainable Apparel* 2015, 3–33 Preprint at https://doi.org/10.1016/b978-1-78242-339-3.00001-7.

function of the skin and the potential of these chemicals to be absorbed into the body are still being researched.[44]

Textiles absorb the sweat and microbes of the skin, which can lead to increased odour generation and bacterial colonisation.[45] An increase in synthetic fibres in textile production has exacerbated odour retention in textiles, microbiome disbalance and pathogenic colonisation of bacteria, which can trigger skin diseases. As a result, a wide range of textile finishes, antimicrobial techniques and bioactive remedies have recently been developed in response to these findings. Yet the toxic nature of some of these chemical and antimicrobial textiles, which are not always effective and are sometimes associated with unwanted side effects, are now being scrutinised due to their unsustainable method of manufacture. It seems that improving the performance of the product or textile is the main focus of innovation, while the performance of the user and how these materials affect the body and environment is neglected. Through research into the skin's co-host, bacteria, we can consider clothing and the body simultaneously. This enables a new connection with nature and can provide wearable solutions to the health of our bodies and environment. Looking more closely at the skin's living ecosystem and natural skin biome may enable manufacturers to reduce the effects of the antibacterial ingredients and toxic cosmetics. Researchers are now looking into the incorporation of healthy skin commensal bacteria into textiles.[46] Designing microbiome-smart textiles can be a novel and alternative way to advance the functionality of clothing and to combat odour development or potential textile-related skin conditions.

The project Skin II—'Probiotic Clothing'—explores the impact of the textile microbiome and highlights the direct involvement of particular microbes on malodour development and skin disease. The project investigates 'microbiome-smart' textiles, in which certain microbes, or their enzymatic potential are applied to textiles to help to produce healthy skin-native communities. The project is a collaboration with Dr Chris Callewaert a microbiologist and skin microbiome expert at Ghent University, Belgium and directly builds on his research. Dr Callewaert was the first to discover

[44] J. Carlsson et al., 'Suspect and non-target screening of chemicals in clothing textiles by reversed-phase liquid chromatography/hybrid quadrupole-Orbitrap mass spectrometry', *Anal. Bioanal. Chem.*, 414, 2022, 1403–1413.

[45] J. Szostak-Kotowa, 'Biodeterioration of textiles', *Int. Biodeterior. Biodegradation* 53, 2004, 165–170.

[46] R. Broadhead, L. Craeye, & C. Callewaert, 'The Future of Functional Clothing for an Improved Skin and Textile Microbiome Relationship', *Microorganisms* 9, 2021.

skin bacterial transplants and use them to solve underarm body odour. This revolutionary research also revealed that the skin microbiome can transfer to textiles, and therefore our clothes microbiome can reflect that of the wearer. This textile and skin microbiome interaction can effect the pH, moisture content, odour generation, and the bacteria and chemical composition on the body." The aim of Skin II was to develop functional performance textiles using a healthy biocompatible organism, that already resides on the body, by encapsulating probiotic bacteria into the fibres of clothing. The encapsulated bacteria are activated when they come into contact with the moisture on our skin, allowing them to dominate other less beneficial bacteria. When designing these probiotics, I strategically placed the active ingredients in areas where you would normally sweat down the back, under the arms and between the breasts. The encapsulated bacteria are associated with reducing body odour, encouraging cell renewal, and improving the skin's immune system. Thus, proving that health and performance benefits can be provided to the wearer without the use of toxic or antimicrobial additives. The project also aimed to create awareness of the importance of this ecosystem on our bodies, known as the skin microbiome.

8.5 Design Approaches

Performance wear promotes the idea that we can prepare ourselves for all contingencies; that our clothes can be completely functional. The aim of many designers of performance clothing is to foster and promote an equitable balance of self-sufficiency and connectivity with the environment.[47] When approaching Skin II, I first considered the body: what it needs and how it functions. When designing clothing, one also has to consider that it is simultaneously a medium of style, technology, and design, and of course, they are all interrelated.[48] Research into the skin microbiome and the science behind bacteria transplantation informed the design process and aesthetics from the beginning. Once I understood which areas of the body I wanted to target, I could narrow down which probiotics to apply. I created a pattern inspired by biofilm of bacteria under the microscope, and then this pattern was then applied to the inside of the garment positioning it as close to the skin as possible (Fig. 8.1).

[47] A. Bolton, *The Supermodern Wardrobe*, V&A Publications: London, 2002, 7–15.

[48] Bolton, *The Supermodern Wardrobe.*

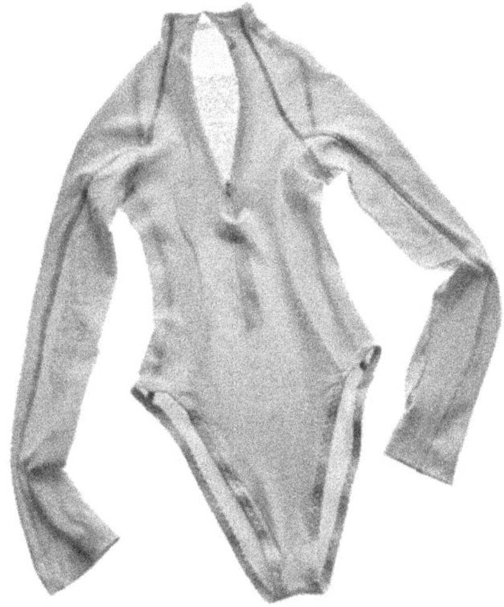

Fig. 8.1 Rosie Broadhead, Skin II Probiotic Clothing by Rosie Broadhead and Dr Chris Callewaert, 2019, Photo © Tom Mannion

The first probiotic garment I made was a bodysuit, pictured in this chapter, that is designed to sit closely to the body, making it easier for the skin and textile interaction which is essential to the performance mechanism. The garment design has an intentional sci-fi aesthetic and was inspired by the 1980s space age era and its impact on visual culture. The futuristic space aesthetic is dated, a sort of past future, as it hasn't substantially changed over the last 50 years. Thus, this paradoxical style draws attention to the project's scientific and technically advanced nature while implying that the material used, bacteria, has always existed on the body—it is both old and new. When exhibited the light grey bodysuit was pressed between two Perspex sheets and illuminated from the back. The light produces a shadow on the areas of the garment where the bacteria had been applied, therefore, making visible the invisible organism living on the textile surface.

In addition to the bodysuit at least 50 t-shirts and base layers have been designed to conduct wear testing trials to monitor the product's performance. Due to the interdisciplinary nature of this project, I also conduct lab testing in a sterile microbiology lab in order to identify the most effective method to encapsulate the bacteria onto fabric, and the best ratio to apply. We also test the wash durability, heat stability and viability of the bacteria over time. These are all important parameters for the long-term viability of bacteria-encapsulated clothing. When working between design and science it's important that I am aware of every stage of the production process from the growing of bacteria to the industrial production. The benefit of being in control of all these stages means I can test and make amendments throughout the process. If I know the industrial requirements of textiles at scale, then I can start to work on these criteria from the early stages in the lab.

8.6 Conclusion

As we tangled and weaved threads throughout this essay and make connections between human and non-human bodies and clothing, loose ends that at first seem trivial turn out to be essential to rethinking the relationship between fabric, body and garment.[49] Quantum physicist and Professor of Feminist studies, Karen Barad, remarks that biological theory in isolation will not suffice when it comes to understanding the body and its relationship with technology.[50] Equally Ursula K. Le Guinn encourages us to redefine technology and science more as a cultural 'carrier bag' rather than a means to control and dominate continuous economic growth.[51] The practise of science can sometimes be perceived as an abstract yet unquestionable power. However, science and culture are intrinsically linked, despite using different methods of communication. The relationship between design, science and technology is an important one, and fundamental for opening new and generative insights for society, and in this case, new ways to interact with our clothing. Hans Ulrich Obrist remarked that scientists must act in an artistic way to communicate their research and position new inventions in the world.[52] When approaching this project, I found that scientific and artistic approaches are not all that different, for example, there is a research and experimental phase in both practices, but different languages are used to express the final outcomes. The aesthetics of my projects are constantly changing in line with the development of technology.

[49] Haraway, *Staying with the Trouble.*

[50] Barad, *Meeting the Universe.*

[51] Ursula K. Le Guin, *The Carrier Bag Theory of Fiction,* 2019.

[52] R. Mackay, Future Art Ecosystem, *Serpentine R&D Platform,* 2020, ISBN 978-1-9086-66-8.

The infancy of some of the biotechnologies I offer a moment of opportunity, a fertile space in which artists and designers can interpret and provide alternative perspectives, potentially designing radical new worlds. Artistic expression can offer a glimpse of what may be possible, not positioned as utopian nor dystopian, but as ambiguous and pregnant with possibility, much like the microbiomes themselves. Bio-design and speculation provide an opportunity and a responsibility to rethink the surfaces that surround and intersect with our bodies. Donna Haraway describes the entanglement of speculative fiction and scientific fact as an important tool for deciding which stories are told and by whom, which concepts are conceptualised, and which systems are systematised. These technologies have a fundamental impact on our future living for both humans and non-humans.[53] We need speculation as well as real-life solutions in order to develop an alternative reality which opens up our perspectives on the challenges ahead.[54] Often speculative design relies on the viewer's feelings around a particular work or subject, allowing space for the consumer to question how something, in this case, clothing, might make a difference.[55]

Thus, microbiome-smart textiles can be a novel and alternative way to shift industries away from antibacterial ingredients and toxic fabric finishes while nurturing healthy relationships between the textile, skin microbiome, and the body. Skin II is an example of how a science and design practise can provide new perspectives on the future of clothing and human health. I continue to work closely with Dr Callewaert and the team at Ghent University to develop and scale these bacteria-based products for the textile and sportswear industry.[56] Most importantly it demonstrates how we might manipulate our biologies through what we wear, and how can manipulate what we wear through our bodies. Our skin and its microbiome are vast, with varying ecologies in different areas of the body. Each of these sites has its own microorganism ecosystem. Therefore, the future of probiotic clothing is developing new garments for different areas of the body for different microbiome-related symptoms.

[53] Haraway, *Staying with the Trouble.*

[54] T. U. Lenskjold, 'Anthony Dunne & Fiona Raby: Speculative Everything', *Artifact* vol. 3 2, 2016, Preprint at https://doi.org/10.14434/artifact.v3i4.22034.

[55] Anthony Dunne & Fiona Raby, *Speculative Everything: Design, Fiction, and Social Dreaming*, MIT Press, 2013.

[56] This could be underwear for female intimate health or a hat for scalp and hair conditions.

References

Barad, K. *Meeting the Universe Halfway: Quantum Physics and the Entanglement of Matter and Meaning.* (Duke University Press, 2007). 220-222.

Bäumel, S. et al. Fifty Percent Human – how art brings us in touch with our microbial cohabitants. Microb. Biotechnol. 11, 571–574 (2018).

Bolton, A. *The Supermodern Wardrobe.* V&A Publications London (2002). 7-15.

Britton, R. A. et al. ProbioticL. reuteriTreatment Prevents Bone Loss in a Menopausal Ovariectomized Mouse Model. Journal of Cellular Physiology vol. 229 1822–1830 Preprint at https://doi.org/10.1002/jcp.24636 (2014).

Broadhead, R., Craeye, L. & Callewaert, C. The Future of Functional Clothing for an Improved Skin and Textile Microbiome Relationship. Microorganisms 9, (2021).

Byrd, A. L., Belkaid, Y. & Segre, J. A. The human skin microbiome. Nat. Rev. Microbiol. 16, 143–155 (2018).

Callewaert, C. et al. Characterization of Staphylococcus and Corynebacterium Clusters in the Human Axillary Region. PLoS ONE vol. 8 e70538 Preprint at https://doi.org/10.1371/journal.pone.0070538 (2013).

Carlsson, J. *et al.* Suspect and non-target screening of chemicals in clothing textiles by reversed-phase liquid chromatography/hybrid quadrupole-Orbitrap mass spectrometry. *Anal. Bioanal. Chem.* 414, 1403–1413 (2022).

Caselli, E. *et al.* Reducing healthcare-associated infections incidence by a probiotic-based sanitation system: A multicentre, prospective, intervention study. *PLOS ONE* vol. 13 e0199616 Preprint at https://doi.org/10.1371/journal.pone.0199616 (2018).

Chow, P. & Ciupa, C. Impregnated Odour Control Products and Methods of Making the Same. *Composites.* U.S. Patent No. 2018/0228164, 16 (2018).

Dayan, N. Skin Microbiome Handbook: From Basic Research to Product Development. (John Wiley & Sons, 2020).

Dunne, A. & Raby, F. *Speculative Everything: Design, Fiction, and Social Dreaming.* (MIT Press, 2013). 155-165.

Gilbert, S. F. A holobiont birth narrative: the epigenetic transmission of the human microbiome. Front. Genet. 5, 282 (2014).

Gilbert, S. 2016. The NEW Body Politic: How Knowledge of Our Bodies Can Affect the Wisdom of Our Policies. *Jefferson Journal of Science and Culture, 1*(4). Retrieved from https://journals.sfu.ca/jjsc/index.php/journal/article/view/45.

Ginsberg, A. D.et al. *Synthetic Aesthetics: Investigating Synthetic Biology's Designs on Nature.* MIT Press, 2017 4-11.

Ginsburg, D. H. Synthetic Competition. *Antitrust and Regulation in the EU and US* Preprint at https://doi.org/10.4337/9781848447394.00006. (2009).

Groll, J. *et al.* Biofabrication: reappraising the definition of an evolving field. *Biofabrication* 8, 013001 (2016).

Haraway, D. J. Staying with the Trouble: Making Kin in the Chthulucene. (2016). 45-51.

Jablonski, N. G. Skin: A Natural History. (University of California Press, 2006). 1-11.

Lyman, M. The Remarkable Life of the Skin: An Intimate Journey Across Our Largest Organ; . (Atlantic Monthly Press, 2020).

Elias, P. M. The skin barrier as an innate immune element. Semin. Immunopathol. 29, 3–14 (2007).

Le Guin, U. K. *The Carrier Bag Theory of Fiction*. (2019). 35–37.

Lenskjold, T. U. 2016. Anthony Dunne & Fiona Raby: Speculative Everything. *Artifact* vol. 3 2 Preprint at https://doi.org/10.14434/artifact.v3i4.22034.

Lin, S.-Y., Chien, S.-C., Wang, S.-Y. & Mau, J.-L. Nonvolatile Taste Components and Antioxidant Properties of Fruiting Body and Mycelium with High Ergothioneine Content from the Culinary-Medicinal Golden Oyster Mushroom Pleurotus citrinopileatus (Agaricomycetes). *International Journal of Medicinal Mushrooms* vol. 18 689–698 Preprint at https://doi.org/10.1615/intjmed-mushrooms.v18.i8.50 (2016).

Lyman, M. The Remarkable Life of the Skin: An Intimate Journey Across Our Largest Organ; . (Atlantic Monthly Press, 2020).Elias, P. M. The skin barrier as an innate immune element. Semin. Immunopathol. 29, 3–14 (2007).

Mackay, R, Future Art Ecosystem *Serpentine R&D Platform* ISBN 978-1-9086-66-8 (2020).

Menon, G. K. & Duggan, M. Strategies for improving the skin barrier by cosmetic skin care treatments. Skin delivery systems: Transdermals, dermatologicals, and cosmetic actives. Blackwell Publishing, Ames 25–42 (2006).

Naik, S. et al. Compartmentalized control of skin immunity by resident commensals. Science 337, 1115–1119 (2012); Lai, Y. et al. Commensal bacteria regulate Toll-like receptor 3-dependent inflammation after skin injury. Nat. Med. 15, 1377–1382 (2009); Pessemier, B. D. et al. Gut–Skin Axis: Current Knowledge of the Interrelationship between Microbial Dysbiosis and Skin Conditions. Microorganisms vol. 9 353.

Niehaus, K.-L. Viability and Efficacy of Probiotics Printed on a Textile Material. (Högskolan i Borås, Akademin för Textil, Borås, Sweden, 2016).

Raman, J., Kim, D.-S., Kim, H.-S., Oh, D.-S. & Shin, H.-J. Mycofabrication of Mycelium-Based Leather from Brown-Rot Fungi. *Journal of Fungi* vol. 8 317 Preprint at https://doi.org/10.3390/jof8030317 (2022).

Robertson, B., Johansson, J. & Curstedt, T. Synthetic surfactants to treat neonatal lung disease. *Molecular Medicine Today* vol. 6 119–124 Preprint at https://doi.org/10.1016/s1357-4310(99)01656-1 (2000).

Rokka, S. & Rantamäki, P. Protecting probiotic bacteria by microencapsulation: challenges for industrial applications. *Eur. Food Res. Technol.* 231, 1–12 (2010).

Salehi *et al.* Current Trends on Seaweeds: Looking at Chemical Composition, Phytopharmacology, and Cosmetic Applications. *Molecules* vol. 24 4182 Preprint at https://doi.org/10.3390/molecules24224182 (2019).

Scharschmidt, T. C. & Fischbach, M. A. What Lives On Our Skin: Ecology, Genomics and Therapeutic Opportunities Of the Skin Microbiome. *Drug Discov. Today Dis. Mech.* 10, (2013).

Schommer, N. N. & Gallo, R. L. Structure and function of the human skin microbiome. Trends Microbiol. 21; 660–668 (2013); Byrd, A. L., Belkaid, Y. & Segre, J. A. The human skin microbiome. Nat. Rev. Microbiol. 16, 143–155 (2018).

Shrimali, K. & Dedhia, E. Microencapsulation for textile finishing. IOSR Journal of Polymer and Textile Engineering 2, 1–4 (2015).

Szostak-Kotowa, J. Biodeterioration of textiles. Int. Biodeterior. Biodegradation 53, 165–170 (2004).

Smet, D. D., De Smet, D., Weydts, D. & Vanneste, M. Environmentally friendly fabric finishes. *Sustainable Apparel* 3–33 Preprint at https://doi.org/10.1016/b978-1-78242-339-3.00001-7 (2015).

Thanhauser, S. *Worn: A People's History of Clothing*. (Pantheon, 2022). xvi.

Tsing, A. L., Bubandt, N., Gan, E. & Swanson, H. A. Arts of Living on a Damaged Planet: Ghosts and Monsters of the Anthropocene. (U of Minnesota Press, 2017). 71–83.

Williams. A., Transdermal and topical drug delivery from theory to clinical practice. Pharmaceutical Press, 2003.

Understanding "Bio" Material Innovations: a primer for the fashion industry, (2020) https://fashionforgood.com/wp-content/uploads/2020/12/Understanding-Bio-Material-Innovations-Report.pdf Accessed 15 October 2022.

CONTROLLING

Fiona Johnstone

The texts and artworks in this section consider selected wearable objects as regulatory apparatuses for the production of disciplined and 'healthy' bodies. Dawn Woolley explores how self-tracking watches facilitate the reframing of fitness as personal responsibility and consumer choice; Alanna McKnight shows how in the late nineteenth century narratives around women's health were shaped and exploited though claims made by corset advertisers; and Lucie Armstrong rethinks office dress and office furniture as a prosthetic extension that shapes the working subject. Whilst these objects belong to different historical periods—McKnight is a historian of the late nineteenth century, whilst Woolley and Armstrong are both artist-researchers whose practices focus on contemporary culture—all objects are significant actants in what Canniford and Bajde describe as 'body centred market assemblages'.[1] Body-centred market assemblages are sets of objects and discourses that shape the social, symbolic and material positioning of the body in a consumption environment; the fitness, fashion and wellness industries are prime examples of body-centred market

[1] Robin Canniford and Domen Bajde, 'Assembling Consumption', in *Assembling Consumption: Researching Actors, Networks and Markets*, ed. Robin Canniford and Domen Bajde (New York: Routledge, 2016), 1–18; Maria Carolina Zanette and Daiane Scaraboto, 'From the Corset to Spanx: Shapewear as a Marketplace Icon', *Consumption Markets and Culture* 22, no. 2 (2019): 183–99.

assemblages where normative ideas about 'healthy' versus 'pathological' bodies are expressed and negotiated.[2]

'Controlling', the one-word gerund verb that brings together these texts and artworks seeks to convey a range of disciplinary techniques that characterise consumer societies. Writing in the late 1970s, Michel Foucault identified biopower as a constituent component in the disciplinary mechanisms of capitalism: 'for capitalist society, it [is] biopolitics, the biological, the somatic, the corporeal, that [matters] more than anything else'.[3] In modern liberal societies, Foucault argued, power was no longer 'absolute' (exercised by the sovereign upon individual subjects), but was instead applied by shaping behaviours on a population level via the normalising disciplinary practices of institutions such as factories, prisons, schools and hospitals. More recently, thinkers such as Byung-Chul Han have shown the limitations of Foucault's framework for understanding contemporary neoliberal constructions of power. Neoliberalism transforms workers into entrepreneurs: everyone is now 'an auto-exploiting labourer in his or her own enterprise', compelled to self-optimise in order to realise their own potential as capital.[4] Whilst biopolitics worked primarily on the body and was focussed on maximising the general health (and therefore fitness to work) of the population by regulating 'reproductive cycles, birth and death rates, levels of general health, and life expectancy',[5] contemporary regimes of power (which Han terms 'psycho-politics') take a subtler form, ensuring that individuals act on themselves so that power relations are interiorised and then experienced as freedom. Han's insights reveal the complexities of disciplinary 'control' in contemporary consumer societies, when 'self-optimization and submission, freedom and exploitation fall into one'.[6]

Dawn Woolley's artwork *Desire Lines* (2022) and accompanying text for this volume 'Desire Lines: Quantified-Self-Portraits Produced with a

[2] Zanette and Scaraboto, 'From the Corset to Spanx: Shapewear as a Marketplace Icon', 183; on 'healthy' versus 'pathological' bodies see Georges Canguilhem, *The Normal and the Pathological*, trans. Carolyn R. Fawcett (Princeton, NJ: Zone Books, 1991).

[3] Michel Foucault, 'The Birth of Social Medicine', in *Essential Works of Foucault 1954–1984*, ed. James D. Faubion, vol. 3 Power (New York: New Press, 2000), 137; cited in Byung-Chul Han, *Psycho-Politics: Neoliberalism and New Technologies of Power* (London and New York: Verso, 2017), 25.

[4] Han, *Psycho-Politics: Neoliberalism and New Technologies of Power*, 5.

[5] Han, *Psycho-Politics: Neoliberalism and New Technologies of Power*, 21.

[6] Han, *Psycho-Politics: Neoliberalism and New Technologies of Power*, 28.

Fitness Tracking Watch' explore Han's conceptualisation of self-tracking devices as apparatuses of biopower in neoliberal societies. *Desire Lines* is a series of linocut prints made by the artist-researcher, visualising data collected from their own fitness tracking watch. In a text that critically engages with the practices of the Quantified Self-Movement, Woolley shows how tracking devices and apps position the attainment of health as an individual choice and personal achievement whilst failing to account for the significance of socioeconomic determinants (such as access to fresh food or safe spaces to exercise). Woolley reimagines geolocational data collected by her tracking watch whilst working at home as a set of spatial diagrams; carved into lino and reproduced as prints, these 'desire lines' present an aesthetic materialisation of her (usually invisible) domestic labours. Fitness tracking devices encourage users to upload personal data via networked apps in order to measure progress or compare one's performance against others: as Han notes, consumers now live in a digital panopticon; data is given away freely, not under duress, but 'out of an inner need'.[7] Data is big business; used to actively steer consumer choices, Big Data offers a new dispositive of domination and control. Acknowledging but ultimately resisting determinist narratives of technological supremacy, Woolley's linocut prints draw attention back to the embodied, haptic and gestural nature of the experience that underpins the data, subverting the intended use of the wearable technology by slowing down the processes that underpin self-tracking and undermining their perceived automatism, efficiency and accuracy.

The corset is popularly imagined as an expression of patriarchal control through female dress; scholarship by Valerie Steele and others has challenged this cultural stereotype, indicating that traditional binaries of oppression versus liberation, fashion versus health are unhelpful and over-simplistic ways of thinking about this semantically complex garment.[8] Alanna McKnight's chapter, "The Shocking History of Electric Corsets", situates itself in relation to the ongoing tensions between bodily control and consumer choice that characterise literature on the corset, as well as a long history of medicalising and pathologizing women's bodies.[9] Rather

[7] Han, *Psycho-Politics: Neoliberalism and New Technologies of Power*, 9.

[8] Valerie Steele, *Corsets: A Cultural History*. (New Hazen: Yale University Press, 2001).

[9] For an accessible history of the pathologization of women's bodies, see Elinor Cleghorn, *Unwell Women: A Journey Through Medicine and Myth in a Man-Made World*. (London: Weidenfeld & Nicholson, 2021).

than addressing the corset itself as object, McKnight explores the rhetoric surrounding it via an emphasis on the visual and material culture of late nineteenth-century corset advertising, with a particular focus on the case of 'electric' corset manufacturer Scott and Harness, revealing the corset as an integral part of late nineteenth-century consumer discourses around health. As McKnight shows, whilst nineteenth-century dress reformers denounced corsets as physically (and often morally and spiritually) harmful, corset advertisers made claims for the curative and health-giving properties of their products: the advertising copy for the 'electric' corset promised to deliver 'an exhilarating, health-giving current to the whole system' which could 'quickly cure' a range of diseases including nervous debility, spinal complaints, rheumatism, paralysis, numbness, dyspepsia, liver and kidney troubles, impaired circulation, constipation and 'all other diseases, peculiar to women'.[10] By invoking a seemingly scientific vocabulary around the relatively new technology of electricity and the vitalist notion of 'Odic force', corset advertisers were able to capitalise on existing anxieties about women's health.

Lucie Armstrong is a photographer whose practice sits at the intersections of fashion and fine art. Her photographic series *Office Exercises* (2018) and accompanying text for this volume explore the health implications of office work, with a particular focus on workplace wellbeing initiatives. Undertaking temp work in an office pre-pandemic (and so before the rise of widespread working from home), Armstrong became interested in exploring the ideological assumptions underlying so-called 'wellness-at-work' poster campaigns. Her performative photographs depict a woman, dressed in a clichéd female office worker's 'uniform' of white blouse, tight black pencil-skirt and heels, enacting a series of poses derived from corporate posters promoting the need for regular movement and exercise for desk-based employees. Office objects are frequently deployed as bodily extensions or prostheses: for example, an office chair that echoes the curve of its user's spine becomes visible as 'an apparatus for establishing workplace discipline'.[11]

[10] Cited by Alanna McKnight in this volume, 256.

[11] Lucy Armstrong, in this volume, 262.

Armstrong's text offers a useful account of practical decisions taken during the making of the work and an articulation of the theoretical framework underpinning the project. Citing Lauren Berlant's observation that 'our bodily lives are shaped pretty significantly'[12] by the demands of work, and drawing on insights from David Harvey, David Graeber and Sarah Sharma, Armstrong explores the health impacts of office-based work in terms of a disciplining of the neoliberal worker as a self-managing subject with responsibility for maintaining their own wellbeing and productivity through self-care and self-management. In particular, Armstrong draws on Sarah Sharma's analysis of the introduction of yoga classes into the corporate workplace; Sharma uses Foucault's work on biopower and worker productivity to demonstrate how such wellbeing initiatives actively reinforce the disciplining of the worker's body to make it productive for desk-based labour. Moreover, employees participating in such activities are not only maximising their corporate efficiency, but also working on themselves, supporting an ideology of personal fulfilment at work. Through both images and text, Armstrong shows how a discourse of self-care, once a radical political gesture of self-preservation in the face of a hostile and unjust society, has become corporatised and co-opted into neo-capitalist ideology.[13]

All of these objects—office dress and furniture, fitness tracking watches, and corsets—draw attention to some compelling intersections between consumer culture and control (broadly defined). The instructive tone of Scott and Harness' corset advertisements ('No Woman Should Be Without One') in the late nineteenth century (addressed in McKnight's essay) anticipates the present-day discourse of personal health responsibility and compulsory self-improvement through self control and consumer choice that is explored at length by Woolley and Armstrong in their artworks and texts. The one-word title of the section, 'Controlling', arguably belies the complexity of the networks of power relations—social, political, and economic—that these objects and their wearers are both entangled within and actively producing.

[12] Lauren Berlant, "Risky Bigness: On Obesity, Eating, and the Ambiguity of 'Health'," in *Against Health: How Health Became the New Morality*, ed. Jonathan M. Metzl and Anna Kirkland (New York: NYU Press, 2010), p. 29; cited by Lucy Armstrong in this volume, 265.

[13] On the origins of self-care as radical political gesture see Audre Lorde, 'Epilogue' in *A Burst of Light and Other Essays* (New York: Ixia Press, 1988) 130–33; see also Johanna Hedva, 'Sick Woman Theory', *Mask Magazine*, no. 24, eds. Hanna Hurr & Ripley Soprano (January 2016).

References

Berlant, Lauren. 'Risky Bigness: On Obesity, Eating, and the Ambiguity of "Health",' in *Against Health: How Health Became the New Morality*, ed. Jonathan M. Metzl and Anna Kirkland (New York: NYU Press, 2010).

Canguilhem, Georges. *The Normal and the Pathological*, trans. Carolyn R. Fawcett (Princeton, NJ: Zone Books, 1991).

Canniford, Robin and Domen Bajde. 'Assembling Consumption', in *Assembling Consumption: Researching Actors, Networks and Markets*, ed. Robin Canniford and Domen Bajde (New York: Routledge, 2016), 1–18.

Cleghorn, Elinor. *Unwell Women: A Journey Through Medicine and Myth in a Man-Made World*. (London: Weidenfeld & Nicholson, 2021).

Foucault, Michel. 'The Birth of Social Medicine', in *Essential Works of Foucault 1954–1984*, ed. James D. Faubion, vol. 3 Power (New York: New Press, 2000).

Han, Byung-Chul. *Psycho-Politics: Neoliberalism and New Technologies of Power* (London and New York: Verso, 2017).

Hedva, Johanna 'Sick Woman Theory', *Mask Magazine*, no. 24, eds. Hanna Hurr & Ripley Soprano (January 2016).

Lorde, Audre. 'Epilogue' in *A Burst of Light and Other Essays* (New York: Ixia Press, 1988), 130–33.

Steele, Valerie. *Corsets: A Cultural History*. (New Hazen: Yale University Press, 2001).

Zanette, Maria Carolina, and Daiane Scaraboto. 'From the Corset to Spanx: Shapewear as a Marketplace Icon', *Consumption Markets and Culture* 22, no. 2 (2019): 183–99.

CHAPTER 9

Desire Lines: Quantified-Self-Portraits Produced with a Fitness Tracking Watch

Dawn Woolley

9.1 Introduction

I am an artist and researcher examining the construction of ideal (gendered) neoliberal subjects in contemporary consumer culture.[1] This began with an examination of gender performance in early works such as The Doll's House (2004) and idealised representations of femininity in The Substitute (2007–8) and Visual Pleasure (2009–10). In my still-life work,

[1] Neoliberalism is an economic system characterised by deregulation and privatisation that extends into social life and influences the way people behave. Neoliberal subjectivity denotes the way that individuals are expected to view themselves as flexible entrepreneurs and health as a personal, rather than social or governmental, responsibility. Individuals also optimise the self to increase productivity and competitiveness in the free-market economy. For in-depth discussion, see: Dawn Woolley, 2022, *Consuming the Body: Capitalism, Social Media and Commodiciation*, London: Bloomsbury, 2022.

D. Woolley (✉)
Leeds Arts University, Leeds, UK
e-mail: dawn.woolley@leeds-art.ac.uk

D. Woolley et al. (eds.), *Wearable Objects and Curative Things*, Palgrave Studies in Fashion and the Body,
https://doi.org/10.1007/978-3-031-40017-9_9

such as Pacifier (2014) and Hysterical Selfies (2015), I attempted to describe the idealised, gendered, ageing body through commodities.[2] Currently I am researching self-tracking practices to understand how these forms of measurement and judgement employ an ideology of health to produce particular neoliberal subjects. By viewing quantification through a queer, feminist lens I hope to draw attention to the inequalities that are concealed by this notion of health. Self-tracking practices also enable me to examine experiences of the neoliberalisation of the body in a manner that resists sexist stereotypes and appearance-based judgements. I wear a fitness tracking watch on my wrist and the information it gleans from my body and its activities are reproduced as a collection of self-portraits that present the self 'as-a-work-of-art',[3] a rich autobiography, and an embodied archive.

In this chapter I discuss some of the positive and negative aspects of self-tracking practices and the Quantified Self movement to outline the position from which I appropriate self-tracking techniques as creative practice-based research methods. My fitness tracking watch, an off-the-shelf, standardising device, records bodily movements and the resulting data are presented as indicators of health. The watch encourages self-optimisation and competition, and data production is characterised by automatism and ease. In contrast, the performances I track do not focus on health or self-improvement but bring attention to hidden labour, often gendered and unpaid, such as admin, cleaning and care. In the series *Desire Lines*, the geolocation diagrams produced when working at home are reproduced in linocut prints. These prints, and my body of work on quantification, aim to contextualise self-tracking data within the personal, social and political environment, undoing the propensity of neoliberal capitalism to present health as a personal responsibility and a consumer choice. Using a phenomenological approach, I describe some of the preliminary findings of this on-going embodied research, including the augmented and outsourced ways of looking at the body, and varying temporalities of self-tracking.

[2] Artworks can be viewed at www.dawnwoolley.com.

[3] Byung-Chul Han, *Psychopolitics: Neoliberalism and New Technologies of Power*, trans. Eric Butler (London: Verso, 2017), 28.

9.2 Quantified Selves

Founded by Gary Wolf and Kevin Kelly, the Quantified Self movement is a self-tracking phenomenon that emerged in the mid-2000s with the development of wearable devices and apps designed to record detailed measurements relating to the users' physical, psychological, and social wellbeing in order to identify problems and anomalies, and change habits.[4] The Quantified Self movement (QSers[5]) aims to 'gain knowledge through numbers' and 'support new discoveries about ourselves and our communities that are grounded in accurate observation'.[6] In an article for *The New York Times* Wolf writes: 'We use numbers when we want to tune up a car, analyze a chemical reaction, predict the outcome of an election. We use numbers to optimise an assembly line. Why not use numbers on ourselves?'[7] QSers use the devices for a variety of reasons including managing chronic health conditions, fine-tuning fitness regimes and tracking moods in order to 'find their own way to personal fulfilment amid the seductions of marketing and the errors of common opinion'.[8] Wolf argues that self-tracking should be viewed as a tool of discovery rather than a tool of optimisation because it focuses on observing and recording details of life.

However, there is a disjuncture between the QSers and the companies that develop the apps and devices, even though many lead QSers work in the companies. Dawn Nafus and Jamie Sherman note that Quantified Self meetings are 'one of the few places where the question of why data matters is asked in ways that go beyond advertising and controlling the behaviors of others'.[9] QSers tend to be sceptical about standardised notions of

[4] Gina Neff and Dawn Nafus, *Self-tracking*, Cambridge, MA: MIT Press, 2016.

[5] QSers attend Quantified Self meetups and conferences, and their interest in self-tracking exceeds the average consumer's engagement with the devices. QSers often have high levels of tech know-how and adapt existing devices for their own means or create their own methods.

[6] Anonymous, 'What is quantified self', *Quantified Self: Self Knowledge Through Numbers*. Available at http://quantifiedself.com/about/ what-is-quantified-self/ (accessed 3 August 2019).

[7] Gary Wolf, 2010, 'The data-driven life', *The New York Times Magazine*, 28 April 2010. Available at http://www.nytimes.com/2010/05/02/magazine/02self-measurement-t.html?_r=0. Accessed 6 May 2022.

[8] Wolf, The data-driven life.

[9] Dawn Nafus and Jamie Sherman, 'This One Does not Go Up To 11: The Quantified Self Movement as an Alternative to Big Data Practice', *International Journal of Communication* 8(2014), 1784–1794, 1788.

health and wellbeing, and Quantified Self meetups focus on the idea that, what is effective and positive for one body may not work for other bodies. Because their self-tracking methods are individualistic they are not amenable to being incorporated into big data commodities. While QSers use off-the-shelf devices but 'see outside the frame that devices set for them' in order to determine their own standards of health, the devices encourage less specialised users (including myself) to accept predetermined benchmarks for health.[10] This is problematic because the devices and apps are predominantly designed by and for white, wealthy male bodies, and this shapes the way that health is measured.[11] Self-tracking equipment also tends to present ideal behaviours as the 'norm' of how most people behave, producing pressure to achieve an ideal that is unattainable for many consumers. For example, apps may penalise an individual for driving rather than walking, without taking into consideration where the individual lives, and whether they have a health condition or children. The devices do not differentiate between individuals who benefit from or lack the social privileges that enable the achievement of 'good health', such as access to healthy food, equipment and safe spaces to exercise.[12] This contributes to an ideology of health that conceals the causal relation between poor health and social inequality.[13] Gina Neff and Dawn Nafus note that this 'gives tremendous power to those who decide what to measure' and burdens the user with 'the work of determining whether their data represents ordinary human variation, a physical problem, or a social belief about health and wellness'.[14] Ideology and measures of health merge, and failure to perform ideal behaviours are presented as a failure to achieve health.

Self-tracking practices are marketed as 'empowering' tools because they put health data in the hands of the consumer, but they do not explain how to interpret the data and use it in a meaningful way.[15] In neoliberal societies that equate health with good citizenship and moral worth, self-tracking practices are becoming influential and pervasive measures that exceed their

[10] Nafus and Sherman, 'This One Does not Go Up To 11', 1793.

[11] Deborah Lupton, *The Quantified Self*, Cambridge: Polity, 2016.

[12] Lupton, *The Quantified Self*, 120.

[13] Lucy Aphramor and Jacqui Gingras, 'Helping People Change: Promoting Politicised Practice in the Health Care Professions', in *Debating Obesity: Critical Perspectives*, eds. Emma Rich, Lee F. Monaghan and Lucy Aphramor, 192–218, New York: Palgrave Macmillan, 2011.

[14] Neff and Nafus, *Self-tracking*, 39.

[15] Neff and Nafus, *Self-tracking*.

original use as tools for self-discovery. They place the responsibility for achieving good health with the individual, and imply that this should be done without medical and state support. In addition, self-tracking devices are increasingly used in employment and insurance contexts that risk producing hierarchies of data inequality.[16] Self-tracking data are becoming 'the very lenses we use to see ourselves and others'.[17]

Byung Chul Han views self-tracking practices as apparatuses of biopower in neoliberal societies. He writes that neoliberal workers are no longer shackled to commodity production processes but are optimised 'along aesthetic lines or in terms of health technology' noting that 'physical optimization means more than aesthetic practice alone: sexiness and fitness represent new economic resources to be increased, marketed and exploited'.[18] The commodified pursuit of health optimises the worker as labour because they have more energy and stamina for work, and as consumers when they buy the latest apps and devices. Han describes the neoliberal consumer as a 'self-as-a-work-of-art': 'a beautiful but deceptive illusion that the neoliberal regime maintains in order to exhaust its resources entirely'.[19] The body is segmented and mapped out by self-tracking devices that medicalise daily life, turning all activities into health activities. For example, in their promotional material Fitbit (a company that developed an early a wearable fitness tracking device in 2009) states that 'fitness is not just about gym time. *It's all the time*'.[20] Every action and minute of the day can be quantified. In one respect, this means that enjoyable social activities, such as dancing with friends, are deemed to be exercise. But it also extends the expectation of achievement and self-improvement into leisure activities, reducing the opportunities for respite from this form of productivity.[21]

Furthermore, self-tracking practices can reinforce the neoliberal view of the body 'as bounded and compartmentalised into separate domains' that can be 'renovated or upgraded' with the purchase of wearable devices,

[16] For discussion of healthism and self-tracking see Woolley, *Consuming the Body*.

[17] Neff and Nafus, *Self-tracking*, 9.

[18] Han, *Psychopolitics*, 25–6.

[19] Han, *Psychopolitics*, 28.

[20] Fitbit band Apple Watch, 2017, quoted in Steffen Krüger, 'The authoritarian dimension in digital self-tracking: Containment, commodification, subjugation', in *Lost in Perfection: Impacts of Optimisation on Culture and Psyche* eds. Vera King, Benigna Gerisch and Hartmut Rosa, 85–104, London: Routledge, 2019, 95 (emphasis original).

[21] Krüger, 'The authoritarian dimension in digital self-tracking'.

apps, diet supplements, health programmes, cryogenic treatments, and blood transfusions.[22] Some psychoanalysts interpret body-labour practices that aim to extend life and conceal ageing as 'attacks' on or 'rebellious acts against the transience of life' and 'secular strategies to protract mortality'.[23] The expectation that self-tracking practices can prolong life is problematic because 'promises of youthfulness and immortality are in opposition to lifelong efforts of integration that are based on the recognition of limitation and transience'.[24] Self-tracking may interrupt this process of integration if it prevents people from accepting their perceived flaws. Through the body's abstraction into numbers, self-tracking and other body practices 'facilitated by technological and medical advancements' may be reactions against 'experiences of alienation or even pathological depersonalisation caused by social excessive demands…that motivate fantasies of omnipotence'.[25] Self-tracking practices may impede the process of integration, but they also produce a feeling of mastery and power, reducing anxiety and distress caused by a social environment that is increasingly competitive and unpredictable. They enable the user to 'outsource' bodily management and the pursuit of health to the technology, and relieve themselves of 'the burden of thinking about it'.[26]

9.3 Embodied Practices and Quantified-Self-Portraits

Self-tracking is criticised by some as a narcissistic activity. To be identified as a narcissist denotes an inability to form functional relationships outside of yourself, creating an enclosed world. Self-portraiture also indicates the formation of a self-contained artistic practice in which external subjects are not required. However, in her discussion of feminist body art practices in the 1970s, Amelia Jones writes that in narcissism, the image (or reflection

[22] Mike Featherstone, 'Body, image and affect in consumer culture', *Body and Society* 16/1 2010, 193–221, 205.

[23] Benigna Gerisch, Benedikt Salfeld, Christiane Beerbohm, Katarina Busch and Vera King, 'Optimisation by knife: on types of biographical appropriating of aesthetic surgery in late modernity', in *Lost in Perfection: Impacts of Optimisation on Culture and Psyche*, eds. Vera King, Benigna Gerisch and Hartmut Rosa, 131–145, London: Routledge, 2019, 135.

[24] Gerisch and King, quoted Gerisch, Salfeld, Beerbohm, Busch and King, 'Optimisation by knife', 136.

[25] Gerisch, Salfeld, Beerbohm, Busch and King, 'Optimisation by knife', 136.

[26] Neff and Nafus, *Self-tracking*, 24.

in water in the original story) produces a distance from the self that allows the individual to see the self as other. The subject of the image is self and other simultaneously, and so the distance that is created collapses, and 'the borders of the frames of identity are imploded'.[27] Jones argues that this paradox of distance and proximity, and the inescapable [gendered, classed, racial] specificity of the performing body, prevents the viewer from reducing the body to an object.

In self-tracking, the individual is subject and object, and scientist and experiment. Wolf writes that 'manoeuvres of self-separation' are also 'techniques of enlightenment':

> Although trackers describe projects explicitly designed to distance themselves from themselves, giving them a picture of their own experiences as if from afar, this is universally understood to be a kind of trick, used by the presenter to awaken awareness, overcome the inertia of habit, and cast off illusion.[28]

Data enables the individual to see the self as other, gaining a different perspective that may produce new knowledge. These methods of quantification can be viewed as creative and embodied practice-led research. Creative practice-led research makes unique contributions to knowledge because it employs tacit and experiential knowledge alongside explicit and exact knowledge.[29] Ben Spatz describes the creative process of embodied research, noting that we receive feedback from the world most clearly 'not when we step away from it to contemplate its totality but when we dive into it to accomplish a specific material task'.[30] In closely examining specific aspects of daily life, embodied practice-led research methods are 'privileged sites for practical encounters with the real and for the concrete enactment of ontological inquiries'.[31] Quantified Self data are unique

[27] Amelia Jones, *Body Art Performing the Subject*, Minneapolis: University of Minnesota Press, 1998, 180.

[28] Gary Wolf, 'The Quantified Self: Reverse Engineering', in *Quantified: Biosensing Technologies in Everyday Life*, ed. Dawn Nafus, 67–72, Cambridge, Massachusetts: MIT Press, 2016, 69.

[29] Elizabeth Barrett, 'Experiential Learning in Practice as Research: Context, Method, Knowledge', *Journal of Visual Art Practice*. 6(2): 2007, 115–124.

[30] Ben Spatz, 'Embodiment As First Affordance: Tinkering, Tuning, Tracking'. *Performance Philosophy*. 2(2): 2021. 257–271 https://doi.org/10.21476/Pp.2017.2261 Issn 2057-7176, 259.

[31] Spatz, 'Embodiment As First Affordance', 164.

because they are particular to and contingent on the physical and social context of one body. QSers idiosyncratic processes of tracking resist generalisation and prevent the data from being meaningfully combined in big data commodities.[32] Nevertheless, the data are rich because they are specific and informed by multiple sources. Dana Greenfield describes self-tracking data used to manage chronic illness as 'deep data' because clinical practices are combined with personal data that are 'probing and fine-grained ... extended and deepened by social stakes hinged to it and its collection'.[33] Furthermore, the specificity of the data and the care that is taken in its collection, enable self-trackers to see things that are overlooked or distorted by clinical methods, providing 'a way to stare back at a clinical gaze whose surveillance probes much but actually sees very little'.[34]

My fitness tracking watch provides data that enable a fine-grained but abstracted view of the self. Distance opens up and collapses. Eric Topol, a medical futurist, says that self-tracking practices produce a 'high-definition human' and that quantification is a 'digitized upgrade of Foucault's anatomo-politics, where the political desires and drivers for better population management are operationalized at the individual level, just finer grained'.[35] By viewing the self as an object of scientific study and gathering data on a range of tangible and intangible bodily attributes, the self-tracking data are 'a window and conduit to interiority' that make visible 'previously indiscernible or unintelligible bodily processes'.[36] The Quantified Self is both high-definition and transparent in this respect. It brings to mind Maurice Merleau-Ponty's description of the translucent object, 'shot through from all sides by an infinite number of present scrutinies which intersect in its depths leaving nothing hidden'.[37] He invites the reader to imagine viewing a lamp from the perspective of the wall

[32] Nafus and Sherman, 2014, 'This One Does not Go Up To 11'.

[33] Dana Greenfield, 'Deep Data: Notes on the *n of 1*', in *Quantified: Biosensing Technologies in Everyday Life*, ed. Dawn Nafus, 123–146, Cambridge, Massachusetts: MIT Press, 2016, 139.

[34] Greenfield, 'Deep Data: Notes on the *n of 1*', 139.

[35] Eric Topol quoted in Greenfield, 'Deep Data: Notes on the *n of 1*', 132.

[36] Gavin J. D. Smith and Ben Vonthethoff, 'Health by numbers? Exploring the practice and experience of datafied health', *Health Sociology Review* 26/1: 2017, 6–21, 12.

[37] Maurice Merleau-Ponty, *The Primacy of Perception*, trans. Carleton Dallery, Evanston, Illinois: Northwestern University Press, 1964, 79.

behind it and the table beneath it. When I view the data visualisations of my movements and heart rate fluctuations produced by my watch, I see myself through the eyes of machines that track me via satellites in space and sensors that record the tiny movements caused by blood pulsing through veins. A vast scale of close proximity and distance is brought into play in embodied quantified-self-portraits that are also disembodied and outsourced. They are indexical self-portraits that trace my movements and bodily processes.

Using Lacanian psychoanalytic concepts, Michael Newman writes that data portraits represent the subject in relation to the real (traces of the senses, a pre-symbolic and pre-imaginary self that cannot be symbolised in language).[38] Discussing Susan Morris' self-tracking artworks *Medication* and *Mood Swings* (2006) Newman notes that data self-portraits are abstracted in a 'double condition of standardization and opacity'.[39] They are non-representational portraits that use a standardised format and do not express narrative information or the likeness of the individual. In *Desire Lines* my activities are represented by lines on a section of a Google map. The activities are standardised and stripped of narrative information by lines that are traces of real movements of the body.

QSers are criticised for valuing numerical data above cues about health and wellbeing deriving from the body—for preferencing the symbolic over the real. However, the data are an 'unsophisticated, intermediate stage towards more augmented senses' that can enable greater self-reflection and a more intuitive understanding of the body when it supplements the information communicated by the body.[40] The data present a self-image that exceeds and extends the ways that the body can view and feel itself.

[38] Michael Newman, 'Decapitations: The portrait, the anti-portrait ... and what comes after?', in *Anti-Portraiture: Challenging the Limits of the Portrait*, eds. Fiona Johnstone and Kirstie Imber, 25–68 London: Bloomsbury, 2020.

Newman writes that portraits that visually resemble the sitter are iconic signs of the imaginary self (an expression of an idealised, whole self), whereas anti-portraits reject the imaginary in favour of the symbolic in word portraits (a self that is constructed through culture and language) or the real in data portraits.

[39] Newman, 'Decapitations: The portrait, the anti-portrait ... and what comes after?', 54.

[40] Tamar Sharon and Dorien Zandbergen, 'From data fetishism to quantifying selves: self-tracking practices and the other values of data', *New Media and Society* 19/11, 2016, Available at https://doi.org/10.1177/1461444816636090. Accessed 12 June 2017.

Kevin Kelly uses the term 'exosenses' to describe the enhanced 'technology-mediated sensations' produced by self-tracking technology when they bring the users awareness to the body and environment'.[41] These haptic and technological 'exosenses' enable the self-tracked body to become increasingly 'visible and sensitive for itself'.[42] Through dis-embodiment I experience an enhanced form of embodiment that knots together the real and symbolic.[43]

Quantification also slows down the pace of life in a world experienced as too fast.[44] Wolf writes that self-tracking practices copy the 'internal machines of biology and psychology and external machines of administration and surveillance' but as a 'handcrafted forgery' that slows down these processes.[45] Slowness and inefficiency can be methods of resistance when performed in societies that champion speed and productivity. For example, fashion, art and medicine each have slowness initiatives that encourage people to purchase clothes that are made to last and resist seasonal trends, and to take their time when viewing art or consulting with a patient. Han writes that information and the accumulation of capital accelerate when gaps and anomalies are erased and so neoliberal societies '[strip] people of interiority, which blocks and slows down communication'.[46] However, he notes that otherness and foreignness impede smooth communication. By reproducing data maps as linocut prints I slow down the processes of tracking and undermine their perceived automatism, efficiency and accuracy. I look intently at the lines that trace my movements, and slowly and imperfectly recreate them as grooves in the surface of the lino. Seduced by the commensurability of data I compare the pace of my activities, expressed in minutes per mile, without the intention of moving faster or working more efficiently. I track without the logic of competition or improvement.

The diagrams produced by my watch are also records of the past. QSers look back when reviewing their data but also simultaneously reach 'into

[41] Kevin Kelly quoted in Neff and Nafus, *Self-tracking*,. 78.

[42] Merleau-Ponty, *The Primacy of Perception*, 126.

[43] A term used by Newman when describing Susan Morris's work as 'a destructive/productive knotting and unknotting, or weaving and unpicking', Newman, 'Decapitations: The portrait, the anti-portrait … and what comes after?', 58.

[44] Wolf, 'The Quantified Self', 72.

[45] Wolf, 'The Quantified Self', 72.

[46] Han, *Psychopolitics*, 9.

the future with intention' when deciding what and how to track.[47] Wolf writes: 'Self-trackers look in two directions at once, dropping reminders along the way in anticipation of returning, like Hansel with his crumbs. As artifacts, collections face backward, but as an activity, collecting is acquisitive and speculative, encompassing the future'.[48] When I choose which data to collect and the parameters for its collection, I imagine the types of information that will be revealed and the comparisons I will make. *Desire Lines* record the time and movement of my tracked activities, and the time and motion of the cutting and printing process, two instances of the past recorded through bodily movement and gesture. I carve into the lino, reproducing the paths that I carve out during my daily activities. Sara Ahmed writes that 'desire lines' is a term used by landscape architects to describe the marks on the ground produced when people 'deviate from the paths they are supposed to follow'.[49] Ahmed is interested in deviations because 'bodies are gendered, sexualized, and raced by how they extend into space'.[50] Drawing on Judith Butler's description of gender as a series of repeated performative acts, Ahmed writes that tendencies of actions are inherited 'effects of histories rather than being originary'.[51] We are orientated towards some objects (which can be physical objects and objects of thought, feeling, judgement and aspiration) and away from others. In choosing to turn in a different direction, other worlds and objects come into view that extend our capabilities.[52] My fitness tracking watch extends the view I have of myself by presenting my movements via satellites. It also shows which objects are brought into close proximity to my body due to the lines I have chosen. I experience my movements as I carry out tasks that were previously unworthy of attention such as cleaning, cooking, doing admin or phoning a sick friend. Tracking these tasks brings attention to the hidden labour I perform. The tasks, frequently performed by women and other marginalised people, are undervalued by capitalist societies but produce infinite surplus-value because they are often unpaid but

[47] Wolf, 'The Quantified Self', 70.

[48] Wolf, 'The Quantified Self', 72.

[49] Sara Ahmed, *Queer Phenomenology: Orientations, Objects, Others*, Durham and London: Duke University Press, 2006, 20.

[50] Ahmed, *Queer Phenomenology: Orientations, Objects, Others*, 5.

[51] Ahmed, *Queer Phenomenology: Orientations, Objects, Others*, 56.

[52] Ahmed, *Queer Phenomenology: Orientations, Objects, Others*, 2006.

support valued labour and the production of profit. Using the standardising measure of minutes per mile, *Desire Lines* draw attention to the time and energy spent on tasks that do not fit into the value systems of neoliberalism or self-tracking. To use Lisa Baraitser's term, they are maintenance activities that are separate from and hidden by temporalities of production.[53] Maintenance time is the 'lateral time of "on-go" that tries to sustain an elongated present' rather than working towards a future achievement.[54] It maintains the material conditions of life 'along with the anachronistic ideals that often underpin them', constituting a form of 'stuck time' that intervenes in 'dominant temporal imaginaries' because time is given and shared rather than 'spent' productively.[55]

9.4 [De]humanised Self-Portraits

Self-tracking practices are tools that extend neoliberal ideologies of health and personal responsibility, ***and*** tools for individualised knowledge production that may be used to challenge neoliberal values and 'look back' at the clinical gaze. Bodies are fragmented and abstracted in data, making it difficult to 'detect the humanity'.[56] Han writes, 'Data and numbers are not narrative; they are additive. Meaning … is based on narration'.[57] According to Han, self-tracking represents a 'Dadaist technology … it empties the self of any and all meaning'.[58] Although intended as a criticism, this description supports the idea that quantified-self-portraits can disrupt social norms and ideals. Dada was a radical left-wing movement initiated by artists who were horrified by the bloodshed of the First World War. They produced nonsensical artworks because society no longer made any sense. In my research I argue that the body and lifestyle ideals that are presented in contemporary consumer culture under the ideology of health are unattainable. They demand a perfect body that is continuously worked on and audited in relation to arbitrary standards that are constantly

[53] Lisa Baraitser, *Enduring Time*, London: Bloomsbury, 2017.

[54] Lisa Baraitser, 2015, Touching Time: Maintenance, Endurance, Care, in *Psychosocial Imaginaries: Perspectives on Temporality, Subjectivities and Activism*, ed. Stephen Frosh, 21–47, Basingstoke: Palgrave, 27.

[55] Baraitser, *Enduring Time*, 49, 50 and 180.

[56] Dawn Nafus. 'Biosensing and Representation', in *Quantified: Biosensing Technologies in Everyday Life*, ed. Dawn Nafus, Cambridge, Massachusetts: MIT Press, 2016, 1–4, 3.

[57] Han, *Psychopolitics* 59.

[58] Han, *Psychopolitics* 60.

shifting.[59] Quantified Self methods seem to contribute to this process; however, they appropriate the tools to produce a 'handcrafted forgery' that is not commensurable to commodity culture as data. In addition, when self-optimisation and competition are not the aims, self-tracking does not contribute to the neoliberalisation of wellbeing. *Desire Lines* represent activities that are not valued in capitalism as data sources or paid labour but are essential to the production of profit. Highlighting time-consuming and sedentary 'housework' demonstrates how domestic labour and caring responsibilities can impede the neoliberal pursuit of health that is modelled on and predominantly achievable for white, wealthy male bodies, while also 'maintaining' life and intervening in dominant temporal ideals of speed and productivity.[60]

The fragmented, abstracted self in self-tracking data, brings to mind the 'deessentialised', 'multiplicitous' body art 'technosubject' that is not definable in 'fixed terms of identity relating to the visual appearance of a singularized, so-called material body'.[61] Jones suggests that deessentialised and incoherent bodies may challenge the modernist idealisation of the 'individual' that tends to devalue women and other marginalised people. By choosing to track my geolocation movements I am able to focus on how the body inhabits space and time instead of attributes that enable objectifying judgements. As self-portraits of real rather than iconic attributes (how I look), my quantified-self-portraits present the body as 'a form of expression, a making visible of [its] intentions' through movements.[62] The optimising intention of self-tracking may impede the process of integration in which an individual is reconciled with the limitations and imperfections of their body; however, my fitness tracking watch enables a focused, disembodied way of looking that diminishes perceived flaws in favour of a more integrated view of myself as a social being and neoliberal labouring subject. My quantified-self-portraits present a picture of an active, moving being, all the more accurate for their chaotic incoherency (Figs. 9.1, 9.2, 9.3, 9.4, 9.5, 9.6, 9.7, 9.8, 9.9, 9.10, 9.11 and 9.12).

[59] Vera King, Benigna Gerisch and Hartmut Rosa (eds), 2019, *Lost in Perfection: Impacts of Optimisation on Culture and Psyche*, London: Routledge.

[60] Baraitser, *Enduring Time*, 49.

Baraitser, *Enduring Time.*

[61] Jones, *Body Art Performing the Subject*, 203–4.

[62] Merleau-Ponty paraphrased in Ahmed, *Queer Phenomenology: Orientations, Objects, Others*, p. 53.

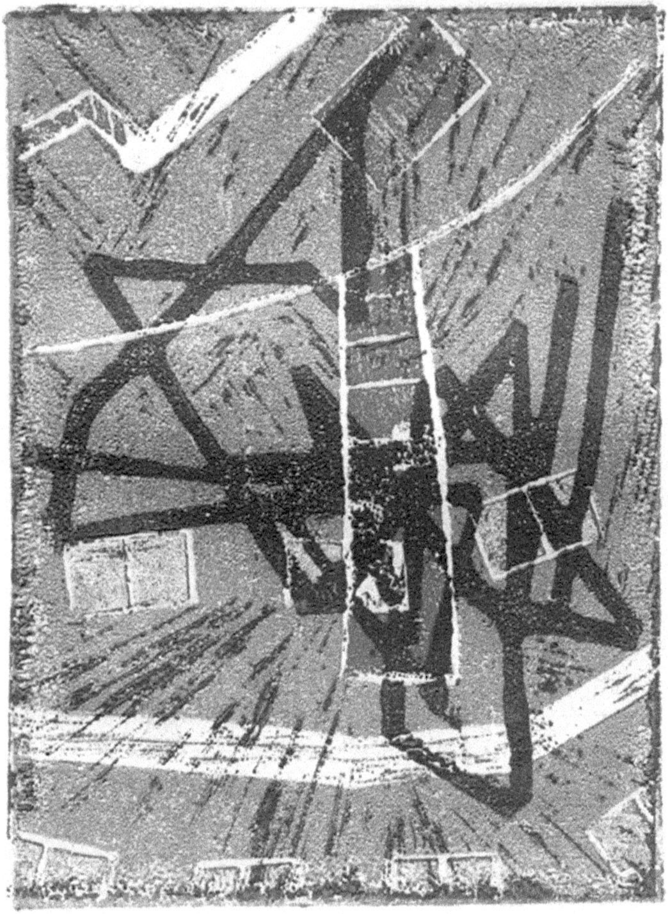

Fig. 9.1 Dawn Woolley, 396.25 minutes per mile (14.04.22 Linocutting and printing), 2022, Linocut print on paper, 22 × 28 cm

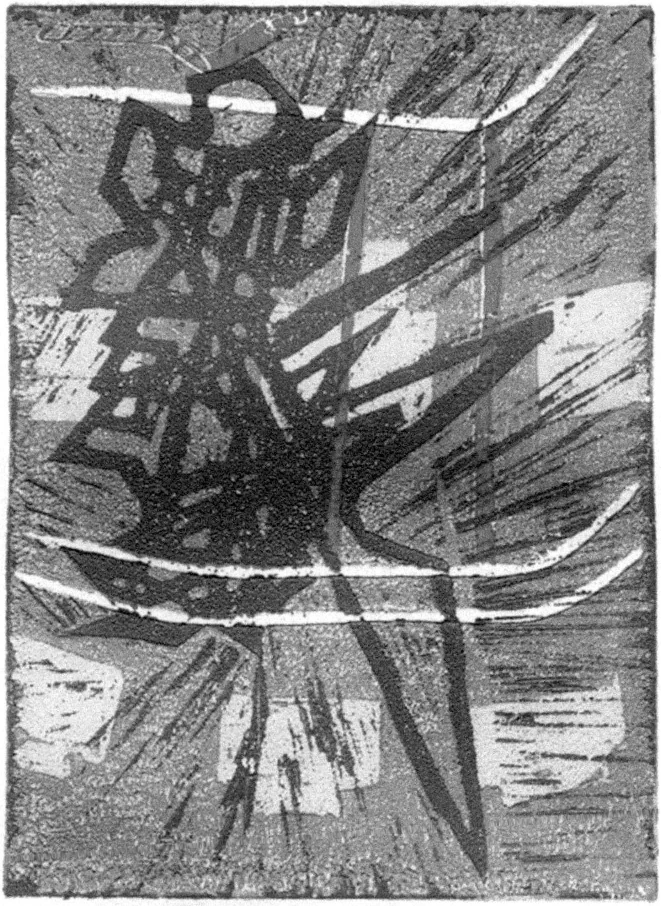

Fig. 9.2 Dawn Woolley, Desire Lines: 49.12 minutes per mile (08.05.22 guinea pig cage cleaning), 2022, Linocut print on paper, 22 × 28 cm

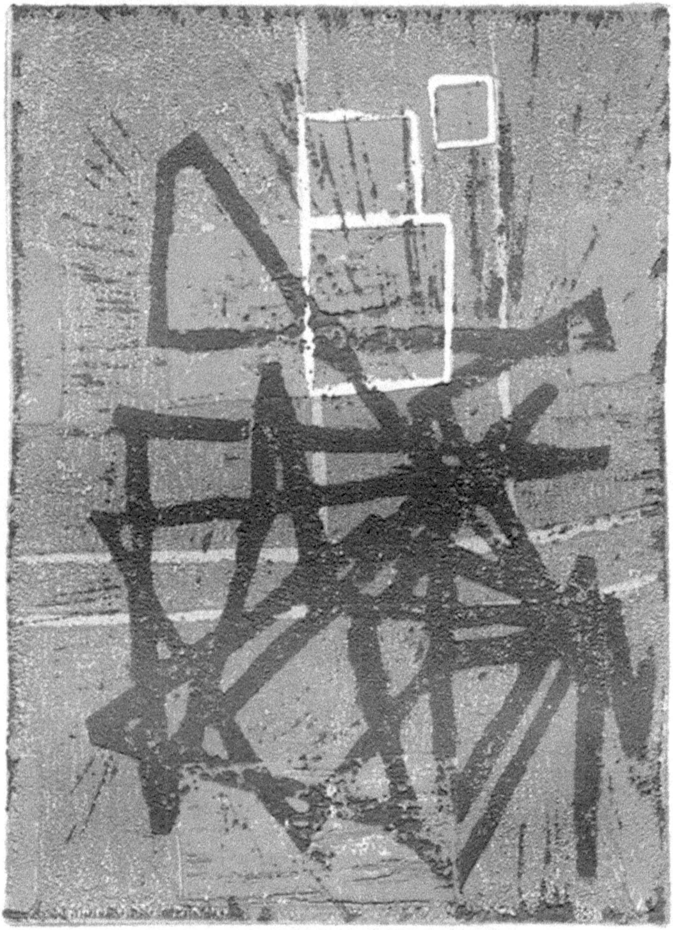

Fig. 9.3 Dawn Woolley, Desire Lines: 3588.89 minutes per mile (09.05.22 book proof reviewing), 2022, Linocut print on paper, 22 × 28 cm

Fig. 9.4 Dawn Woolley, Desire Lines: 3822.33 minutes per mile (02.08.22 phoning a sick friend), 2022, Linocut print on paper, 22 × 28 cm

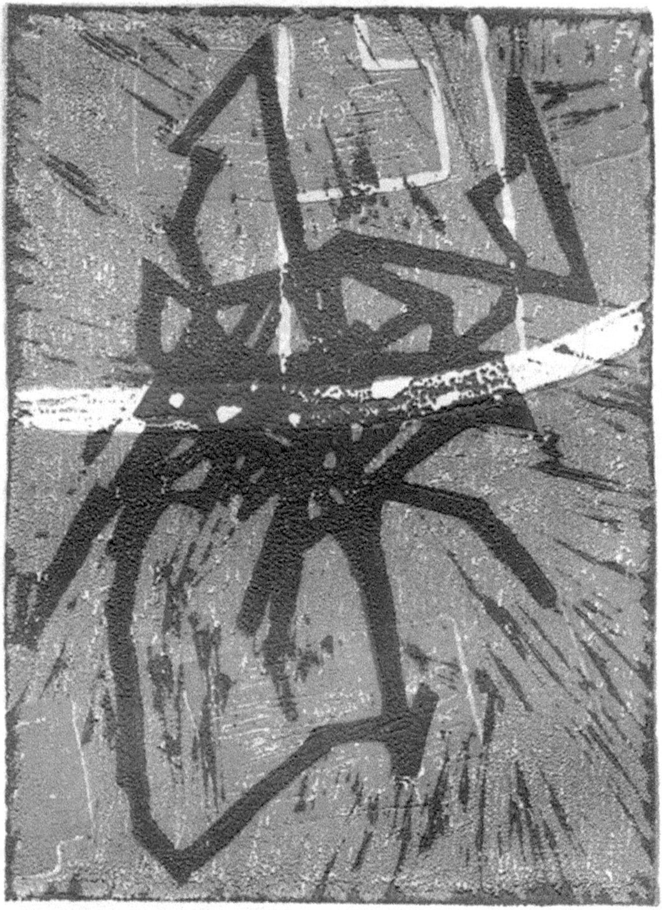

Fig. 9.5 Dawn Woolley, Desire Lines: 189.04 minutes per mile (06.08.22 cooking meal), 2022, Linocut print on paper, 22 × 28 cm

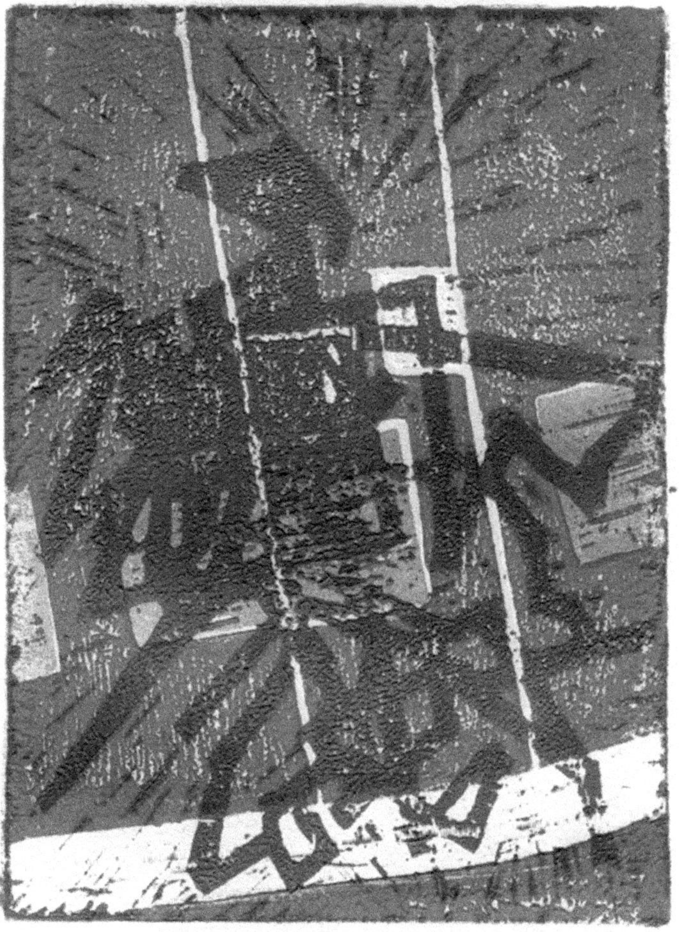

Fig. 9.6 Dawn Woolley, Desire Lines: 109.02 minutes per mile (21.08.22 moving furniture), 2022, Linocut print on paper, 22 × 28 cm

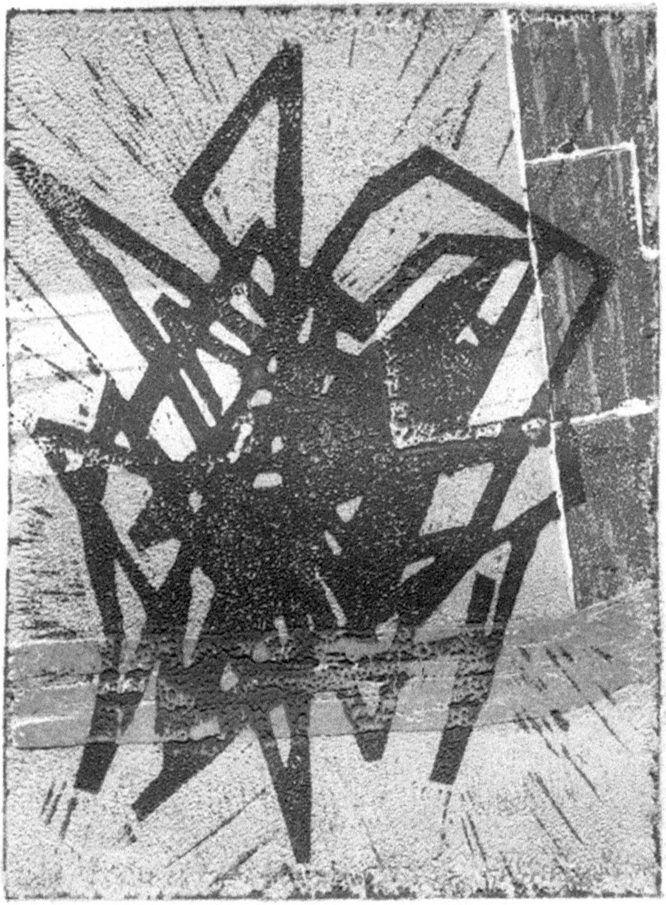

Fig. 9.7 Dawn Woolley, Desire Lines: 217.01 minutes per mile (21.08.22 admin), 2022, Linocut print on paper, 22 × 28 cm

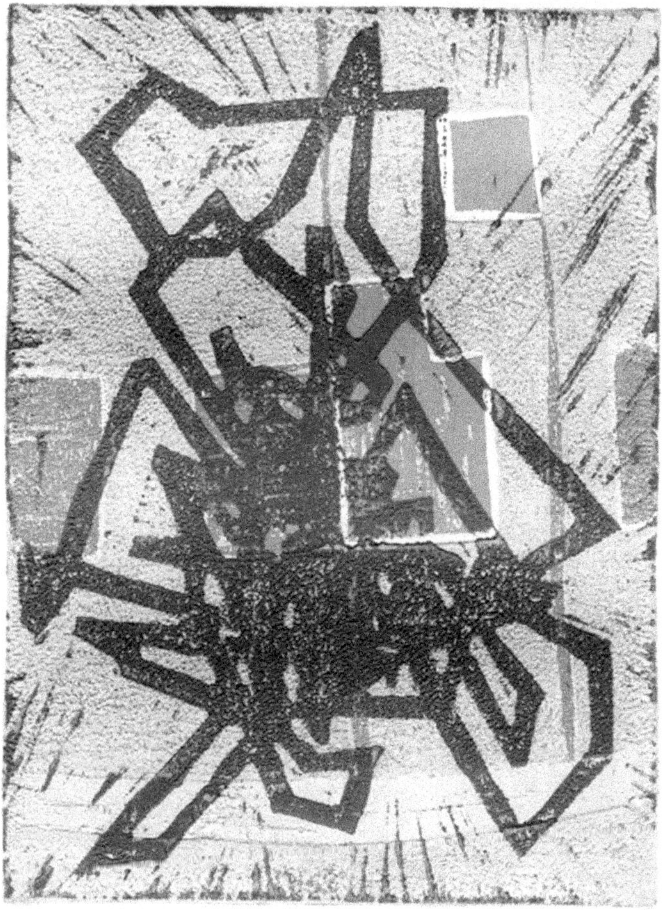

Fig. 9.8 Dawn Woolley, Desire Lines: 32.09 minutes per mile (22.08.22 washing up), 2022, Linocut print on paper, 22 × 28 cm

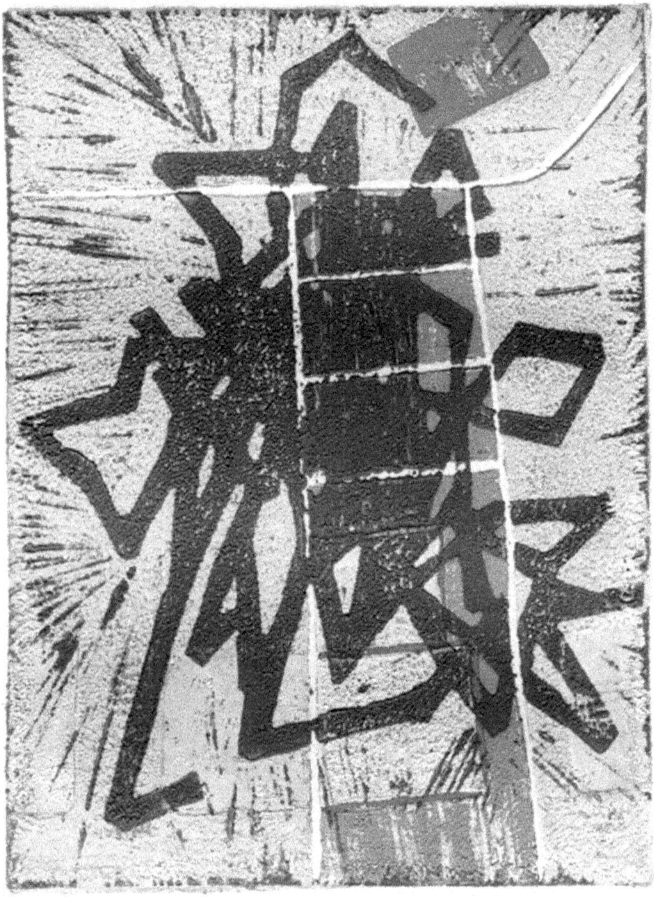

Fig. 9.9 Dawn Woolley, Desire Lines: 158.33 minutes per mile (23.08.22 studio work), 2022, Linocut print on paper, 22 × 28 cm

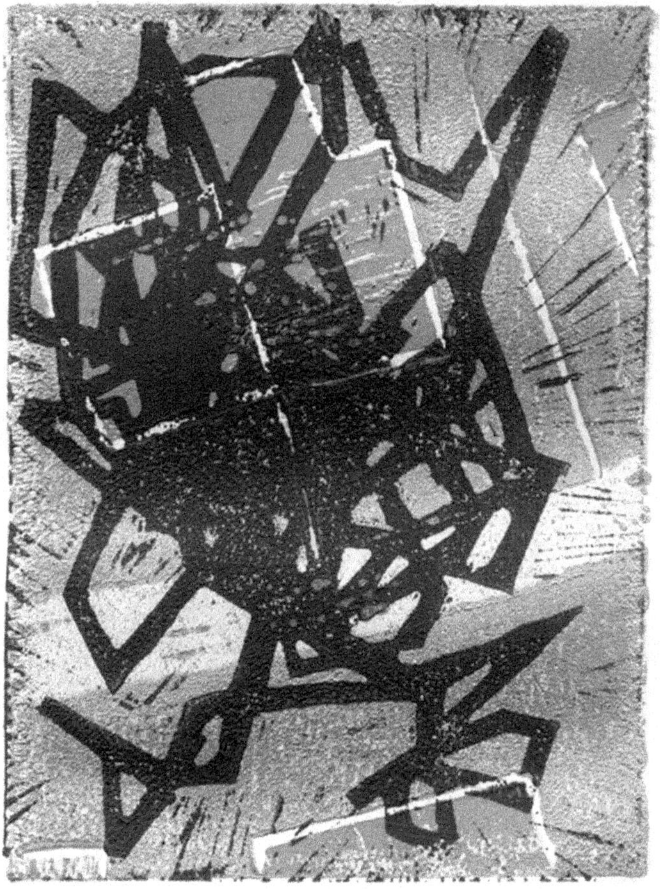

Fig. 9.10 Dawn Woolley, Desire Lines: 67.02 minutes per mile (23.08.22 hanging washing out), 2022, Linocut print on paper, 22 × 28 cm

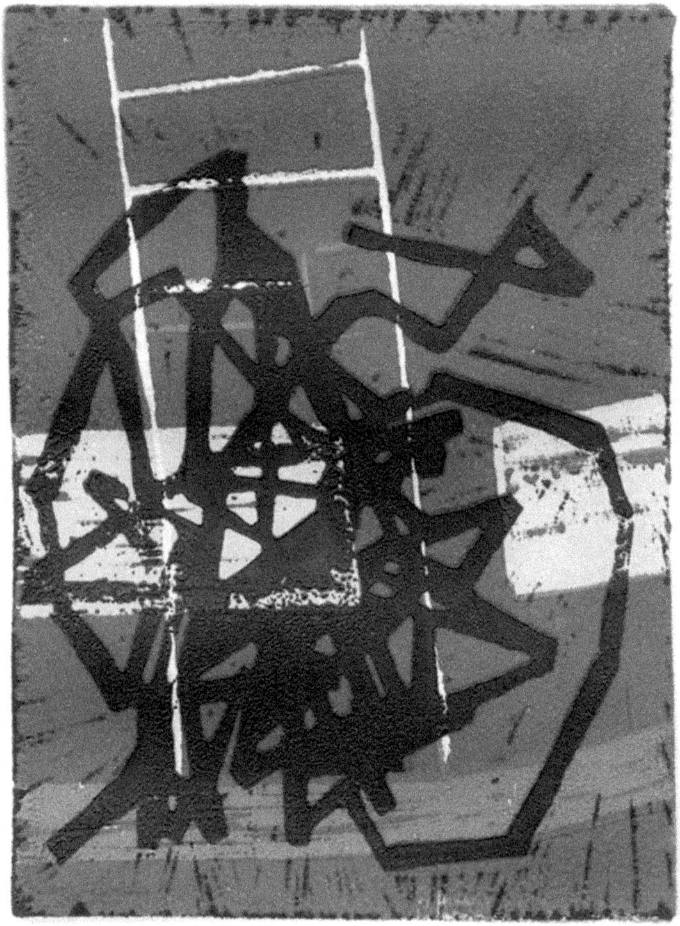

Fig. 9.11 Dawn Woolley, Desire Lines: 93.32 minutes per mile (10.09.22 leg waxing), 2022, Linocut print on paper, 22 × 28 cm

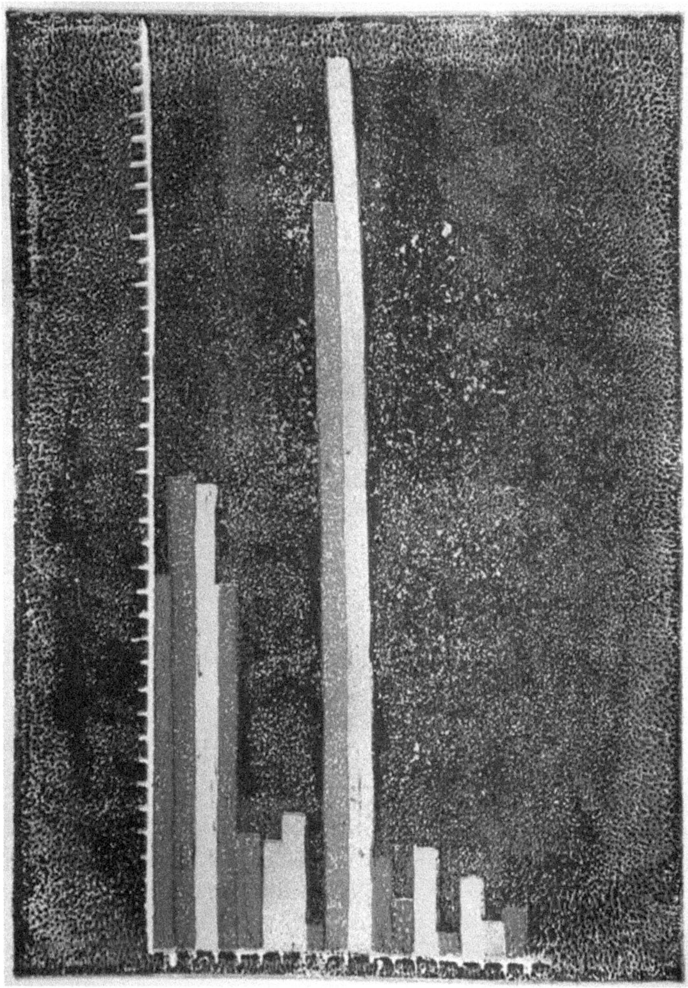

Fig. 9.12 Dawn Woolley, Desire Lines: Bar Chart (Tracked Activities April–September), 2022, Linocut print on paper, 35 × 50 cm

References

Ahmed, Sara. *Queer Phenomenology: Orientations, Objects, Others*. Durham and London: Duke University Press. 2006.

Anonymous. n.d. 'What is quantified self'. *Quantified Self: Self Knowledge Through Numbers*. Available at http://quantifiedself.com/about/what-is-quantified-self/ (accessed 3 August 2019).

Aphramor, Lucy and Jacqui Gingras. 'Helping People Change: Promoting Politicised Practice in the Health Care Professions'. In *Debating Obesity: Critical Perspectives*, eds. Emma Rich, Lee F. Monaghan and Lucy Aphramor, 192–218. New York: Palgrave Macmillan. 2011.

Baraitser, Lisa. *Enduring Time*, London: Bloomsbury. 2017.

Baraitser, Lisa. Touching Time: Maintenance, Endurance, Care. In *Psychosocial Imaginaries: Perspectives on Temporality, Subjectivities and Activism*, ed. Stephen Frosh, 21–47, Basingstoke: Palgrave. 2015.

Barrett, Elizabeth. 'Experiential Learning in Practice as Research: Context, Method, Knowledge'. *Journal of Visual Art Practice*. 6(2): 2007. 115–124.

Featherstone, Mike. 'Body, image and affect in consumer culture'. *Body and Society* 16/1: 2010. 193–221.

Gerisch, Benigna, Benedikt Salfeld, Christiane Beerbohm, Katarina Busch and Vera King. 'Optimisation by knife: on types of biographical appropriating of aesthetic surgery in late modernity'. In *Lost in Perfection: Impacts of Optimisation on Culture and Psyche*, eds. Vera King, Benigna Gerisch and Hartmut Rosa, 131–145. London: Routledge. 2019.

Greenfield, Dana. 'Deep Data: Notes on the *n of 1*'. In *Quantified: Biosensing Technologies in Everyday Life*, ed. Nafus, Dawn, Cambridge, Massachusetts: MIT Press. 2016.

Han, Byung-Chul. *Psychopolitics: Neoliberalism and New Technologies of Power*. Trans. Eric Butler. London: Verso. 2017.

Johnstone, Fiona, and Kirstie Imber. 'Introducing the Anti-Portrait'. In *Anti-Portraiture: Challenging the Limits of the Portrait*, ed. Fiona Johnstone and Kirstie Imber. London: Bloomsbury. 2020.

Jones, Amelia. *Body Art Performing the Subject*, Minneapolis: University of Minnesota Press. 1998.

King, Vera, Benigna Gerisch and Hartmut Rosa (eds). 2019. *Lost in Perfection: Impacts of Optimisation on Culture and Psyche*. London: Routledge.

Krüger, Steffen. 'The authoritarian dimension in digital self-tracking: Containment, commodification, subjugation'. In *Lost in Perfection: Impacts of Optimisation on Culture and Psyche*, eds. Vera King, Benigna Gerisch and Hartmut Rosa, London: Routledge. 2016.

Lupton, Deborah. *The Quantified Self*, Cambridge: Polity. 2016.

Merleau-Ponty, Maurice. *The Primacy of Perception*. Trans. Carleton Dallery. Evanston, Illinois: Northwestern University Press. 1964.

Nafus, Dawn. 'Biosensing and Representation'. In *Quantified: Biosensing Technologies in Everyday Life*, ed. Dawn Nafus, 1–4. Cambridge, Massachusetts: MIT Press. 2016.

Nafus, Dawn, and Jamie Sherman. 'This One Does not Go Up To 11: The Quantified Self Movement as an Alternative to Big Data Practice'. *International Journal of Communication* 8: 2014. 1784–1794.

Neff, Gina, and Dawn Nafus. *Self-tracking*. Cambridge, MA: MIT Press. 2016.

Newman, Michael. 'Decapitations: The portrait, the anti-portrait ... and what comes after?'. In *Anti-Portraiture: Challenging the Limits of the Portrait*, ed. Fiona Johnstone and Kirstie Imber. London: Bloomsbury. 2020.

Sharon, Tamar, and Dorien Zandbergen. 'From data fetishism to quantifying selves: self-tracking practices and the other values of data'. *New Media and Society* 19/11. 2016. https://doi.org/10.1177/1461444816636090.

Smith, Gavin J. D., and Ben Vonthethoff. 'Health by numbers? Exploring the practice and experience of datafied health'. *Health Sociology Review* 26/1. 2017.

Spatz, Ben. 'Embodiment As First Affordance: Tinkering, Tuning, Tracking'. *Performance Philosophy*. 2(2): 2021. 257–271. https://doi.org/10.21476/Pp.2017.2261 Issn 2057-7176.

Wolf, Gary. 'The Quantified Self: Reverse Engineering'. In *Quantified: Biosensing Technologies in Everyday Life*, ed. Dawn Nafus. Cambridge, Massachusetts: MIT Press. 2016.

Wolf, Gary. 'The data-driven life'. *The New York Times Magazine*, 28 April 2010. http://www.nytimes.com/2010/05/02/magazine/02self-measurement-t.html?_r=0.

Woolley, Dawn. *Consuming the Body: Capitalism, Social Media and Commodification*. London: Bloomsbury. 2023.

CHAPTER 10

The Shocking History of Electric Corsets

Alanna McKnight

In the late nineteenth century, women's bodies were both medicalized and pathologized: positioned as a problem to be cured, while women's fashionable dress was blamed for numerous illnesses (see Matthews David 2017). At the same time research had begun into the potentials of electricity, which was by no means the ubiquitous commodity that it is today. Electricity promised a multitude of medical applications, engaging the imagination of both the medical community and the general public, creating a cultural fixation on electricity and electric cures. Almost as soon as legitimate physicians had begun to theorize and experiment with electricity's potential to heal and stimulate, 'quacks' followed, looking to use this emerging technology to exploit the naïve and chronically ill Victorian public. Enterprising con artists promoted a range of electrified or magnetized products which they claimed would increase health and stimulate the body. Among these were corsets, garments that dress reformers and doctors alleged caused a myriad of illnesses affecting women.

A. McKnight (✉)
Toronto, ON, Canada
e-mail: alanna.mcknight@torontomu.ca

D. Woolley et al. (eds.), *Wearable Objects and Curative Things*, Palgrave Studies in Fashion and the Body,
https://doi.org/10.1007/978-3-031-40017-9_10

This chapter examines the development of the electric corset, in the context of narratives around women's health including those developed by the dress reform movement, and standard corset marketing. The idea that corsets caused a myriad of health problems was prevalent during this period. Corset manufacturers sought to address these concerns through the production of models specifically for health, through targeted advertising campaigns which extolled the health-giving properties of their products and equally through the invention of novel products such as of the electric corset. The makers of electric corsets promised to cure a range of ailments afflicting modern women, from vaginal prolapse to congestion of the blood to stupidity,[1] many of which, the dress reform movement claimed were induced by corsets. George A. Scott and Cornelius Harness used the novelty of electricity to sell their products; capitalizing on the pathologization of women's bodies and women's own anxieties around their health. This chapter explores the development and marketing of Scott and Harness' electric corsets, juxtaposing advertisements with those of Dr. Warner, a trained doctor who made and marketed some of the most popular corsets at the end of the nineteenth century.

10.1 Corsets, Medicine, and Electricity in the Nineteenth Century

Valerie Steele opens her book *Corsets: A Cultural History* (2001) with the statement, 'The corset is probably the most controversial garment in the entire history of fashion'.[2] Though the specific areas of compression or enhancement have changed over the centuries, women have worn corsets for over 400 years. The corset's primary function remains to support and shape the wearer's body: creating a fashionable silhouette and a smooth foundation for outer dress. The curative or harmful properties of corset wearing have been subject to multiple controversies and misconceptions. Many of these contemporary misconceptions[3] stem from WB Lord's 1865 pseudo-historical book *The Corset and The Crinoline* which presented corsets as harmful garments and the women who wore them foolish slaves to

[1] Alanna McKnight. 'The Kase of Kim Kardashian's Korset' in *Fashion Studies* 3:20 (2020).

[2] Valerie Steele. *Corsets: A Cultural History*. (New Haven: Yale University Press, 2001): 1.

[3] Including the myth of the 16-inch waist, and the alleged medieval origins of corsets as a punishment for a misbehaving wife.

fashion.[4] The continuation of this narrative is evident in both Victorian and more contemporary critiques of women, clothing and consumption. For example, Roberts' 1977 article 'The Exquisite Slave' argues that women's dress was frivolous and made women submissive and inactive noting that based on the medical information of the time, corsets were to blame for many of women's illnesses.[5] Similarly, Leigh Summers's *Bound to Please: A History of Victorian Corsets* (2001), explicitly states that the book aims 'to identify and tease out the ways that corsetry oppressed women, physically and emotionally', suggesting that corsets not only caused physical illnesses but were also to blame for the decline of women's emotional wellbeing'.[6] More recently, Rebecca Gibson in *The Corseted Skeleton: A Bioarchaeology of Binding* (2020) has sought to disprove the myth that corsets caused a myriad of illnesses, through examining the skeletal remains of women who wore corsets both to determine the level of damage caused by corsetry and to locate evidence of the illnesses that corsets were alleged to have caused.[7] This chapter is thus situated amongst a divided body of literature that sees the corset both as a social evil, squeezing the life out of women in the nineteenth century, and as a benign garment that has been used as a scapegoat for multiple ailments.

Women's bodies in the nineteenth century were a site of both neglect and confusion for the medical profession. As Elinor Cleghorn writes in *Unwell Women*, 'Medicine constantly reflected and enforced Victorian social ideals of womanhood and femininity, and, as a rule, it was dominated by men'.[8] The nature of Victorian medicine framed women as

[4] The first popular monograph on the corset

[5] Hélène Roberts. 'The Exquisite Slave: The Role of Clothes in Making the Victorian Woman', in *Signs* 2:3 (Spring, 1977).

In a response, in the same 1977 edition of the journal *Signs* Kunzle calls Roberts's position 'antifeminist' arguing that it was not the corset that made women weak and submissive, but the lifestyle imposed on them, through multiple pregnancies, household duties, and a culture obsessed with the 'sacred maternal'.

[6] Leigh Summers. *Bound to Please: A History of the Victorian Corset.* (London: Berg, 2001): p. 5.

[7] Kunzel, 572. Five years after this academic argument, Kunzel published *Fashion and Fetishism*, which examines the practice of tightlacing, a form of body modification that uses specially designed corsets to slowly reduce the waist. Tight lacing is often conflated with the regular practice of corsetry. Images of tight lacers are used for shock value to illustrate arguments against the practice.

[8] Elinore Cleghorn. *Unwell Women: Misdiagnosis and Myth in a Man-Made World.* (New York: Dutton Press, 2021): p. 97.

perpetually unwell, largely because of their reproductive organs.[9] Indeed, the reproductive functions of a woman defined her character, position, and value, and could be influenced by any number of nervous disorders.[10] Because corsets put pressure on the abdomen there was concern about their impact upon women's reproductive capacity, alongside rhetoric that corsets might exacerbate women's perceived pre-existing proclivity toward emotional volatility and disease. The idea that women were naturally weak and prone to illness was used to justify the suggestion that corsets could act as both a fashion item and a cure.

In *The Body in Pain*, Elaine Scarry highlights the ways that artifacts may replace the functions of the body, which may result in a reversal of interior body with the exterior body through projection. While Scarry uses the way the lens on a microscope replicates and enhances the function of the eye's lens to illustrate this idea,[11] the corset creates something akin to an exoskeleton, a wearable carapace, aiding in posture by supporting the wearer's body from the outside. For example, writing in the popular press, Havelock Ellis argued that women were too feeble to support their bodies through their own strength[12] and it might be preferable 'if she went always on all fours. It is because the fall of the viscera in woman when she imitated man by standing erect induced such profound physiological displacements ... that the corset is morphologically essential'.[13]

These sentiments were largely based in eugenicist rhetoric and critics of corsets feared that they would lead to the decline of the white middle class.[14] Women's health was perceived to be fragile and was pathologized as existing with a de facto 'extreme nervous susceptibility'.[15] In addition, modern life, with its increased urbanization, trains, automobiles, as well as telegraphs making the world smaller, was thought to cause nervous

[9] Cleghorn, *Unwell Women*, 99.

[10] Mary Poovey. 'Scenes of an Indelicate Character: The Medical "Treatment" of Victorian Women' in *The Making of the Modern Body: Sexuality and Society in the Nineteenth Century* Gallagher and Laqueur eds. (Berkeley: University of California Press, 1987): 146.

[11] Elaine Scarry. *The Body in Pain: The Making and Unmaking of the World.* (Oxford: Oxford University Press, 1985): 283.

[12] Jill Fields. 'Fighting the Corsetless Evil: Shaping Corsets and Culture, 1900–1930' in *The Journal of Social History*, 33:2 (1999): 358.

[13] Havelock Ellis, 'An Anatomical Vindication of the Straight Front Corset,' Current Literature, February 1910, pp. 172–174.

[14] Alanna McKnight, 'Palpably Ugly or Beauty of their Form?: Corsets in Toronto Periodicals, 1871–1914' in *Popular Communication* 18:4 (2020).

[15] Poovey, 'Scenes of an Indelicate Character', 146.

disorders among women (and men).[16] Though many of these alleged causes for mental illness were powered by electricity, advertisements for electric corsets seemed to imply that these ill effects could be countered through the use of electrical cures. Indeed, doctors in the late nineteenth century used electrotherapy to treat many illnesses specific to women, such as fibroids, dysmenorrhea, uterus displacement (hysteria), menopause, and neurosis. Electrotherapeutic treatment involved placing galvanized rods on the abdomen, lower back, or even inserted into the body.[17] Despite the fact that many people did not trust this treatment, and viewed it as quackery, electrotherapy soon overtook surgery as the standard treatment for many women's problems.[18,19] Despite the public's ambivalence around the clinical use of galvanization, manufacturers of 'quack' medical products, such as Scott and Harness, were able to capitalize on the trend for electrical medical devices. It was in this context that electric corsets were marketed as a panacea to women's ailments.

10.2 A History of the Electric Corset

The idea for an electric corset was developed by George A. Scott. Born into a family of brush manufacturers in Lansingburgh, New York,[20] Scott moved to Florence, Massachusetts, in 1866 to help convert Littlefield and Parsons, a former maker of Daguerreotype cases who were struggling after the Civil War, into a brush factory: the Florence Manufacturing Co. In 1874, Scott traveled to London to act as sales agent for the Florence Manufacturing Co. and to set up a new company manufacturing brushes, frames, and hand mirrors.[21] By 1877, Scott had, with Englishman Cornelius Bennett Harness,[22] set up London Pall Mall Electric

[16] Lisa Appignanesi, *Mad, Bad and Sad: A History of Women and the Mind Doctors from 1800 to the Present* (London: Virago, 2009).

[17] Cleghorn, *Unwell Women.*

[18] Eventually, treatment for women's mental health, which was inextricably linked with reproductive health, was taken to an extreme conclusion through the invention of Electro-Convulsive Therapy (ECT).

[19] Cleghorn, *Unwell Women.*

[20] Robert Waits. *The Medical Electricians: Dr. Scott and his Victorian Colleagues in Quackery.* (Sunnyvale: J-IV-IX, 2013).

[21] Waits, *The Medical Electricians.*

[22] With Harness initially working as a salesman, and eventually assuming the role of manager.

Association.[23] The London Pall Mall Electric Association sought to capitalize on the growing trend of medical electrical devices marketing products such as the 'Dr. Scott Pure Bristle Electric Hairbrush'[24] claimed to cure headaches and neuralgia in two to five minutes.[25]

At the time, products produced by other medical electricity companies often used Pulvermacher's batteries. These batteries, developed in the 1840s, consisted of zinc and copper wire wrapped around a wooden rod, with one end of each wire entering one end of the wood, the other end terminating in a loop, creating a miniature galvanic battery, activated by soaking the battery in a solution of water and vinegar.[26] The batteries were messy and acrid smelling, so despite claims of miraculous cures, medical devices using this form of electricity were not popular. Scott realized that he could capitalize on the demand for medical electrical goods and avoid using Pulvermacher's batteries by using magnets instead. The principle behind magnetic clothing was to impart a magnetic force to the iron in the blood of the wearer, in hopes of increasing circulation and blood purity[27] and at the time, magnetic garments were made to target specific sites of the body: belts, knee braces, ankle, and wrist wraps. However, Scott chose not to brand London Pall Mall Electric Association's goods as magnetic, instead using the term 'electric', so that his products would not be confused with those of other companies that made curative clothing with magnets. In using the term electric, Scott sought to imply medical competence and distance Pall Mall Electric Association from the use of magnets, which had already been dismissed as quackery by many consumers and medical professionals.

With Scott's earlier products garnering success for the Pall Mall Electric Company, he decided to manufacture an 'electric' corset. Like the earlier magnetic brushes, these corsets were not in fact electric. Since the 1820s steel boning had been commonly used as replacement for whale bone in corsets.[28] It was therefore relatively simple for Scott to manufacture a fashionable corset containing slightly magnetized steel bones. The design

[23] Waits, *The Medical Electricians*, 61.

[24] By branding himself as a benevolent doctor, Scott, like many purveyors of "quack" medical cures coaxed consumers into a false sense of security.

[25] Waits, *The Medical Electricians*, 62.

[26] Iwan Rhys Morus. *Shocking Bodies: Life, Death, & Electricity in Victorian England.* (Gloucestershire: The History Press, 2011): 108.

[27] Waits, *The Medical Electricians*, 148.

[28] Steele, *Corsets*, 43.

featured copper and zinc bands, which were exposed to the skin through open spaces in the lining, creating a galvanic current when in contact with the wearer's natural perspiration.[29] However the electric corset possessed a particular design flaw; the creation of galvanic current relied upon skin contact, yet women never wore corsets against their bare skin, instead wearing a chemise underneath to help keep the corset clean. Although it is doubtful that Scott believed the electric corset would in fact be efficacious, this oversight highlights the pitfalls of men attempting to capitalize on women's bodies without engaging with their lived experiences.

In fact, Pall Mall Electric Association did not manufacture the corsets themselves, but rather purchased lots of corsets wholesale and then replaced the original boning with the magnetized steel, added their label, and sold them at double the cost of a regular corset.[30] This high-profit margin afforded Scott the ability to invest in advertising. In 1879, Scott returned to New York to establish the Pall Mall Electric Association in New York and embarked on a large-scale advertising campaign. At the time, small periodicals survived largely on advertising revenue, as a result, he was able to advertise widely and in a variety of publications.[31] By 1881, the presence of Scott's advertising campaigns in newspapers and periodicals was so ubiquitous that a satirical advertisement was published in The Washington Tribune, mocking Scott and his claims of greatness.[32]

In 1881, Scott sold the London part of Pall Mall Electric Company to Cornelius Harness, along with the exclusive rights to sell the electric brushes. In August of 1881, Harness had established The Medical Battery Co. Ltd., to exclusively sell his own versions of electric medical devices. Initially The Medical Battery Co. had competed with Pall Mall Electric Association for customers. However, following the acquisition of the London part of Pall Mall Electric Company, Harness merged the companies.[33] Concurrently, Harness was devoting less and less of his company's finances to advertising Scott's products and instead began producing men's electric belts under his new brand name. Unlike Scott's electric Corset the Harness belt did not include magnetized steel but contained currents produced by zinc and copper elements.[34] Further positioning

[29] Waits, *The Medical Electricians*, 67.
[30] Waits, *The Medical Electricians*, 67.
[31] Waits, *The Medical Electricians*, 68.
[32] Waits, *The Medical Electricians*, 74.
[33] Morrus, 138.
[34] Waits, *The Medical Electricians*, 78.

himself and his company as direct competitors to the Pall Mall Electric Association, in 1883, Harness also opened the Electropathic Association offices two streets away from Scott's New York office and by 1889, was using the Pall Mall Electric Association's Oxford Street headquarters and showroom both to attract potential customers through daily displays of free electrical entertainment and to treat customers using the company's electric 'cures'.[35]

Although Harness had copied Scott's successful business model, the Medical Battery Company was embroiled in controversy: receiving multiple complaints from dissatisfied customers, including one lawsuit in 1892, in which a customer asked for a refund and was sued in retaliation. The customer counter-sued, stating that the belt he purchased not only neglected to cure his hernia but also 'chafed the skin and caused an eruption'.[36] The suit was not decided in Harness' favor, not because the belt was ineffective and the claims of the healing properties were fraudulent, but because the salesman had been mis-represented as a medical expert. This defeat in court resulted in a slew of suits and countersuits for The Medical Battery Company and Cornelius Harness.

10.3 Corset Advertising

The field of advertising developed in parallel to the field of 'science'-based commodities. Early examples of quack remedy advertising and use of recommendations by medical professional in adverts, for a range of ailments including toothache and the plague, were created in the 1650s, and grew in number by the 1690s with the growth in popularity of newspapers.[37] At this time, classified adverts tended to be text based and contain only factual information, however, 'pseudo-medical' and 'cosmatick' adverts pioneered persuasion methods.[38] In the UK in the 1850s, the abolition of the Advertisement Tax and Stamp Duty on adverts contributed to an increase in newspaper circulation and advertising, however, 'sellers of pills, adornments and sensational literature' continued to produce most of the adverts.[39] Like the electric corset, the majority of goods subjected to large-

[35] Morus. *Shocking Bodies*, 183.

[36] Waits, *The Medical Electricians*, 193.

[37] Raymond Williams, 2005, *Culture and Materialism*, London: Verso.

[38] Williams, *Culture and Materialism*, p. 172.

[39] Williams, *Culture and Materialism*, p. 172.

scale advertising and branding were 'fringe products and novelties', and this continued until the end of the nineteenth century when advertising became a widely used practice.

The makers of goods, such as the electric corset, took full advantage of the developments in print advertising to advertise their products. For many inventors of the period, filling their advertisements with information that at least sounded scientific helped them to win the trust of the consumer.[40] Indeed, 'The introduction of scientific discourse into advertising was innovative and novel, creating an artificial demand for products on the basis that trusting consumers thought that they would improve their lives'.[41] Companies used promises of health and wellbeing to differentiate themselves from their competitors, and often used false testimonials from medical professionals to add authority to their claims. This proliferation of scientific information, such as infographics, 'facts', and quotes from doctors and scientists, may have been incomprehensible to a general audience, but succeeded in creating a perceived need for devices to aid bodily health.[42] In relation to contemporary advertising but relevant to this examination of historical adverts, Judith Williamson writes that scientific terms and ideas are included in adverts in order to make the consumer 'feel *knowing* but deprive him of *knowledge*'.[43] Adverts, such as those for electric corsets connote '*science*, facts, *seriousness*', representing 'the whole miraculous system of science' without helping the consumer to understand what the commodity does and how (or if) it works.[44]

Rapid advances in technology and manufacturing also allowed fashionable dresses to be more widely accessible, with faster changes to fashionable cuts and styles. Corsets were marketed for specific uses, such as cycling, office work, and functions, including to improve or preserve health. In the context of this rapidly changing and competitive market, manufacturers needed to stay at the cutting edge, first producing

[40] Takahiro Ueyama. *Health in the Marketplace: Professionalism, Therapeutic Desires, and Medical Commodification in Late-Victorian London.* (Palo Alto: The Society for the Promotion of Science and Scholarship, 2010).

[41] Lauren O'Hagan. 'Blinded by Science? Constructing Truth and Authority in Early Twentieth Century Virol Advertisements' in *History of Retailing and Consumption* 7:2 (2021): 164.

[42] Ueyama, *Health in the Marketplace*; O'Hagan, 'Blinded by Science?'.

[43] Judith Williamson, *Decoding Advertisements: Ideology and Meaning in Advertising.* 15th ed. London: Marion Boyars, 2010, 116 (emphasis original).

[44] Williamson, *Decoding Advertisements.* 118 (emphasis original).

alternatives to whale bone and then to steel, novel lacing solutions, and elastic panels. Consumers were bombarded with advertisements declaring the latest development in corset technology, including in the late nineteenth century, the electric corset.

Corsets were the first item of clothing that was advertised on a large scale and by the 1890s, print advertising for corsets featured in most Western newspapers and women's magazines.[45] Indeed, Summers argues that corset advertisements in the nineteenth and twentieth centuries were 'the forerunners to the sexual objectification of women in the public realm in the twentieth century'.[46] These advertisements frequently included an illustration of a corset on its own or a woman in a corset, and accompanying text. Corset marketing text often focused on issues that the advertisers felt were of a concern for women, promising elegance and comfort in corsets that would not stress the body. More practically, advertisements promised that corsets were unbreakable and adjustable, and that corset care and laundering would be less strenuous.[47]

The first corset company to undertake large-scale marketing campaigns was The Warner Brothers Corset Co. headed by Dr. Lucien Warner, who, unlike Scott and Harness, was a medical doctor.[48] The Warner Bros. Corset Co. was a pioneer in corset advertising in the 1870s and continued to lead the industry into the twentieth century. The Warner Bros. Corset Co. revolutionized corset advertising in Britain and North America by glamorizing corsets and promising transformation through the use of the products. The Warner Bros. Corset Co. also tailored advertisements to appeal to distinct groups of women, depending on the publication in which the advertisement was placed (Fig. 10.1).[49]

This advertisement from an 1886 edition of *Harper's Bazaar* features illustrations of 'The Four Most Popular Corsets in America', made by Warner Bros. At this time dress reformers and doctors specifically targeted women with arguments about the potential dangers of corset wearing and manufacturers often used advertisements to counter these narratives and reassure potential customers that their products were not harmful. At the time of this advertisement, Dr. Warner manufactured 12 different styles,

[45] Summers, *Bound to Please*.
[46] Summers, *Bound to Please*, 173.
[47] Steele, *Corsets*.
[48] Summers, *Bound to Please*.
[49] Summers, *Bound to Please*.

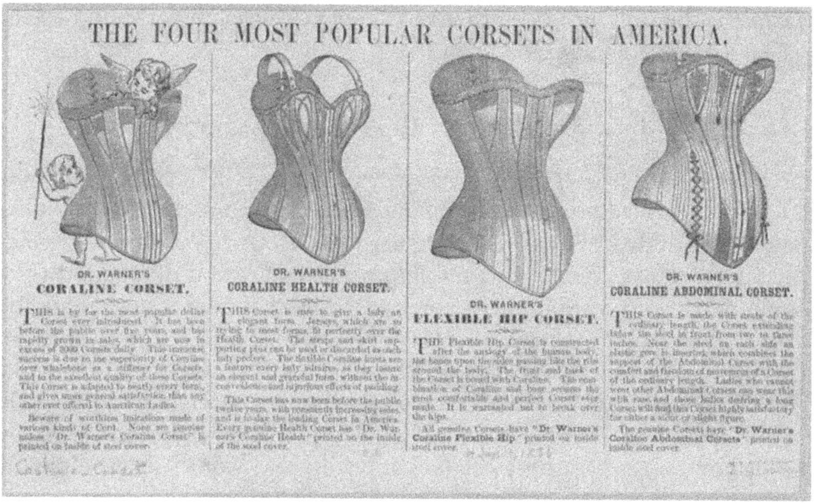

Fig. 10.1 'The four most popular corsets in America' New York Public Library Digital Collections. Accessed July 16, 2022. https://digitalcollections.nypl.org/items/510d47e0-fcba-a3d9-e040-e00a18064a99

giving a broad range of options to a diverse population of women. The advertisement features four of these models and the text describes the features of each corset, implying that the key to a comfortable corset was that it must fit the body, acknowledging that there is a wide range of women's bodies. Warners also used this advertisement to extol the virtues of their patented boning solution Coraline, an alternative to baleen and steel made from plant-based materials which allegedly made corsets more flexible, and easier to wear. This boning innovation was prominently featured in his advertising, with promises of health, and comfort because it gave firm and flexible support, and greater durability because it did not break, like whale and steel, and it did not rust like steel. Also present in this ad are putto. Steel and Summer suggest that their presence in corset advertising represents healthy babies, since medical professionals advised against the dangers of pregnancy and tight lacing.[50] However, while it may be easy to read symbolism into such a sexually and morally charged

[50] Steele, *Corsets*; Summers, *Bound to Please*.

garment, the presence of putti acted simply as an identifiable and established icon of polite sensibility and taste.[51]

10.4 Dr. Scott's Electric Corset, 1883

An 1883 edition of Harper's Magazine, contains a verbose, full-page advertisement, featuring a corset filling a large section of the left half of the page, surrounded by text. Like regular (non-electric) corset advertising, the advert draws attention to the improved quality and durability of the commodity, with the following words are printed in bold text to guide the eyes of the reader: 'A HANDSOME LINE OF ELECTRIC CORSETS', 'ABSOLUTELY UNBREAKABLE', 'Electric', 'Unbreakable' (again), and 'Better Material'. The advert also promises a 'graceful and attractive figure' and 'true French shape'. The advertisement begins and ends by listing the range of prices available, implying that women from different socioeconomic backgrounds who experience ill health can receive the benefits of wearing an electric corset. Whereas Dr Warner's Corset advert offers a number of corset designs for different needs, Dr Scott's electric corset presents the similar or identical models design with variations that are targeted toward different income levels. For example, for wealthier women, the higher priced corsets came in four colors: pink, blue, white, and dove, and are made of the finest French sateen (Fig. 10.2).

Secondary to promises of quality, are scientific explanations and justifications of the product. Though the advertisement does not explain the 'science' behind the product, the corsets are said to be 'constructed on a scientific principle, generating an exhilarating, health-giving current to the whole system'. The text claims the corset will 'quickly cure' nervous debility, spinal complaints, rheumatism, paralysis, numbness, dyspepsia, liver and kidney troubles, impaired circulation, constipation, 'and all other diseases, peculiar to women, particularly those of sedentary habits'. In addition, 'they also become, when constantly worn, equalizing agents in all cases of extreme fatness or leanness'. Thus, the advertisement suggests that Scott's eclectic corsets can aid a plethora of ailments and improve appearance in relation to body shape.

Interestingly, the advert also claims that the corset is capable of 'imparting the system with the required amount of Odic Force which Nature's

[51] Jon Stobart. 'Selling (through) Politeness: Advertising Provincial Shops in Eighteenth Century Britain' in Cultural and Social History 5:3 (2008).

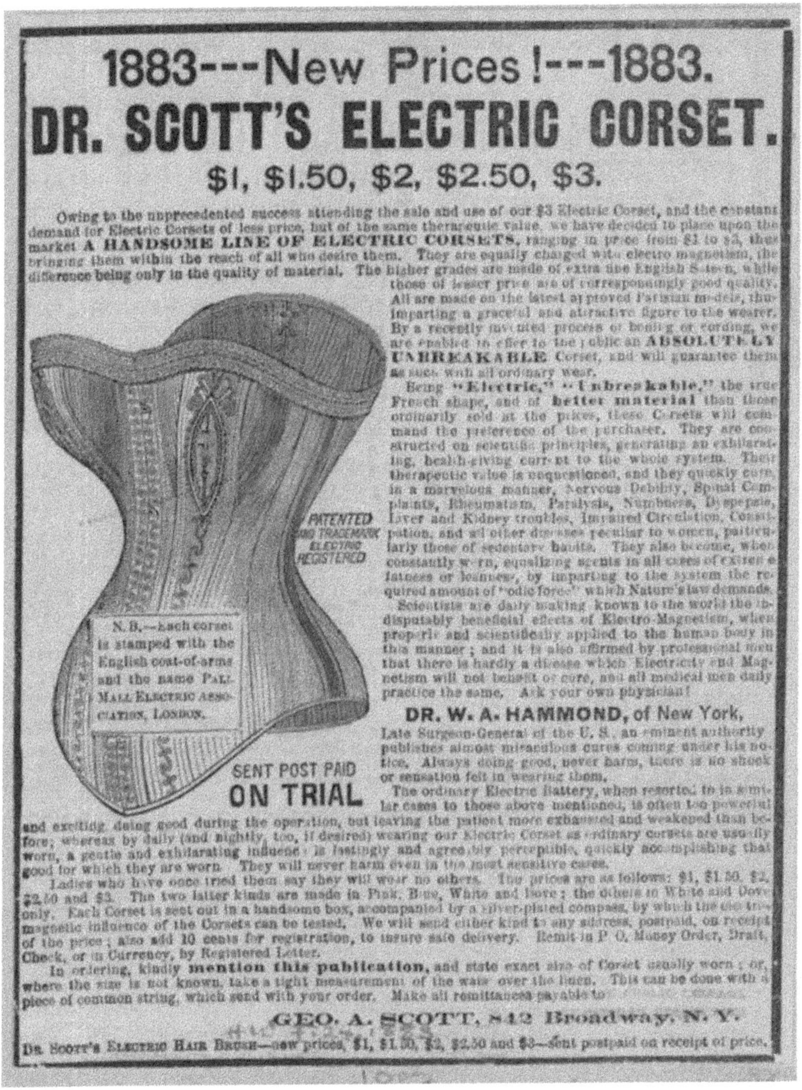

Fig. 10.2 'Dr. Scott's Electric Corset'. *Harper's Weekly: A Journal of Civilization*. (New York: Harper's Weekly Co., 1883). Retrieved from the Digital Public Library of America, http://digitalcollections.nypl.org/items/510d47e0-fcc0-a3d9-e040-e00a18064a99. (Accessed August 24, 2021)

law demands'. The concept of Odic force[52], an invisible force that permeates all living things, was hypothesized by Dr. Karl von Reichenbach, a German scientist and industrialist, in the mid-1800s.[53] In 1883, readers of *Harpers* were unlikely to know about Reichenbach's theory of Odic force, or the new and burgeoning science around electricity and magnetism, and so the advert may have appeared credible. Indeed, the newness of knowledge about the therapeutic value of electricity is foregrounded in a paragraph stating that 'Scientists are daily making known to the world the indisputably beneficial effects of Electro-magnetism, when properly and scientifically applied to the human body'. The advertisers were so confident in this claim that they advise readers to consult their own physicians about the myriad of illnesses electricity can cure. To further legitimize the scientific veracity of the garment, the adverts state that each customer will receive a silver-plated compass 'by which the electromagnetic influence of the corset can be tested'. The inclusion of a free compass, a scientific device that is easy for a consumer with no scientific knowledge to use was a clever marketing tactic that seems to support the scientific claims of the adverts. To further allay concerns about the potential harm an electric corset could cause, the advertisement reassures the consumer that the corset is 'always doing good, never harm'. Furthermore, the wearer will not feel a shock or sensation, apart from a gentle and exhilarating uplift, 'even in the most sensitive cases'. Toward the bottom of the page 'Dr. W.A. Hammond', the late Surgeon-General of the United States, is introduced as an eminent authority, who publishes 'almost miraculous cures coming under his notice'. Dr. Hammond had in 1872 published a translation of *Electricity in its Relations to Practical Medicine* by German doctor Moritz Meyer. Dr. Hammond was frequently cited in Scott's advertisements, and sued Scott in 1887 for libel, so it is likely that this endorsement was fraudulent.[54]

[52] Scott's use of Odic force might be compared the cooption of the eastern philosophical idea of Qi new age hucksters, which is similarly used to sell yoni eggs, or copper bracelets, in contemporary consumer societies.

[53] Karl von Reichenbach. *The Odic Force: Letters on Od and Magnetism*. (London: Hutchinson & Co, 1926).

[54] Waits, *The Medical Electricians*.

10.5 Harness' Electric Corset, 1892

Dr. Cornelis Harness advertised his electric corsets widely, reaching a diverse readership, and this advert from the 31st December 1892 edition of the *Penny Illustrated Paper and Illustrated Times* is a pertinent example. *Penny Illustrated Paper and Illustrated Times* catered to a general lower to low-middle-class readership and the illustrated nature of the paper did not require the customer to have advanced reading comprehension, however, the advertisement itself contains a lot of text. The advertisement begins with a headline declaring 'Ladies in all Stations of Life should send at once for HARNESS' ELECTRIC CORSET'. Below this, capitalized subheadings state, 'Beautifully Designed', 'Scientifically Constructed', and 'Comfortable to Wear'. The right side of the advert shows an Illustration of a beautiful and buxom woman in a corset, with the words 'Don't delay. Send at once. Try it', located between her body and the margin. Immediately next to the woman's breasts is a frame containing text, underlined for emphasis, stating 'for Health, Comfort, and Elegance'; language that reiterates the subheadings of the advert and is common to corset adverts more generally.[55] The advertisement works on two levels, the placement, spacing, and word choice surrounding the image place the reader at ease, as even with a cursory perusal of the page, they are met by rhetoric and imagery familiar from other corset advertisements, whilst the words 'don't delay' 'send at once' and the short staccato sentences are intended to create a sense of urgency. Apart from the small zig-zagged lines (lightning bolts) around the hips denoting electricity, the image of the woman does not differ greatly in terms of design or appearance from regular corset advertisements. Unique to this advert, however, is the inclusion of an illustration of 'The Electropathic and Zander Institute',[56] a tactic 'perfectly calculated to reassure potential customers of the establishment's respectability' (Fig. 10.3).[57]

In the bottom of the advert a headline states 'Specially designed corsets for children'. Corsets for children were not uncommon, though were

[55] Steele. *Corsets.*

[56] The Electropathic and Zander Institute building was named for Harness' acquisition of patents by Gustav Zander, a Swedish inventor. Zander was renowned in Europe, and Harness used this connection to capitalize on Zander's reputation. Customers were encouraged to visit the site and exercise on Zander's machines and attend consultations to determine which of Harness' devices were best suited to treat their ailments.

[57] Morus, *Shocking Bodies*, 184.

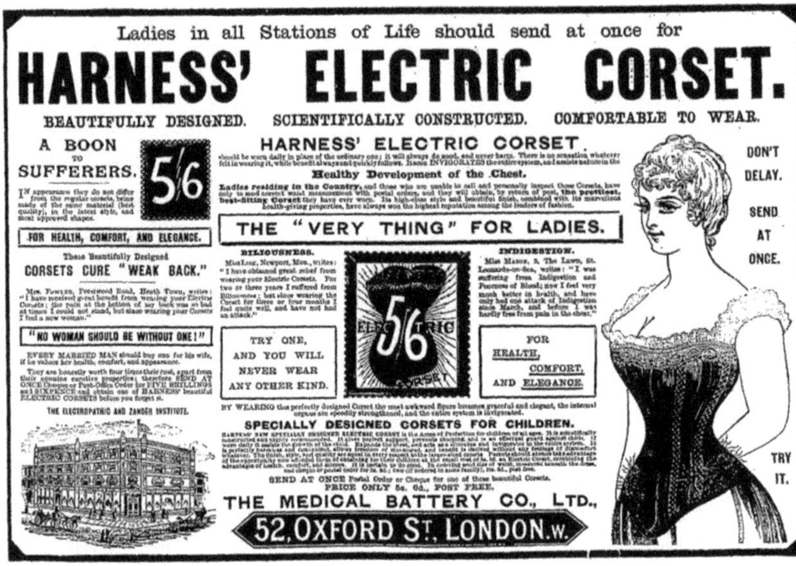
Ladies in all Stations of Life should send at once for
HARNESS' ELECTRIC CORSET.
BEAUTIFULLY DESIGNED. SCIENTIFICALLY CONSTRUCTED. COMFORTABLE TO WEAR.
A BOON TO SUFFERERS.
5/6
HARNESS' ELECTRIC CORSET.
Healthy Development of the Chest.
THE "VERY THING" FOR LADIES.
DON'T DELAY.
SEND AT ONCE.
FOR HEALTH, COMFORT, AND ELEGANCE.
These Beautifully Designed
CORSETS CURE "WEAK BACK."
"NO WOMAN SHOULD BE WITHOUT ONE!"
THE ELECTROPATHIC AND ZANDER INSTITUTE.
BILIOUSNESS.
INDIGESTION.
TRY ONE, AND YOU WILL NEVER WEAR ANY OTHER KIND.
FOR HEALTH, COMFORT, AND ELEGANCE.
SPECIALLY DESIGNED CORSETS FOR CHILDREN.
SEND AT ONCE Postal Order or Cheque for one of these beautiful Corsets.
PRICE ONLY 5s. 6d., POST FREE.
THE MEDICAL BATTERY CO., LTD.,
52, OXFORD ST., LONDON. W.
TRY IT.

Fig. 10.3 'Harness' Electric Corset'. *The Penny Illustrated Paper and Illustrated Times*, 31 December 1892. The Miriam and Ira D. Wallach Division of Art, Prints and Photographs: Picture Collection, The New York Public Library

generally not worn before the onset of puberty, and were not as heavily boned, often using cording instead.[58] Like corsets worn by adults, they were not necessarily overly tight, provided a smooth foundation for fashionable dress, and can be compared to training bras of the late twentieth century in terms of personal sartorial rituals into adulthood. The Harness electric corset, however, makes claims similar to that of a regular corset for children, declaring it 'gives perfect support, prevents stooping', and is 'an effectual guard against chills'. The text offers no indication of how the latter claim is achieved, but it asserts that this product combines 'the advantage of health, comfort, and science'.

Like the two adverts previously discussed, The Medical Battery Co., adverts used familiar visual cues and key terms, 'Health, comfort, and elegance', to sell their wares. However, unlike the adverts discussed earlier, this advert includes testimonials from customers claiming that the Harness

[58] Steele. *Corsets.*

electric corset cured their weak back, biliousness, and indigestion. Although there is no explanation for how or why the corset cured these ailments, the three testimonials state that the wearers 'feel quite well', 'feel very much better in health', and 'feel like a new woman', privileging the voice of female consumers rather than the opinions of male professional endorsers.[59] The advertisement goes into detail about the corset construction, its quality and 'approved' shapes, but there is no technical information about how the corset is electrified, how it produces health benefits including 'speedily' strengthening 'the most awkward figure', 'the internal organs', and invigorating 'the entire system' so that the customer must trust the testimonials allegedly provided by satisfied customers.

10.6 Conclusion

The attempts of Scott and Harness to capitalize on health anxieties relating to women's bodies fit within the broader tradition of women's medical advice and corset marketing. As Scott and Harness invested in marketing their electric corsets, manufacturers of regular corsets also mounted ambitious advertising campaigns. Advertisements for corsets and electric corsets ran concurrently with articles about dress reform in newspapers, journals, and magazines.[60] Dress reformers argued that women's health and wellbeing suffered because of their clothing. Corsets, in particular, were deemed to be responsible for a wide variety of ailments, including prolapsed vaginas and stupidity.[61]

More common ailments, experienced by women, like weak back and indigestion, were also alleged to be caused by corsets, and reformers shared these views in newspapers and lecture halls in order to encourage women to stop wearing them. Concurrently, the same newspapers and magazines published advertisements for corsets that contradicted these claims and included fashion columns informing readers about which corsets most fit in with current styles. Electric corsets were presented as a cure to many of the same ailments that reformers claimed were caused by wearing corsets. The claims by Scott and Harness that their corsets could cure extreme fatness or leanness and work against nervous debility, spinal complaints, rheumatism, paralysis, numbness, dyspepsia, liver and kidney

[59] Albeit fraudulently, as in the case of Dr Scott's electric corset advert.

[60] McKnight, 'Palpably Ugly or Beauty of their Form?'.

[61] McKnight, 'Palpably Ugly or Beauty of their Form?'.

troubles, impaired circulation, constipation, and all other diseases specific to women, particularly those with sedentary habits, are reflections of the contemporary medical and anti-fashion discourse of the time.

Scott and Harness were the first to apply electric belt technology to women's corsets. Their competitors, such as Scrivner, Gill & Co., Harry Lobb, and Ashworth Bros., exploited a general array of medical problems with belts, throat and lung protectors, knee caps, wristlets, and other wearable electric cures. However, the electric corset targeted women's medical complaints specifically. The electric corset claimed to cure all the issues for which conventional corsets were blamed, and afforded women an opportunity to continue to wear fashionable dress without worry. Equally, the promises of health and comfort presented in Scott and Harness's advertisements were similar to those made by manufacturers of regular corsets. Thus, the electric corset presented both a convenient and profitable solution: a garment for women who did not want to discard their fashionable undergarments, which offered the possibility of both fashionable figure and improved health.

In the nineteenth century, numerous entrepreneurs sought to exploit the mysterious power of electricity and capitalize on anxiety around women's health and bodies, selling dubious products that claimed to cure a myriad of illnesses. At a time when women's bodies and natural functions were widely pathologized, 'science' and the popular association between electricity and nervous vitality, enabled marketers to present some garments as a 'cure' and cause of good health.[62] The development and marketing strategies of the electric corset thus provide a case study of the intersections of marketing, emerging technologies, and quack medicine. The electric corset makes visible the ways that the pathologization of women's bodies in the nineteenth century, alongside the emergence of the science of electricity facilitated the development of fraudulent curative things which claimed to cure women of illnesses of modernity and sate the desire for fashionability and for health.

References

Appignanesi, Lisa, *Mad, Bad and Sad: A History of Women and the Mind Doctors from 1800 to the Present* (London: Virago, 2009)

[62] Ueyama, *Health in the Marketplace.*

Barker, A.T. and I.L. Freeston. 'Medical Applications of Electric and Magnetic Fields' in Electronics and Power, October (1985): pp. 757–760.

Cleghorn, Elinore. *Unwell Women: Misdiagnosis and Myth in a Man-Made World*. New York: Dutton Press, 2021.

Fields, Jill. 'Fighting the Corsetless Evil: Shaping Corsets and Culture, 1900–1930' in *The Journal of Social History*, 33:2 (1999): 355–384.

Gallagher, Catherine, and Thomas Laqueur. *The Making of the Modern Body: Sexuality and Society in the Nineteenth Century*. Berkley: University of California Press, 1987.

Gibson, Rebecca. *The Corseted Skeleton: A Bioarchaeology of Binding*. New York: Palgrave Macmillan, 2020.

Kevles, Daniel. 'Struggles for Truth: Scientists, Hucksters, and Charlatans in Nineteenth-Century America' in Social Research: An International Quarterly 85:4 (2018): pp. 863–887.

Martschukat, Jurgen. 'The Art of Killing by Electricity: The Sublime and the Electric Chair' in The Journal of American History 89:3 (Dec. 2002): pp. 900–921.

Matthews David, Alison. *Fashion Victims: The Dangers of Dress Past and Present* (2017) London: Bloomsbury.

McKnight, Alanna. 'The Kurious Kase of Kim Kardashian's Korset' in Fashion Studies 3:20 (2020a).

McKnight, Alanna. 'Palpably Ugly or Beauty of their Form? Corsets in Toronto Periodicals, 1871–1914' in *Popular Communication* 18:4 (2020b): pp. 301–312.

Meyer, Moritz. *Electricity in its Relations to Practical Medicine*, trans. Dr. William A. Hammond. New York: Appleton & Co., 1872.

Morus, Iwan Rhys. 'Bodily Disciplines and Disciplined Bodies: Instruments, Skills and Victorian Electrotherapeutics' in *Social History of Medicine* 19:2 (2006): pp. 241–259.

Morus, Iwan Rhys. 'No Mere Dream: Material Culture and Electrical Imagination' in *Centaurus* 57:3 (2015): pp. 173–191.

Morus, Iwan Rhys. 'The Measure of Man: Technologizing the Victorian Body' in *Science History*, 37 (1999): pp. 249–282.

Morus, Iwan Rhys. 'The Two Cultures of Electricity: Between Entertainment and Edification in Victorian Science' in *Science and Education* 16 (2007): pp. 593–602.

Morus, Iwan Rhys. *Shocking Bodies: Life, Death & Electricity in Victorian England*. Stroud, Gloucestershire: The History Press, 2011.

Murison, Justine. 'Quacks, Nostrums, and Miraculous Cures: Narratives of Medical Modernity in the Nineteenth-Century United States' in *Literature and Medicine* 32:2 (Fall 2014): pp 419–440.

Piccolino, Marco. 'Animal Electricity and the Birth of Electrophysiology: The Legacy of Luigi Galvani' in *The Brain Research Bulletin* 46:5 (1998): 381–407.
O'Hagan, Lauren. 'Blinded by Science? Constructing Truth and Authority in Early Twentieth Century Virol Advertisements in *History of Retailing and Consumption* 7:2 (2021): 162–192.
Steele, Valerie. *Corsets: A Cultural History.* New Haven: Yale University Press, 2001.
Stobart, Jon. 'Selling (through) Politeness: Advertising Provincial Shops in Eighteenth Century Britain' in Cultural and Social History 5:3 (2008), 316.
Summers, Leigh. *Bound to Please: A History of Victorian Corsets.* Oxford: Berg Press, 2001.
Thomas de la Pena, Carolyn. *The Body Electric: How Strange Machines Built the Modern America.* New York: New York University Press, 2003.
Ueyama, Takahiro. *Health in the Marketplace: Professionalism, Therapeutic Desires, and Medical Commodification in Late-Victorian London.* Palo Alto: The Society for the Promotion of Science and Scholarship, 2010.
Von Reichenbach, Karl. *The Odic Force: Letters on Od and Magnetism.* London: Hutchison and Co, 1926.
Waits, Robert. *The Medical Electricians: Dr. Scott and his Victorian Colleagues in Quackery.* Sunnyvale: J-IV-IX, 2013.

CHAPTER 11

Office Exercises

Lucie Armstrong

Office Exercises (2018) is a photographic series that explores the mental and physical impact of office work, with a particular focus on office wellness initiatives (Fig. 11.1). Produced before the Covid-19 pandemic (and so focussed on the corporate work environment rather than the home office) *Office Exercises* developed out of my experiences in a variety of temporary office jobs. Undertaking office work with an awareness that my presence there was transitory, I was able to view the work space through the eyes of a visitor (albeit a working one) (Fig. 11.2). Standing at a photocopier and enacting the same monotonous tasks over and again, I began to feel as though I was literally acting the role of an office worker, with the office the stage for my performance. The daily routines, consisting of repetitive physical movements and recurring conversations, transformed the environment into a theatre of productivity counterbalanced by an undercurrent of inertia.

Corporate posters advocating for the benefits of regular physical movement at work provided me with a set of visual reference points for my own photographic exploration of office 'wellness' culture. These posters

L. Armstrong (✉)
Leeds Arts University, Leeds, UK
e-mail: lucie.armstrong@leeds-art.ac.uk

D. Woolley et al. (eds.), *Wearable Objects and Curative Things*, Palgrave Studies in Fashion and the Body,
https://doi.org/10.1007/978-3-031-40017-9_11

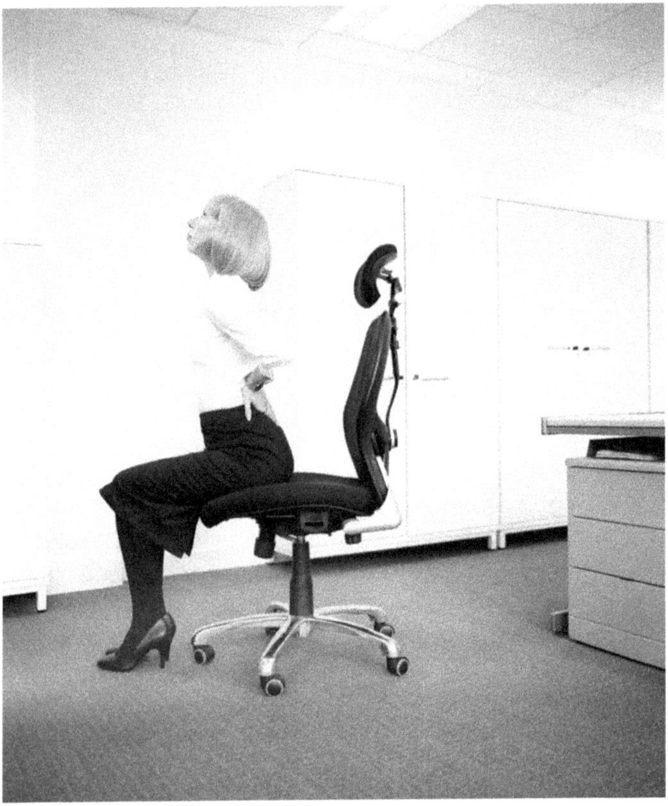

Fig. 11.1 Lucie Armstrong, *Office Exercises* I, 2018. (Photograph © Lucie Armstrong)

typically depicted employees holding poses designed to stretch the body out of its usual seated posture, with a striking number of positions incorporating the office chair as a physical extension of the worker's form. A highly symbolic object, the office chair acts as a cultural signifier of the many factors that make the office an absurd and potentially harmful environment for body and mind. Whilst the office chair can sometimes act as a tool for subversion and rebellion (exemplified by occasional outbursts of wild spinning or chair-based races with colleagues), it is first and foremost an apparatus for disciplining the normative corporate subject. With these illustrations of 'office exercises' as my source material, and with access to

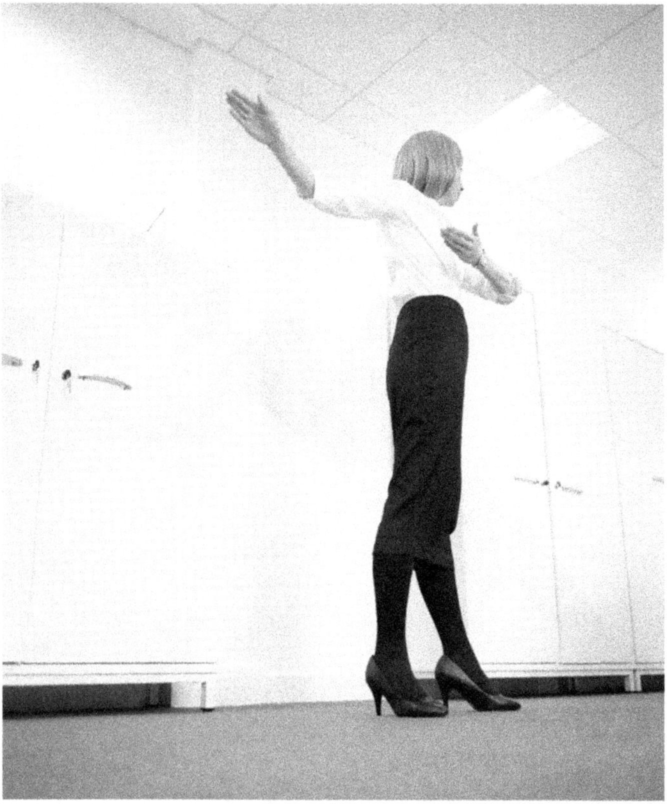

Fig. 11.2 Lucie Armstrong, *Office Exercises* II, 2018. (Photograph © Lucie Armstrong)

an office space that was closed for the weekend, I worked with a model to choreograph poses, producing a series of absurdist performative photographs.

This chapter offers an account of the influences and theories underpinning the project, and describes how the work was made. Although *Office Exercises* was not produced as a fashion editorial (which would have required the inclusion of varied and styled looks) the visual language and sequencing of fashion images influenced the making of the photographs (Fig. 11.3). This chapter therefore focuses on two significant connections between *Office Exercises* and the contemporary fashion image: the office

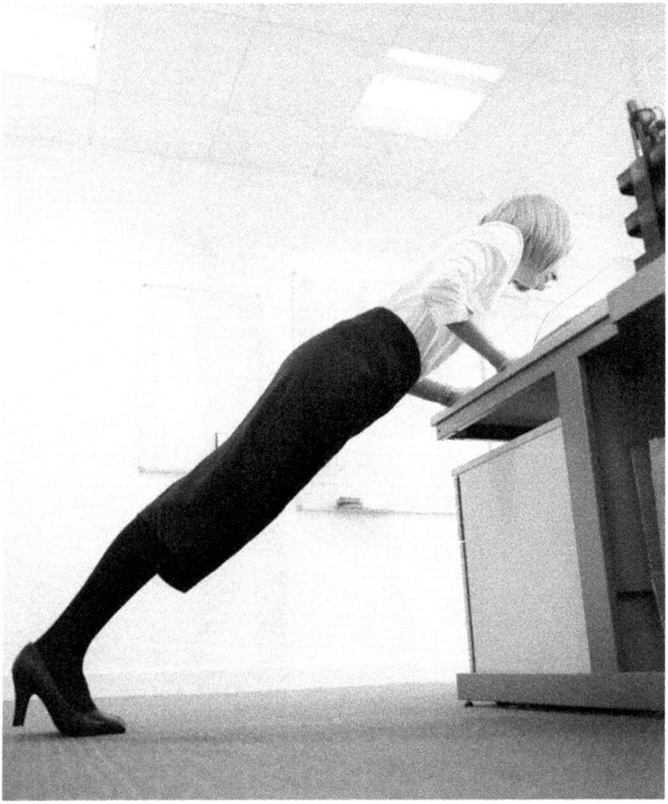

Fig. 11.3 Lucie Armstrong, *Office Exercises* III, 2018. (Photograph © Lucie Armstrong)

environment as a popular fashion shoot location, and a performative approach to bodily posture (Fig. 11.4).

11.1 Wellness in the Workplace

The office chair can be viewed as an apparatus for establishing workplace discipline. Sarah Sharma has analysed sedentary work and the introduction of yoga classes in the corporate workplace, drawing on Foucault's argument about how postures of the worker's body are limited and controlled

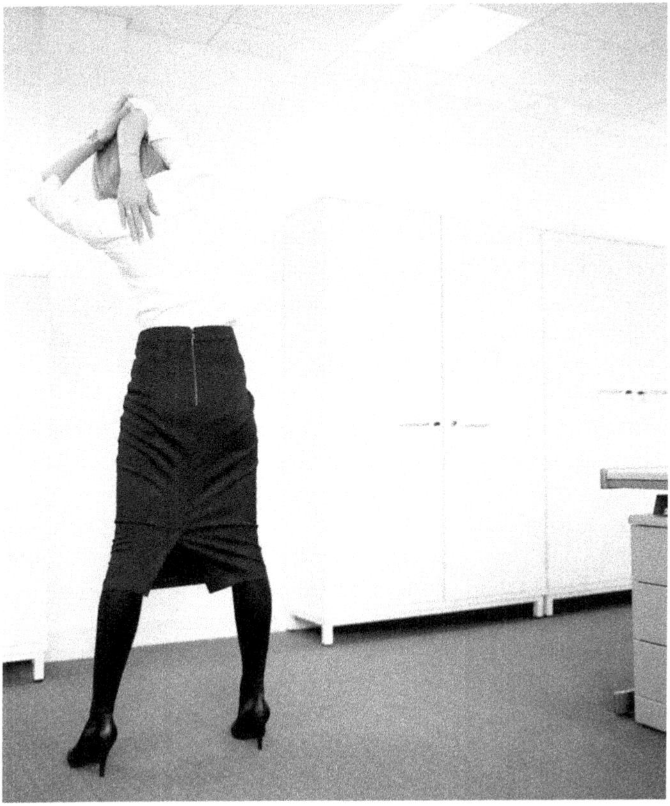

Fig. 11.4 Lucie Armstrong, *Office Exercises* IV, 2018. (Photograph © Lucie Armstrong)

to ensure speed and efficiency.[1] The office chair fulfils a role of quiet enforcement, positioning the body to enhance productivity. Sharma observes that the body remains active when it is seated: 'Even while sitting in front of screens, bodies are transmitting information: moving, sharing, connecting, and creating it'.[2]

[1] Sarah Sharma, *In the Meantime: Temporality and Cultural Politics*, Durham and London: Duke University Press, 2014.

[2] Sharma, *In the Meantime: Temporality and Cultural Politics*, p. 94.

The health impacts of sedentary work are well established: inactivity and sitting for long periods of time are associated with raised risks of obesity, type 2 diabetes, some types of cancer and shortened life expectancy.[3] Vybarr Cregan-Reid notes that two hours spent in the sitting position significantly reduces blood flow and blood sugar levels, and that even for those achieving the recommended levels of daily activity, long periods spent seated can undermine the benefits of regular exercise.[4] The promotion of physical movement in the office space might initially be considered a positive intervention by employers to improve the work environment for their employees. However, standing up and exercising periodically throughout the day is unlikely to combat the health issues linked to sedentary work, suggesting that office wellness initiatives may be little more than a panacea.

However, such programmes may achieve other less obvious outcomes. Reviewing the use of advertisements to promote corporate yoga classes, Sharma notes that a professional image is maintained during the yoga classes. The workers are dressed in office attire, sitting at their desks in a cross-legged yoga pose. A clock behind them highlights that although a change of task has taken place, they are still working to a scheduled time frame. The worker might view the yoga class as an opportunity to take a break from work and devote some time and headspace to themselves. However, they remain in the workplace, saving time that might otherwise be used travelling to another location, and using their lunch break to improve their health and mental wellbeing, potentially improving their stamina and concentration for work. Sharma writes that employers bring yoga into the workplace as a means to 'take further disciplinary control over the worker's body by mobilizing time differently'.[5] This mobilisation is created by offering 'a new experience of time within the confines of a sedentary life' and a 'renewed sense of time' for the employee.[6] This adaptation of the work day to incorporate wellness activities helps to maintain a system of compliance and normalisation within the workforce.[7] The overworked employee views their employer as caring about their workers'

[3] NHS, '*Why we should sit less*,' https://www.nhs.uk/live-well/exercise/exercise-guidelines/why-sitting-too-much-is-bad-for-us/.

[4] Vybarr Cregan-Reid, '*Primate Change: How The World We Made Is Remaking Us*' https://play.google.com/books/reader?id=XcJWDwAAQBAJ&hl=en_GB.

[5] Sharma, *In the Meantime: Temporality and Cultural Politics*, p. 95.

[6] Sharma, *In the Meantime: Temporality and Cultural Politics*, p. 84.

[7] Sharma, *In the Meantime: Temporality and Cultural Politics*.

'total selves—physical, material, and spiritual well-being'.[8] In return, the employer benefits from an agreeable and productive workforce. The system of compliance to which office yoga contributes goes beyond the employees' acceptance of a work-life imbalance that is skewed to prioritise work, enrolling them as responsible citizens in the neoliberal work environment. The employees are not only working on their designated office tasks but also working on themselves. The notion that personal fulfilment can be achieved at work maintains a cycle of productivity and a workforce eager to excel.[9]

The responsible citizen is also discussed by Katherine Teghtsoonian, who notes that a good citizen is expected to 'take responsibility for making choices that ensure they will be able to contribute as healthy, productive members of their workplaces and communities'.[10] The responsibility for good health is placed with the worker, not with the employer (who actually has the means to make changes to the environment and structure of the working day). Teghtsoonian's analysis, based on emerging health policy relating to depression in a Canadian workplace, finds that employees are expected to care for themselves outside of work time in order to optimise their ability when in work. She writes 'Rather than directing their energies to organizational or political change, "responsibilized" employees diagnosed mentally ill are exhorted instead to undertake the work of self-care and self-management'.[11] Time associated with personal freedom is increasingly absorbed by the requirements of the workplace, now designated for rest and recovery, rather than for pursuing interests and aspirations unconnected to paid employment.

Lauren Berlant has also articulated how our 'bodily lives are shaped pretty significantly' by the demands of work.[12] Citing David Harvey, she writes that in capitalist societies sickness is defined as being unable to work, and that 'many arguments for exercise and healthy eating do not focus on cultivating better health: they're about having more energy to be

[8] Sharma, *In the Meantime: Temporality and Cultural Politics*, p. 84.

[9] Sharma, *In the Meantime: Temporality and Cultural Politics.*

[10] Katherine Teghtsoonian, 'Managing Workplace Depression: Contesting the Contours of Emerging Policy in the Workplace,' *in Contesting Illness: Process and Practices*, ed. Pamela Moss and Katherine Teghtsoonian, p. 72.

[11] Teghtsoonian, '*Managing Workplace Depression*', p. 72.

[12] Lauren Berlant, '*Risky Bigness: On Obesity, Eating, and the Ambiguity of 'Health*,' in Against health: How Health Became the New Morality, ed. Jonathan M. Metzl and Anna Kirkland, p. 29.

more productive'.[13] The act of taking responsibility and the stresses of everyday life exhaust 'our practical sovereignty', and as a result, people are 'tired from work, tired from being good, tired from being overwhelmed by the demands of production and the reproduction of life'.[14] Berlant argues that this mental exhaustion leads employees to develop habits that cause and exacerbate health problems. For example, pressed for time and lethargic, many workers choose to remain at their desks during their lunch breaks, avoiding the expense of energy 'it takes to manage the sociality of lunch and rest along with giving the body what it needs'.[15] Workers may also eat unhealthy, comforting food as a form of self-medication for fatigue and an opportunity to 'become absorbed in the present', providing pleasure and enabling them 'to *feel* more resilient in the everyday'.[16] Gaining weight may be viewed as a form of negotiation of workplace stress and an 'effect of the intensity with which so many people need more and more mental health vacations from their exhaustion'.[17] The daily compliance of the worker, in the hope of achieving 'the good life', is an on-going pursuit with no end in sight.[18]

Instead of maintaining the body in a posture that is productive for work, the office chair can become a site of mental and physical decline. Whilst some individuals may enjoy their jobs, this is not the case for all: for many workers, worry about the value and purpose of work and life is a daily activity that may contribute to mental health issues. David Graeber discusses the rise of pointless jobs, in which workers feel that they are devoting their days to tasks that are valueless and unnecessary[19]: whilst the jobs that Graeber analyses are not limited to office-based roles, the uniformity and ubiquity of office work makes it an exemplar of repetitive and unengaging white-collar labour in the UK. Graeber writes: 'It's not just an assault on the person's sense of self-importance but also a direct attack on the very foundations of the sense that one even *is* a self. A human being unable to have a meaningful impact on the world ceases to exist'.[20] Boring and demoralising work denies workers full subjectivity as valued,

[13] Berlant, 'Risky Bigness', p. 28.
[14] Berlant, 'Risky Bigness', pp. 27 and 30.
[15] Berlant, 'Risky Bigness', p. 28.
[16] Berlant, 'Risky Bigness', p. 27.
[17] Berlant, 'Risky Bigness', p. 27.
[18] Berlant, 'Risky Bigness', p. 32.
[19] Graeber, *Bullshit Jobs*, London: Penguin Books, 2019.
[20] Graeber, *Bullshit Jobs*, pp. 83–84.

contributing members of society, often with debilitating consequences for their health.

In conversations with my office colleagues, I discovered that many people spent time at work imagining a different way of life: anxiety caused by the inability to pursue an alternative, and feelings of boredom, frustration and entrapment were common. I too experienced the office environment as a space of perpetual introspection and self-analysis, enabled by the repetitive nature of the tasks (such as data entry) that I was required to perform. When my brain was not used for complex activities, it quickly wandered to reflect on why my time was consumed by pointless labour that prevented me from pursuing more creative endeavours. As a result of this, I would feel anxious and unhappy, which quickly led to the desire for a mental health holiday.[21] *Office Exercises* was a reaction to this experience.

11.2 Office Spaces and Attire in Fashion Photography

Many employers have dispensed with strict (gendered) dress guidelines; for example, Virgin Atlantic now allow employees to wear either skirts or trousers and no longer require female crew members to wear make-up.[22] However, many office workers choose to wear formal office attire and in *Office Exercises* these recognisable garments help to reinforce the absurdity and futility of office wellbeing initiatives. The white buttoned shirt and the knee-length pencil skirt, both closely associated with office dress, can be uncomfortable to sit down in for eight hours a day. These garments are also impractical when performing office exercises and it seems unlikely that typical office attire was considered when devising these initiatives. Furthermore, such workwear would be extremely uncomfortable and restrictive if worn when performing the yoga poses that feature in the posters described by Sharma. It seems that the exercises are promoted without the expectation that they can actually be performed.

Office Exercises reference the static poses of workplace wellness posters, recreating them for the camera as though the model is mid-task. The restrictive nature of the garments is noticeable: the shirt rises and untucks

[21] Berlant, 'Risky Bigness'.

[22] Sirin Kale, 'Why should I have to work on stilts': the women fighting sexist dress codes,' https://www.theguardian.com/lifeandstyle/2019/jul/11/why-should-i-have-to-work-on-stilts-the-women-fighting-sexist-dress-codes, accessed.

itself. Each pose was held for a prolonged period of time to allow the photographs to be adequately framed, focussed and lit: counterintuitively, the model experienced physical discomfort undertaking an action intended to be a health-improving activity. The photographs therefore performatively reproduce the paradoxical notion of wellness in office environments. Each exercise culminated in a fixed moment perfected through many repetitions: this approach to making the images echoes the monotonous daily grind of tasks that inspired the project.

In fashion photography, as in *Office Exercises*, the office environment is a space where stylised workers are pushed and pulled into uncomfortable and contorted positions, symbolising the expectation of compliant workplace behaviour. There is also an aspect of subversion in the use of the office in these scenes: fashion photographs frequently create a work space in which no office work actually happens. For example, Isabelle Wenzel—an artist using performance, photography and moving image and predominantly working in self-portraiture—creates and holds 'an impossible position' captured with the camera's self-timer function.[23] As a trained acrobat, Wenzel is able to transform her body into sculptural forms: this is a key aspect of her practice, focusing on the expressive force of the body rather than the face or identity of the subject. Her earlier works, shown as part of Wenzel's 2010 solo exhibition, 'Building Images' at Kunst Kapel, Amsterdam and Virtueei Museum Vuidas, Amsterdam, explored the conventional visual tropes of the office environment, with office-wear and props used in absurdist constructed images that imply frustration and repetition. One photograph features Wenzel in a crouched pose that looks uncomfortable and potentially painful. Wenzel holds a stack of lever-arch files behind their back in a contorted pose. Another image shows Wenzel dressed in a knee-length skirt, opaque tights and heels, balancing on a chair with their back on the seat area and their legs held up and positioned above the head. Papers fill the space between their chest and legs, covering the face and arms: they are literally drowning in paperwork. In each image by Wenzel, office paraphernalia both support and hinder the body in its contorted poses. The poses resemble yoga postures taken to absurd extremes, beyond wellness and into physical collapse: indeed, the series could be considered as a humorous response to the office yoga posters that Schama discusses.

[23] Isabelle Wenzel, 'About' https://www.isabelle-wenzel.com/.

11.3 Performative Poses in Fashion Photography

Working with a model or models and focusing on the sculptural form of the body, this method (used by Wenzel and in *Office Exercises*) has been a common motif in fashion photography during the last two decades. In 2017, curator and writer Shonagh Marshall and photographic director Holly Hay produced a multi-faceted project titled *Posturing: Photographing the Body in Fashion*. The project includes an exhibition, film and book exploring a new aesthetic vision in fashion photography that asks the question 'what is this new landscape, in which glamour and opulence have been superseded by humour and absurdity?'[24]

Works by Charlie Engman are included in *Posturing*, providing key examples of how the body is presented through a performative and absurdist lens in contemporary fashion photography. An editorial for *Dazed* magazine in 2014 shows a model creating exaggerated shapes with their body in a manner that seems at odds with the spacious outdoor environments they are acting within. The model rolls on the ground while their arms and legs are positioned in static poses: they run in different directions and seem to fall backwards and stumble for no reason. An editorial for issue 5 of *Alla Carta* magazine, also 2014, presents a series of images that contain the traditional components of fashion photography—garments, props and location—but focuses on the gesturing body as the subject of the images. In this series, the face of the model is not shown as the body bends and turns, interacting with objects within an interior space. At times the body is almost unrecognisable as a body.

An important feature of the *Posturing* approach to fashion photography is the active participation of the model in the construction of the fashion image. Maisie Skidmore and Holly Hay discuss this in the *British Journal of Photography*, stating that photographers now look for models who can collaborate in making the image. Photographers ask models to forget what they have learned about posing for the camera and instead participate in an approach in which the photographer and models are both performing, working together to draw out new and different movements in the image.[25]

[24] Maisie Skidmore, 'Posturing—a new vision of the body in fashion', https://www.1854.photography/2018/04/posturingfashion/.

[25] Skidmore, 'Posturing'.

The expressive use of the body is also evident in advertising media. In Adidas x Marimekko, shot by Laura McCluskey, the sportswear fashion brand aligns its identity with ideas of freedom and unity through movement and posturing of the body. Photographs and videos created for the brand's campaign show people moving as a group and individually to create expressive shapes with their bodies. McCluskey has previously worked with a number of dancers to produce a personal project exploring feelings of unrest and anxiety.[26] The photographic series captures improvised dance, freezing the subjects in time as they perform complex and fluid movements with their bodies. These images formed the photobook, *The Blue Above* published in 2019.

The use of performance in fashion imagery has grown in popularity, creating the need for movement directors in production teams, a title that is now frequently seen in the credits of fashion editorials and campaigns. Ryan Chappell, a dancer and choreographer, describes their role as a movement director as helping to develop a collaborative experience between the photographer and model. Chappell also works with people through their Movement+ development programme which provides mentoring centred around breaking down psychological barriers through movement. Chappell emphasises the importance in the ability to embody emotions and in having a strong connection between mind and body.[27]

The growth of the use of performance in fashion photography aligns with an increase in photographers communicating their own experience through their creative practice. Performance and choreography are used as a method to translate and express aspects of the self. For example, *The New Black Vanguard* by Antwaun Sargent (first published in 2019, and followed by international exhibitions) highlights the growing influence of black photographers in contemporary fashion image-making.[28] Arielle Bobb-Willis, one of the photographers featured in *The New Black Vanguard*, creates photographic images that express their personal experience regarding identity and mental health. For the viewer, the awkward positions of the (often faceless) subjects in Bobb-Willis' photographs may seem uncomfortable, conveying insecurity and fear. In contrast to the use

[26] 'Laura McCluskey, Blue Above', *Guest Editions*, https://guesteditions.com/products/blue-above-regular-edition.

[27] Martin Onufrowicz, 'Ryan Chappell: What does a Movement Director do', https://1granary.com/fashion-image/ryan-chappell-what-does-a-movement-director-do/.

[28] Aperture, *The New Black Vanguard: Photography between Art and Fashion, Curated by Antwaun Sargent. Aperture.* https://aperture.org/exhibition/the-new-black-vanguard.

of brightly coloured garments, the model's body moves and pauses in poses that aim to visualise the photographer's struggle with mental health. When discussing their work in the *British Journal of Photography*, Bobb-Willis describes how the body of the model symbolises the part of themselves that was in a state of depression and the emotionally uncomfortable experiences they have been positioned in.[29] Sarah Kent notes the inclusion of or allusion to mental health issues in fashion photography has increased in recent years, due to the 'rise of social media and a shifting cultural and political landscape [...] catapulting such conversations into the mainstream'.[30]

Locating fashion editorials in realistic, if not banal, scenes and scenarios, may also enable photographers to engage with personal experience and everyday life more explicitly in their work. For example, Pascal Gambarte's photograph of a 'woman in a crab pose on a corporate office desk for *Marfa Journal*' is described by Hay and Marshall as 'a move away from fantastical sets and towards the domestic sphere'.[31]

11.4 Conclusion

The emergence of the angled and twisted figure in fashion imagery, alongside the use of realistic scenarios, could be interpreted as a reaction to the idealisation of the overworked individual and the growth of mental health issues in relation to work. The office environment and contorted poses of the body enable fashion photography to imply that the continuation of everyday life depends on individuals adapting to uncomfortable and awkward positions. Holding a crab pose atop a desk while clad in the latest fashion is a logical exaggeration of the worker in office attire attempting a cross-legged yoga position while seated on their office chair. As this chapter argues, the discomfort caused by some types of work is both physical and mental. As fashion photographers continue to highlight individual and cultural experiences of anxiety and distress, my own photographic practice has continued to communicate issues around mental health by visualising manifestations of anxiety. My current creative outputs are

[29] Marigold Warner, 'Arielle Bobb-Willis' darker shade of bright', https://www.1854.photography/2018/05/arielle-bobb-willis-darker-shade-of-bright/.

[30] Sarah Kent, 'Fashion's Long Road to Inclusivity', https://www.businessoffashion.com/articles/news-analysis/fashions-long-road-to-inclusivity/.

[31] Skidmore, 'Posturing—a new vision of the body in fashion'.

influenced by experiences of the fear of missing out (on life) and how this has become normalised in capitalist societies. I continue to examine the anxiety that is caused by the difficulty in regulating or maintaining work-life balance and the on-going hope of attaining the elusive good life.[32] The ubiquity of temporary and zero-hour contracts and the normalisation of pointless and unfulfilling jobs keep many individuals trapped in the cycle of precarious and demoralising work which produces precarious mental and physical health. *Office Exercises*—and in particular the office chair—symbolise the absurd paradox of workplace wellbeing. Twenty minutes of chair yoga during a lunch break will not alleviate the impact of eight hours of sedentary work. Such activities are distractions at best, enrolling workers in a regime of compliance in which they accept responsibility for the detrimental effects of their labour on their health. Subversive acts like office chair racing may be the 'mental health vacations' that workers really need to counter the debilitating tedium of the work.[33] However, office health and safety guidelines are unlikely to permit them.

References

Aperture, n.d. *The New Black Vanguard: Photography between Art and Fashion, Curated by Antwaun Sargent. Aperture.* https://aperture.org/exhibition/the-new-black-vanguard.

Berlant, Lauren, "Risky Bigness: On Obesity, Eating, and the Ambiguity of 'Health'," in *Against health: How Health Became the New Morality*, ed. Jonathan M. Metzl and Anna Kirkland, New York and London: New York University Press (2010).

Cregan-Reid, Vybarr, '*Primate Change: How The World We Made Is Remaking Us*'. London: Hachette UK, 2018. Google Play, https://play.google.com/books/reader?id=XcJWDwAAQBAJ&hl=en_GB.

Graeber, David, *Bullshit Jobs*. London: Penguin Books, 2019.

Guest Editions, '*Laura McCluskey, Blue Above*'. Guest Editions. https://guesteditions.com/products/blue-above-regular-edition.

Isabelle Wenzel, 'About'. *Isabelle Wenzel*. https://www.isabelle-wenzel.com/.

Kale, Sirin, 'Why should I have to work on stilts': the women fighting sexist dress codes'. *The Guardian*, July 11, 2019. https://www.theguardian.com/lifeandstyle/2019/jul/11/why-should-i-have-to-work-on-stilts-the-women-fighting-sexist-dress-codes

[32] Berlant, 'Risky Bigness'.

[33] Berlant, 'Risky Bigness'.

Keaney, Magda, 'Does Fashion Photography matter?' *Frances Corner*, March 16, 2015. https://www.francescorner.com/does-fashion-photography-matter-by-magda-keaney/.

Kent, Sarah, 'Fashion's Long Road to Inclusivity'. *Business of Fashion*, October 7, 2019. https://www.businessoffashion.com/articles/news-analysis/fashions-long-road-to-inclusivity/.

Maynard, Margaret, 'The Fashion Photograph: An Ecology', in *Fashion as Photograph*, ed. Eugenie Shinkle, London: IB Taurus & Co Ltd. (2008): 56

NHS England, 'Mental Health'. *NHS England*. https://www.england.nhs.uk/mental-health/.

NHS UK, 'Why we should sit less'. *NHS UK*, Last reviewed November 22, 2019. https://www.nhs.uk/live-well/exercise/exercise-guidelines/why-sitting-too-much-is-bad-for-us/.

Onufrowicz, Martin, 'Ryan Chappell: What does a Movement Director do'. *1Granary*, December 1, 2021. https://1granary.com/fashion-image/ryan-chappell-what-does-a-movement-director-do/.

Sharma, Sarah, *In the Meantime: Temporality and Cultural Politics*. Durham and London: Duke University Press, 2014.

Skidmore, Maisie, 'Posturing—a new vision of the body in fashion'. *British Journal of Photography*, April 3, 2018. https://www.1854.photography/2018/04/posturingfashion/.

Stoppard, Lou, 'The Fashion Image after Nan Goldin', *Aperture*, June 24, 2020. https://aperture.org/essays/fashion-photography-after-nan-goldin/.

Teghtsoonian, Katherine, 'Managing Workplace Depression: Contesting the Contours of Emerging Policy in the Workplace', in *Contesting Illness: Process and Practices*, ed. Pamela Moss and Katherine Teghtsoonian, Toronto, Buffalo and London: University of Toronto Press (2008).

Warner, Marigold, 'Arielle Bobb-Willis' darker shade of bright'. *British Journal of Photograph*, May 21, 2018. https://www.1854.photography/2018/05/arielle-bobb-willis-darker-shade-of-bright/.

COMMUNICATING

Paula Chambers

Things communicate with us all the time: we share information with the objects and materials around us in an ongoing loop of what Karen Barad has termed intra-action, a dynamic process of exchange between the human and the non-human.[1] When an electric kettle boils we hear (and see) the bubbling of water, we see steam rising from the pouring lip, we hear the click as the mechanism cuts out, we understand that the water has boiled and can now be poured for that reviving cup of tea or reassuring cup of hot chocolate. When we lift the kettle off its stand it has weight; with experience we can guess how much water is in the kettle without having to look. We understand other properties of the kettle too, the moulded (often) plastic body and handle tells us about its manufacture, the base with heat element has a lead that plugs into a socket in the wall that we understand as being powered by electricity which travels (as if by magic) through copper wires, and so on. The same sort of communication loop happens with the clothes we wear, for example, that itchy wool jumper we know has been made from the shorn and processed coat of a sheep; or for example with the soil in our garden as we plant spring bulbs, we know it is full of worms and other organisms helpful for breaking down decaying matter. We may not know clearly how certain processes work, or how or from where certain materials or manufactured objects appear, but we do in fact have a very sophisticated way of understanding what it is these things are telling us, about themselves, about ourselves and about the

[1] Karen Barad, *Meeting the Universe Halfway: Quantum Physics and the Entanglement of Matter and Meaning*. Durham: Duke University Press, 2007, 141.

world more widely. Objects speak of the things that they are, and of all the things that we know about things like them, a process Sara Ahmed terms *co-perceived*.[2] Developing Heidegger's philosophy of things whereby the thing is always becoming, the thing communicates an ***in-order-to*** Ahmed identifies as the tendency of objects, objects or things understood as what they do, yet also what they allow us to do, the thing communicates 'capacities that are open to the future'.[3] Barad's concept of intra-action is one which enables us to understand our relationship with things as being the process through which agency is shared between bodies, human and non-human, processes of communication that go both ways.

In *The Language of Things*, Hito Steyerl asks 'What if things could speak? What would they tell us? Or are they speaking already and we just don't hear them? And who is going to translate them?'[4] Steyerl reminds us that the materialist understanding of commodities as a condensation of social forces is one that Walter Benjamin interpreted as objects consisting of tensions, forces, and hidden powers, which keep being exchanged,[5] an idea which is in many ways what Barad was also explaining and expanding upon with her concept of intra-action, but perhaps is also closely linked to animism and other forms of magical thinking. Michael Taussig proposes that storytelling animates things, and that through certain media, and at certain times, things assume the task of the storyteller, at these intersectional moments materialist and spiritual philosophies reconcile and reinforce one another.[6] Although Taussig was discussing film and fictional narrative, he situated this animating principle within the things themselves. The things analysed and contextualised in the following chapters each in their own way animate ideas and forms of relationality through processes of communication. Their specific and individual thingness speaks of and to their time, their maker, their wearer, their performers, producers, actors and agents. The Crazy Jane hat, the Maria medallion; wounds, holes, text, language and script; votives and charm bracelets, an assemblage of ideas, objects and things that are not just an aggregate of individual traits, nor an

[2] Sara Ahmed, *Queer Phenomenology: Orientations, Objects, Others*, Durham and London, Duke University Press, 2006, 30.

[3] Ahmed, *Queer Phenomenology*, p. 46.

[4] Hito Steyerl, *The Language of Things*, Transversal Texts. June, 2006, https://transversal.at/transversal/0606/steyerl/en (accessed 20th January 2023).

[5] Steyerl, *The Language of Things*, np.

[6] Michael Taussig, *The Stories Things Tell and Why They Tell Them* in *The Corn Wolf*. University of Chicago Press, 2015, 22.

accumulation of specific properties but are rather the always-becoming things identified by Heidegger, the materialisation of processes of communication that go both ways.[7]

Returning to our boiling kettle and that reviving cup of tea or reassuring cup of hot chocolate, and considering Steyerl's question of translation in more depth, we can consider that there are other channels of communication open here too. We translate experiences and emotions through things and objects, or they translate for us. The souvenir or memento becomes a holder of memory; that childhood teddy bear that offered comfort and consolation (an object identified by Winnicott as transitional) is the kind of 'object[s] we can experience as both within and outside of the self'.[8] Sherry Turkle writes that objects communicate social relations, they reveal themselves as gifts and as networks, 'the object is animated by the network within it'.[9] Turkle identifies and contextualises a series of things she calls evocative objects, things that speak of the vast structure of recollection, subjective, communal, social, cultural and historical. These types of things are object as facilitator, often of affect (of mourning, of love, of joy, of trauma or despair, etc.), but can also be a facilitator of learning, or of fear (amongst other emotive recollections). There is an intimacy to these types of things: they share a relationship to the body as intra-action. The Crazy Jane hat and the Maria medallion analysed and contextualised in Anna Jamieson's chapter are objects that communicate on several levels: they speak to the wearer of certain societal expectations, and act as a moral warning, yet they also communicate outwards too, conveying subtle social and cultural codes about the wearer's class, fashionability and emotional sensibility. These objects are associative symbols that take the role as facilitator of affect via a subtle network of object materiality and subjective agency. Like an actor who breaks a monologue to address the audience, these multiple channels of communication are understood simultaneously by all parties, yet are not directly acknowledged as being so. Each plays their own part, aware of the role of the other, yet bound by convention to adhere to the prescribed script.

Katharina Ludwig's play without a play *(Ad)dressing Wounds—A Trauma in Seven Act(or)s*, communicates through its form as much as its content. The structure, use of language and narrative flow mimics that of

[7] Ahmed, *Queer Phenomenology*, 36.

[8] Sherry Turkle, *Evocative Objects: Things We Think With*. MIT Press, 2007, 314.

[9] Turkle, *Evocative Objects*, 312.

theatrical performance, yet these assumed channels of (mis)information are misleading in this particular context, for the real communication takes place in the holes and gaps in the text which act like pauses for breath or thinking space. Communication here is both physical and temporal, this is language that materialises Taussig's intersectional moments where storytelling animates things at the same time as things assume the task of the storyteller.[10] Garry Barker's handmade votives and charms communicate in a call-and-response format; processes of conversing, imagining, making, giving, healing and returning can be understood as a literal materialisation (a coming-into-being) of individual's health-related experiences. These are objects as the congealed residue of performance and agency as proposed by Alfred Gell.[11] The agency of artist as maker, of the responder who relates their health concerns then receives a charm or votive, and the agency of the object itself as it first materialises, then assuages the dis-ease of the responder. All of the objects in the following chapters, human and non-human, can be co-perceived: they speak to us of the things that they are, and of all the things that we know about things like them.[12] The language these objects and things speak is that of mutual exchange, whereby processes of communication animate the dynamic exchange of properties and forces as intra-action.

References

Ahmed, Sara. *Queer Phenomenology: Orientations, Objects, Others*, Durham and London, Duke University Press, 2006.

Barad, Karen. *Meeting the Universe Halfway: Quantum Physics and the Entanglement of Matter and Meaning*. Durham: Duke University Press, 2007.

Gell, Alfred. *Art and Agency: An Anthropological Theory.* Oxford: Oxford University Press, 1998.

[10] Taussig, *The Stories Things Tell and Why They Tell Them* in *The Corn Wolf.*

[11] Alfred Gell, *Art and Agency: An Anthropological Theory.* Oxford University Press, 1998, 67.

[12] Ibid., p. 30.

Steyerl, Hito. *The Language of Things*. Transversal Texts. June, 2006 https://transversal.at/transversal/0606/steyerl/en (accessed 20th January 2023).
Taussig, Michael. '*The Stories Things Tell and Why They Tell Them*' in *The Corn Wolf, 15–30*. Chicago: University of Chicago Press, 2015.
Turkle, Sherry. *Evocative Objects: Things We Think With*. Cambridge, Massachusetts: MIT Press, 2007.

CHAPTER 12

Votives and Charm Bracelets: Materialising Health-Related Experiences Through 'Sacred' Objects

Garry Barker

Votives promise a connection between everyday human existence and psychical or spiritual experience. The concept of a physical artefact acting as an intermediary between the embodied individual and the quasi-divine has historically taken many forms, including charms and tokens worn to ward off evil and ensure good spiritual and physical health.[1] As an artist, my practice aims to give material form to people's psychological relationships with their bodies; to do this, I frequently incorporate votive objects into my working process. My practice responds to themes that emerge from one-on-one conversations with project participants: physical outcomes include ceramics, drawing, printmaking, painting, wallpaper design, textiles, writings, installation and game design, often exhibited alongside

[1] Ittai Weinryb (ed.), *Ex Voto: Votive Giving Across Cultures* (New York: Bard Graduate Center, 2016).

G. Barker (✉)
Leeds Arts University, Leeds, UK

D. Woolley et al. (eds.), *Wearable Objects and Curative Things*, Palgrave Studies in Fashion and the Body,
https://doi.org/10.1007/978-3-031-40017-9_12

more performative work involving face-to-face conversations akin to the exchanges that one might have with a fortune teller or tarot reader. My recent work focuses on participants' lived experiences of physical and mental health in relation to ageing, an experience that I myself share.[2]

This chapter contextualises my use of votives and charms to articulate and materialise health-related narratives, with particular focus on two projects: a commission in 2021 for *Beyond Measure?*, a programme exploring research and evidence in culture and health; and a more recent exploration of the votive possibilities offered by very small images and objects, using the charm bracelet as a device for mediating between everyday reality and wish fulfilment.

* * *

Religious folk charms are still used as votive offerings in many Catholic societies and charms worn on the body have operated as mediation devices between the human and the divine for millennia. Charm bracelets today are often regarded primarily as fashion accessories, yet decorative charms may also have personal significance for the owner, commemorating life events, invoking good luck, or providing a focus in times of joy, illness, self-discovery or sadness: arguably, the charm bracelet today performs a function similar to votives within ancient animist practices.[3] I understand the rising popularity of Milagros or 'miracle' charms—once designed to be pinned to objects of devotion in a shrine, but now advertised for clip-on charm bracelets—as a sign of spiritual need in a post-religious society[4]: these fashionable objects offer rich source material for an artistic enquiry into the contemporary reinvention and re-positioning of votive forms. As Jessica Hughes points out in her work on the 'object biography' of votives,

[2] Garry Barker, 'Drawing Age', *Drawing: Research, Theory and Practice* 5, no. 2 (2020): 351–361; Garry Barker, 'Is It To Feel Each Limb Grow Stiffer, Is It To Feel The Full Potential Of A Life?' *TRACEY* 15, no.1 (2021): 1–17; Garry Barker, 'In Conversation,' *Shine Magazine*, 2022, https://www.shinealight.org.uk/inconversation-garrybarker. Accessed 9 September 2022; Garry Barker, Life Hacks for Limited Futures, 2020 https://lifehacksforlimitedfutures.wordpress.com/author/garrybarker69/. Accessed 9 September 2022.

[3] Jade Albert and Kai Hackney, *The Charm of Charms* (London: Abrams, 2005); Deborah Alun-Jones and John Ayton, *Charming: The Magic of Charm Jewelry* (London: Thames and Hudson, 2005).

[4] Robert Shanafelt, 'Magic, miracle, and marvels in anthropology', *Ethnos* 69, no. 3 (2004): 317–340.

in modern societies the votive form has had continued significance as a site for transactional processes that operate between one realm and another, between the everyday and concepts of luck, spiritual need and religious belief.[5]

Over an extended period, I have used my practice to explore object-making in relation to the ways in which humans think and feel about their ageing bodies. I have made drawings and objects that consider my personal experience of ageing and respond to my own changing form. I have also made work in one-to-one dialogue with a series of older individuals reflecting on their ageing bodies and exploring ways in which their feelings about ageing might be visualised or materialised: through these conversations, a visual language emerged out of iterative methods of working with drawing materials and clay, and was subsequently refined in response to feedback from my interlocutors.[6] The research resulted in a range of visualisations of externalised feelings about the body, exhibited at Workshop Press Gallery, Leeds, in 2019–2020.

However, there were still questions relating to the agency of the objects and images produced. How can artefacts of this sort be used? Could these objects be used as tools for materialising, manifesting and externalising interior thought processes? Bruno Latour observes that objects themselves are the result of a process of negotiation between the material world and humans.[7] This notion of object agency is echoed in Clark and Chamber's concept of the extended mind; Johnson's work on embodiment and thought as inseparable from the physical world in which we are embedded; and the work of Jane Bennett and Karen Barad who have both highlighted a 'material turn' in relation to our understanding of ourselves and our relationship with the world.[8]

[5] Jessica Hughes, 'Fractured Narratives: Writing the Biography of a Votive Offering', in *Ex Voto: Votive giving across cultures*, ed. Ittai Weinryb (New York: Bard Graduate Center, 2016), 23–48.

[6] For further information on this process, see Garry Barker, 'Drawing the Embodied Mind: A Project Report on Research Into Interoception', *PSIAX #5 Estudos e reflexões sobre desenho e imagem* 5 (2021): 17–24.

[7] Bruno Latour, *Reassembling the Social: An introduction to actor-network-theory*, Oxford: OUP, 2007.

[8] Andy Clark and David Chalmers, 'The Extended Mind', *analysis* 58, no. 1 (1998): 7–19; Mark Johnson, *Embodied Mind, Meaning, and Reason: How Our Bodies Give Rise to Understanding*, Chicago and London: University of Chicago Press, 2021; Jane Bennett, *Vibrant Matter*, New York: Duke University Press, 2010; Karen Barad, *Meeting the Universe Halfway*, New York: Duke University Press, 2007.

12.1 Beyond Measure?

An opportunity arose to test some alternative directions for my practice when I was awarded a *Beyond Measure?* Micro Commission in 2021.[9] The commission involved making a series of images (a set of cards) designed to facilitate conversations with people who, for a variety of reasons, found it hard to talk about their health problems and as a result had struggled to fully articulate their symptoms and experiences to health professionals, often with repercussions for their clinical care. As a foundation for this new work, I drew on my existing body of ceramic and drawn responses to older bodies: these provided a starting point for a collective process of visualising the body in a way that incorporated somatic feelings and tried to dissolve the boundaries between things, representing boundaries as permeable membranes that are constantly in movement, rather than making fixed, centralised images that rely entirely on external visual representations. The theoretical underpinning for this work was informed by my research on Markov blankets.[10] The Markov blanket is a hermeneutic used by statisticians as a concept for mediating the porous and arbitrary boundary between the known and the unknown, order and chaos and it proposes flexible thresholds as models for realisation instead of solid and permanent borders between things.[11] This means that a clearly defined form is an inappropriate visual metaphor for somatic feelings (because we don't quite know what those feelings are or where they begin and end).

My earlier work (making contemporary votives in response to people's experiences of pain or loss) had engaged with conversations about possible uses for images of internal feelings of discomfort or anxiety.[12] For this new project, participants (including people from 25 different community centres, religious groups, women's support groups, community voluntary workers, older people's groups and men's groups) suggested that the resultant images might act as intermediaries between 'ordinary' people

[9] *Beyond Measure?* https://beyond-measure.mailchimpsites.com/. Accessed 12 September 2022.

[10] http://fineartdrawinglca.blogspot.com/2021/07/paul-klee-and-markov-blankets.html.

[11] Michael Kirchhoff, Thomas Parr, Ensor Palacios, Karl Friston, and Julian Kiverstein, 'The Markov blankets of life: autonomy, active inference and the free energy principle', *Journal of The Royal Society Interface* 15 (2018): 20170792.

[12] E-J Graham and Garry Barker, 'Making Votives; Pain and Practice', *The Votives Project*, September 15 2020, https://thevotivesproject.org/2020/09/15/making-votives/; accessed 15 September 2022.

(like themselves) and 'higher' forces including medical professionals and gatekeepers in benefits offices. As part of the process I showed participants votive images and explained how they were used: these images, participants agreed, could serve as intermediaries between themselves, their self-knowledge and the challenging and inimical situations that they often found themselves facing. Historically a votive was an object placed in a sacred place for religious purposes, made and displayed in order to communicate with invisible supernatural forces that might bring about positive change for the person making an offering.[13] Votives were, as Graham states, associated with 'healing' rather than 'curing', implying that these objects were made to assist in the psychological task of dealing with a challenging life experience (such as illness or misfortune) rather than necessarily provide a cure.[14] This distinction was important to the way in which I conceived the commission: I didn't want to find myself operating as a sort of faith healer, nor did I want to inadvertently frame ageing as inherently pathological.

Working in dialogue with individuals, initially side-by-side in a ceramics studio and then moving to Zoom meetings when Covid-19 restrictions prevented us from meeting in person, I produced a range of drawn and printed images and ceramic objects (e.g. see Fig. 12.1, a votive object made in response to one individual's experience of lung disease). By setting out the rules of engagement at the beginning of every session, I ensured that participants understood that I was working with them as an artist, rather than as a psychic or homoeopathic practitioner or other spiritual or mental health expert. My role was thus explicitly framed as facilitatory rather than necessarily curative. I explained to each participant that everyone has something to say about how they felt about their bodies; I then showed existing pieces and told stories about them so that people could get an idea of how individual issues could be made widely relatable. As we talked, I listened whilst drawing and making (predominantly with clay); as the drawings and objects evolved, the participant would offer verbal feedback on whether the representation was an accurate representation of their experience. I suggested to each participant that they might regard this process as akin to the collaborative production of a portrait; the

[13] Weinryb, *Ex Voto*, 51.

[14] Emma-Jayne Graham, 'Mobility impairment in the sanctuaries of early Roman Italy,' in *Disability in Antiquity*, ed. Christian Laes, London and New York: Routledge, 2016, 264–282; 252.

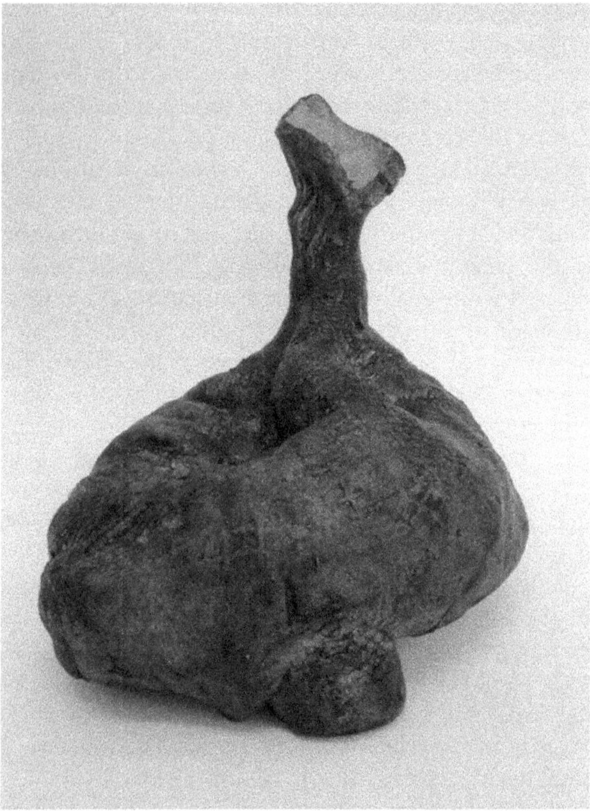

Fig. 12.1 Garry Barker, Votive object made in response to lung disease, 2019. Ceramic 38 × 20 × 17 cm (Photo © Sally Robinson)

anti-mimetic qualities of the resulting 'portraits' (or indeed anti-portraits) means that nobody other than the artist and the participant need ever know what bit of a body belonged to whom.[15] Through this process, participants were able to understand why, as an artist, I needed people's stories to ensure that the work was purposeful and of practical value in helping others come to terms with their own body issues.

[15] On the anti-portrait, see Fiona Johnstone and Kirstie Imber, 'Introducing the Anti-Portrait' in *Anti-Portraiture: Beyond Likeness and Identity*, ed. Fiona Johnstone and Kirstie Imber, London and New York: Bloomsbury, 2020, 1–24.

Invited to consider the potential agency of these contemporary votives, participants felt that such objects might offer a sense of control. To explore this further, we developed rituals surrounding the exchange of objects. Sometimes a ritual was built into the object itself: some objects were made so that they could function as candles; others were made to be broken, displayed or buried. Some participants liked the idea that pain could be trapped in a ceramic object and then destroyed when it was smashed. Others wanted to see their pain (physical or emotional) externalised or put on display: this offered a way of taking control over it. Some gave their objects back to me; they simply wanted the pain to go away. A form of magic ritual emerged from the process: inspired by Andrew Wilburn's definition of magic as a process involving the co-mingling and overlapping of concepts,[16] I came to think of this as quantum 'spooky action at a distance'.[17] Through this process, the participant's awareness of an inner body pain (interoception) became associated with a correspondence concept: a connection between an invisible but tangible thing—for instance a pain in one's foot—became linked to an intermediary representation that connected both foot and pain. The overlapping of different processes of representation (both the *look* of things and the *feeling* of things) alongside an association with a ritual (such as the lighting of a candle), created the opportunity for participants to invest belief in the agential power of objects. As the project evolved, a complex relationship developed between ritual action, object manipulation, an emerging belief system, and a private relationship with objects that relied on a materialist framework.[18]

Some of these hand-held objects had been crafted as a response to loneliness; after further conversations with the person they had been made for, we decided that something more intimate and personal was needed. I returned to the studio and made some tiny ceramic pieces, small enough to be put in a purse (Fig. 12.2). The feedback was positive: small enough to be rolled between a finger and thumb, these diminutive objects were able to function as touch talismans.

[16] Andrew Wilburn, *Materia Magica: the Archaeology of Magic in Roman Egypt, Cyprus, and Spain*, Ann Arbour, Michigan: University of Michigan Press, 2012.

[17] Albert Einstein, *Born-einstein Letters 1916–1955: Friendship, Politics and Physics in Uncertain Times*, Basingstoke and New York: Palgrave Macmillan, 2014. 158.

[18] For a materialist framework, see the quantum arguments developed by Karan Barad in *Meeting the Universe Halfway*; and Graham Harvey on contemporary animism in *Animism: Respecting the Living World*, New York: Columbia University Press, 2005.

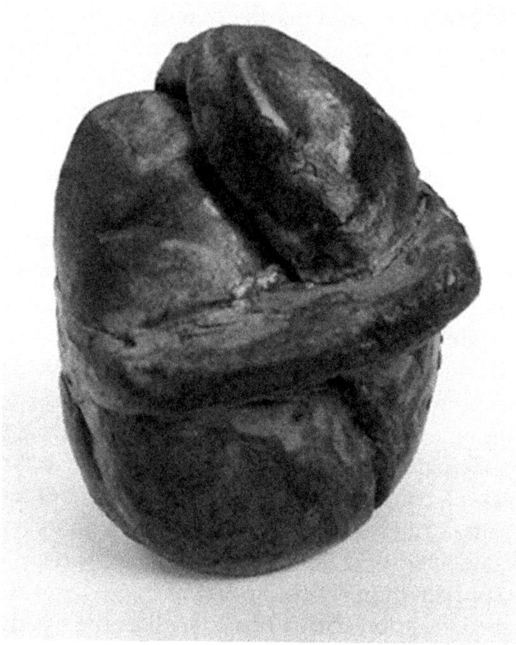

Fig. 12.2 Garry Barker, Votives for loneliness, 2020. Ceramic 7 × 5 × 5 cm. (Photo © Sally Robinson)

These experiments led to the collaborative design and production of a set of 52 cards intended for use in community settings to help initiate conversations about people's health and wellbeing (Fig. 12.3): these were distributed to a list of interested Leeds community groups, accompanied with guidelines for use. The card designs relied heavily on imagery developed during the votive-making sessions; early informal feedback suggested that the cards were engaging and useful in opening out people's stories about their bodies and how they thought about them. When in-person social gatherings were restricted due to the onset of the Covid-19 pandemic in early 2020, I collaborated with a web developer on an online version: however, feedback from users suggested that this was a poor substitute for human interaction.[19]

Whilst Covid-19 caused my work on the *Beyond Measure?* project to stall, the situation occasioned a period of self-reflection. I became more

[19] Garry Barker, artist's website: https://garrybarkeronline.com/project/votive-cards-as-story-prompts/. Accessed 16 September 2022.

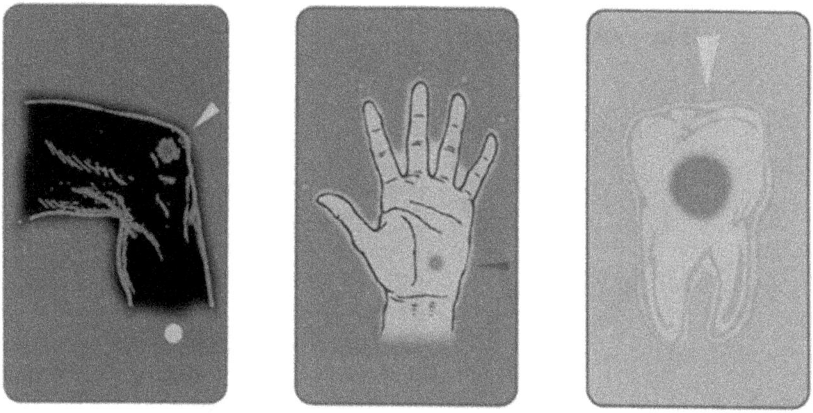

Fig. 12.3 Garry Barker, Examples of card designs (Knee pain, hand pain and toothache), 2021. Various sizes. (Photo © Garry Barker)

aware of the relationship between votive-type objects, sympathetic magic and the use of amulets and charm bracelets as forms of psychic protection. It was clear to me that votive-type objects were somehow charged by people's experiences of pain or strong emotions such as grief. These were powerful things and I did not want to lose the sense of agency that was emerging from these encounters; in particular, I was keen to focus on the positive aspects of protection and coping with illness that earlier manifestations of these ideas had evidenced.

The card designs were simplified to brightly coloured images: this had been part of their success. As the programme for *Beyond Measure?* was drawing to an end, the participants and I decided to design a badge using a similar design process to help people communicate their decision to be vaccinated against Covid-19. The wearing of objects that protect the body from an invisible threat and communicate the wearer's affiliation with a belief creates a form of agency: people use such objects to equip themselves with a form of psychic protection and to visibly signal that they belong to a community of people who support vaccination. The design process looked at mediaeval pilgrim badges as well as enamel badges worn by football supporters and hikers. The final badge design (Fig. 12.4) was accepted and distributed by local health professionals and worn by those who wanted to celebrate their vaccination.

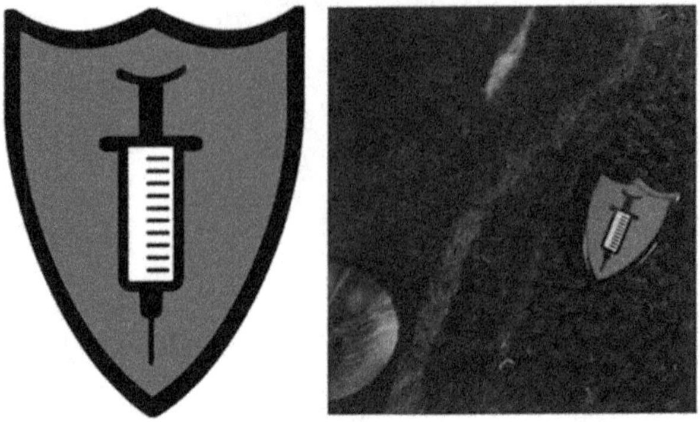

Fig. 12.4 Garry Barker, Design for enamel badge and image of the badge being worn, 2020. (Photo © Garry Barker)

This process caused me to rethink how the objects that I made might help people to engage with images of the imagined somatic body that I had been working with previously. Consequently, I decided to take my exploration of the relationship between the internal body and externalised objecthood in a new direction, experimenting with the possibility of wearing small sculptures of concretised psychological states.

This work would be presented on the site of our skin: skin is our most basic protection from invisible dangers, such as germs and viruses; it has historically and culturally been the thing that 'keeps the body inviolate'.[20] In times of belief in animism in particular, external events could emanate from the essence or spirit of a particular animal, thing or place[21]; these often invisible 'spiritual' contacts were by many cultures and over long periods of time negotiated using amulets or charm bracelets designed to form a psychic line of defence or communication channel.[22] Worn around neck, wrists and ankles, amulets and charms are intended to protect the parts of the body—lips, hands and feet—that are in constant contact with what some societies regard as 'unclean' or 'tainted' surfaces. Charms and

[20] Steven Connor, *The Book of Skin*, Ithaca, New York: Cornell University Press, 2004, 10; on skin, germs and viruses see Frank O. Nestle, Paola Di Meglio, Jian-Zhong Qin, and Brian J. Nickoloff, 'Skin immune sentinels in health and disease', *Nature Reviews Immunology* 9, no. 10 (2009): 679–691.

[21] Harvey, *Animism*.

[22] Sheila Paine, *Amulets: a world of secret powers, charms and magic*, London and New York: Thames & Hudson, 2004, 10.

amulets are intermediary things, sitting between the body and the world, as Alun-Jones & Ayton point out: both a barrier and a sensor, they recognise and stop the entry of invisible forces into the body.[23] Just as medical gloves, masks and other protective items place a barrier between us and the invisible threat of the Covid-19 virus, amulets and charm bracelets claim to offer protection from the invisible threat of spiritual damage, operating in a similar way to traditional votives by helping the wearer to cope emotionally with the anxiety-inducing experience of an invisible viral threat.[24]

Within contemporary global culture amulets and charms have a number of different functions. They might serve as a spiritual focus for the wearer, be used as magic charms, or work to ward off evil; they have been essential to the signification of tribal identity and are now used to develop and signify individual identity.[25] These various roles are ontologically nested, their operations refracted and embedded, with no clear distinction between a bracelet brought as a religious item, a fashion statement, a good luck charm, or as a way to reinforce a growing sense of identity. Indian and Chinese traditions of amulet and charm use continue, existing alongside celebrity image-construction using the self-same items: the capitalist system has embraced these various responses to our unsettling world.[26] In India women still refer to the ancient Solah Shringar Vedic texts that set out why and how women ought to adorn themselves.[27] Husain & Khalid point out that bangles, bracelets, armlets as well as ankle bells and finger rings are suggested adornments for the promotion of good health and wellbeing; in particular, ornaments are worn to protect orifices and body extremities so that energies that move through certain parts of the body,

[23] Alun-Jones and Ayton, *Charming*.

[24] Garry Barker, 'Revealing the invisible: The virus is looking at you', *Journal of Visual Political Communication* 7, no. 1 (2019): 61–87.

[25] Alun-Jones and Ayton, *Charming*.

[26] Jahanzeeb Qurashi, 'Commodification of Islamic religious tourism: from spiritual to touristic experience,' *International Journal of Religious Tourism and Pilgrimage* 5, no. 1 (2017): 89–104; Prabhjot Kaur, and Ruby Joseph 'Women And Jewelry-The Traditional and Religious Dimensions of Ornamentation' *Coherence* 3 (2012): 39–49; Jiayu Wu, 'Research on the Application of Chinese Traditional Auspicious Elements in Modern Jewelry Design,' *Frontiers in Humanities and Social Sciences* 2, no. 3 (2022): 9–13; Lee Barron, 'Postmodern theories of celebrity,' in *Routledge Handbook of Celebrity Studies*, ed. Anthony Elliott, London and New York: Routledge, 2018; 58–72.

[27] Ved Bhatnagar, *Shringar-the Ras Raj: A Classical Indian View*, New Delhi: Abhinav Publications, 2004.

both from internal and external sources, can be controlled.[28] This ancient belief exists alongside contemporary ideas of charm bracelet use, such as lucky charms and charms that celebrate important life moments, such as births or an affiliation with a particular interest group. The rising popularity of Milagros or 'miracle' charms both within Catholic societies and amongst the more agnostic elements of various populations, points to a continuing set of belief systems that have embedded within them aspects of 'magical' protection, whereby objects can be used to effect change. A set of beliefs that are eroded by more secular awareness, and which in turn begin to affect the attitudes and thoughts of people seeking spiritual awareness from other cultures. Traces of religion and folklore are to be found in several contemporary charm designs for jewellery, as Ceri Houlbrook points out when referring to contemporary jewellery charms that have been added to bracelets.[29]

The wearing of contemporary charms as jewellery is locked into multitudes of individual and collective responses to a fluid matrix of influences and historical continuities. As well as capitalist marketing drives to encourage us all to buy 'spiritual' charm bracelets, there are still millions of people who wear charm bracelets because they genuinely believe that they will help protect them from evil. All these various approaches and associations however intersect in a compacted moment that is shaped around a particular wrist or an ankle. For some the wearing of a charm bracelet is a clear protection from evil and the energies of black magic, for others a chance to harness a lucky streak, or to give some form to the chaos of everyday life, for others a fashion statement or sign of belonging to a particular tribe. Charm bracelets and similar jewellery are materialised ideas and emotions, thoughts and feelings cast in metal, laid into resin, lodged in small stones or twisted into knotted cords.

With these multiple and complex contemporary usages of charm bracelets in mind, I decided to develop a new body of work that would follow on from the *Beyond Measure?* programme. Initially converting images of votive sculptures into flat-coloured prints, I began by making charms for Italian-style bracelets (two-dimensional images on flat modular links), before exploring the possibilities of shallow relief charms to be attached to a chain-link bracelet (Figs. 12.5 and 12.6).

[28] Nazim Husain and Mohd Khalid, 'Aesthetic Significance of Solah Shringar (Sixteen Ornaments) in Unani Medicine', *J. Complement. Altern. Med. Res* (2021), 69–81: 75.

[29] Ceri Houlbrook, 'The Love-Lock Charm: Folklore and Fashion', *Tradition Today* 1, no. 9 (2020): 23–32.

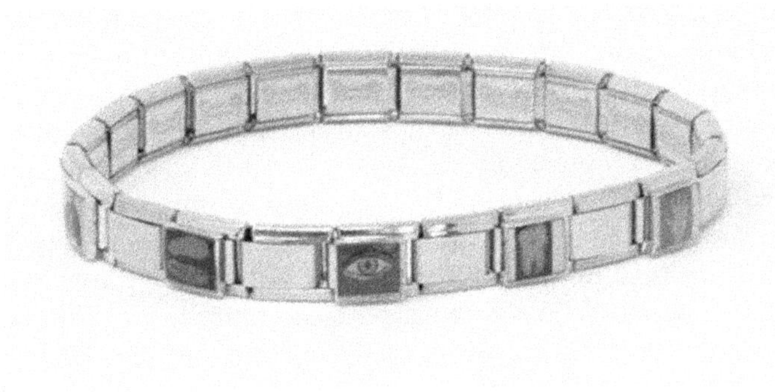

Fig. 12.5 Garry Barker, Italian-style charm bracelet with resin embedded 'votive charms', 2021. (Photo © Sally Robinson)

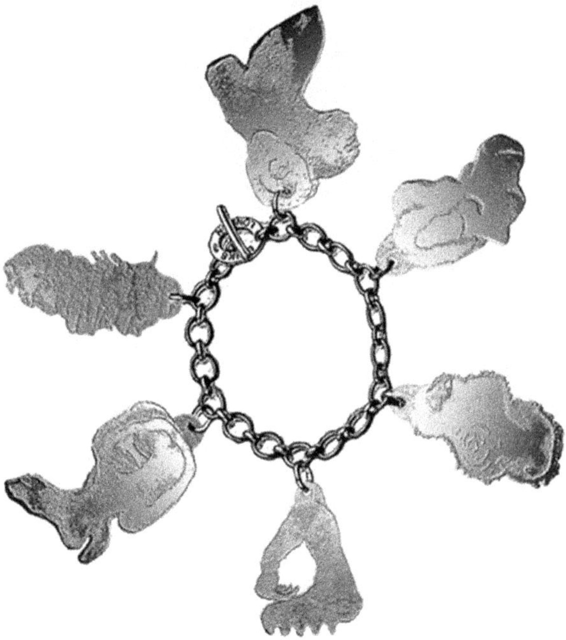

Fig. 12.6 Garry Barker, Bracelet with attached shallow relief sculptures based on somatic images of human bodies, 2021. (Photo © Garry Barker)

Much of my work, including these charm bracelets, is informed by my ongoing research into the concept of interoception—the conscious and non-conscious sense of the internal state of the body. Human experience of the bodily interior is based partly on external observation and partly on other forms of perceptual information such as proprioception (the body's ability to sense self-movement).[30] Perceptions of internal organ function (such as heartbeat and respiration) are linked to the autonomic nervous system (which is largely non-conscious), as well to the production of psychological experience.[31] I see size and scale as significant in expressing the externalisation of interior experience; small items, like jewellery, invoke a feeling of intimacy.[32]

Conceived as small sculpture, jewellery offers an ideal medium for visualising the relationship between the interior and exterior of the body as a conjoined set of forms: by (re)conceptualising people's bodies as exhibition spaces for small sculptural objects, artworks and individuals become entangled in an intimate relationship. Writing on the curative and protective power of amulets in the early modern world, Annie Thwaite notes the significance of portability, which underscores such objects' 'fundamental relationship with the body'.[33] In her work on Tetela amulets in equatorial Africa, Heather Marie Akou highlights the closely entwined relationship between fashion and ritual when considering the multifunctionality of bracelets originally intended for healing purposes.[34] The idea of making charms as both tiny sculptural reliefs and two-dimensional images, as in an Italian style charm bracelet, that could have more than one meaning for a

[30] Lisa Feldman Barrett, Karen S. Quigley, Eliza Bliss-Moreau, and Keith R. Aronson, 'Interoceptive sensitivity and self-reports of emotional experience', *Journal of Personality and Social Psychology* 87, no. 5 (2004): 684.

[31] Oliver G. Cameron, 'Interoception: the inside story—a model for psychosomatic processes', *Psychosomatic Medicine* 63, no. 5 (2001): 697–710; Dieter Vaitl, 'Interoception', *Biological psychology* 42, no. 1–2 (1996): 1–27; Sahib S. Khalsa and Rachel C. Lapidus, 'Can interoception improve the pragmatic search for biomarkers in psychiatry?' *Frontiers in psychiatry* 7, no. 121 (2016), n.p.

[32] On size and scale in relation to human experience see Pasqualini, Isabella, Maria Laura Blefari, Tej Tadi, Andrea Serino, and Olaf Blanke, 'The architectonic experience of body and space in augmented interiors,' *Frontiers in Psychology* 9, no. 375 (2018), n.p.; and Craig, Arthur D. *How Do You Feel?* Princeton NJ: Princeton University Press, 2014.

[33] Annie Thwaites, 'A History of Amulets in Ten Objects,' *Science Museum Group Journal*, 11 (2019): n.p.

[34] Heather Marie Akou, 'Tetela amulets: Re-interpreting a medical anthropology collection as a fashion benchmark,' *International Journal of Fashion Studies*. 6, no. 2 (2019): 163–180.

user, was powerfully reinforced by my reading of Thwaites and Akou: I hoped that my small wearable sculptures might signify a conjunction between the everyday and the 'other', functioning like votives but also be seen as 'simply' fashion items, depending on the changing needs of the wearer. I hoped that the wearer would hold a charm between their fingertips, allowing them to externalise and release feelings of pain, loss or anxiety. However at the same time, I hoped that a wearer would be able to wear the object simply because they liked it. This situation is of course something every jewellery designer takes for granted, but for myself—coming from a tradition of making objects for both site specific and gallery spaces—it has been a thoughtful transition. For both myself and the individuals that I worked with, the holding and touching of tiny relief sculptures and images has generated new understandings of somatic and psychical experience. The philosopher Timothy Morton has described the phenomenology of the human-artwork encounter as 'some kind of mind-meld-like thing that takes place ... if I try to reduce it [the experience] to the artwork or me, I pretty much ruin it'.[35] Both nourished by and actively generative of object-human relationships, these 'curative' objects and images highlight the 'inescapable entanglement' of human and non-human things.[36]

References

Akou, Heather Marie. 'Tetela amulets: Re-interpreting a medical anthropology collection as a fashion benchmark'. *International Journal of Fashion Studies* 6, no. 2 (2019): 163-180.

Albert, Jade & Kai Hackney. *The Charm of Charms*. London: Abrams, 2005.

Alun-Jones, Deborah, and John Ayton. *Charming*. London and New York: Thames & Hudson, 2005.

Barad, Karen. *Meeting the Universe Halfway: Quantum Physics and the Entanglement of Matter and Meaning*. New York: Duke University Press, 2007.

Barker, Garry. 'Paul Klee and Markov Blankets'. Accessed September 26, 2022a. http://fineartdrawinglca.blogspot.com/2021/07/paul-klee-and-markov-blankets.html.

Barker, Garry. 'Drawing Age.' *Drawing: Research, Theory, Practice* 5, no. 2 (2020): 351-361.

[35] Timothy Morton, *All Art is Ecological*, London: Penguin, 2021, 59.

[36] Barad, *Meeting the Universe Halfway*, 3.

Barker, Garry. 'Drawing the Embodied Mind: A Project Report on Research Into Interoception'. *PSIAX# 5 ESTUDOS E REFLEXÕES SOBRE DESENHO E IMAGEM* 5 (2021a): 17–24.

Barker, Garry. 'Is It To Feel Each Limb Grow Stiffer, Is It To Feel The full Potential Of A Life?' *TRACEY* 15, no. 1 (2021b): 1-17.

Barker, Garry. 'Revealing the Invisible: The Virus is Looking at You'. *Journal of Visual Political Communication* 7, no. 1 (2019): 61–87.

Barker, Garry. n.d.-a 'Votive Cards as Story Prompts.' Accessed June 22, 2022. https://garrybarkeronline.com/.

Barker, Garry. 'Garry Barker: In Conversation'. *Shine Magazine*, March 2022b, Accessed June 22, 2022: https://www.shinealight.org.uk/inconversation-garrybarker.

Barker, Garry. n.d.-b Life Hacks for Limited Futures. Accessed January 18, 2022. https://lifehacksforlimitedfutures.wordpress.com/author/garrybarker69/.

Barrett, Lisa Feldman, Karen S. Quigley, Eliza Bliss-Moreau, and Keith R. Aronson. 'Interoceptive sensitivity and self-reports of emotional experience'. *Journal of Personality and Social Psychology* 87, no. 5 (2004): 684-697.

Barron, Lee. 'Postmodern theories of celebrity'. In *Routledge Handbook of Celebrity Studies*, edited by Anthony Elliott, 58-72. London and New York: Routledge, 2018.

Bennett, Jane. *Vibrant Matter*. New York: Duke University Press, 2010.

Beyond Measure? Accessed December 8, 2021. https://beyond-measure.mailchimpsites.com/garry-barker.

Bhatnagar, Ved. *Shringar-the Ras Raj: A Classical Indian View*. New Delhi: Abhinav Publications, 2004.

Cameron, Oliver G. 'Interoception: the inside story—a model for psychosomatic processes'. *Psychosomatic Medicine* 63, no. 5 (2001): 697-710.

Clark, Andy, and David Chalmers. 'The Extended Mind'. *Analysis* 58, no. 1 (1998): 7-19.

Connor, Steven. *The Book of Skin*. Ithaca: Cornell University Press, 2004.

Damasio, Antonio. *The Feeling of What Happens: Body, Emotion and the Making of Consciousness*. London: Vintage, 2000.

Einstein, Albert. *Born-Einstein Letters 1916-1955: Friendship, Politics and Physics in Uncertain Times*. Basingstoke and New York: Palgrave Macmillan, 2014.

Etsy. Accessed January 8, 2022: https://www.etsy.com/uk/listing/294268647/hindu-bracelet-charm-bracelet-buddhist?epik=dj0yJnU9VVR3bGlJOXp0RUViWjBPaVROUkVFdzdJUVVRMmJ0RlkmcD0wJm49RTh2RUJsNTdkLXB4YzhnamFrUFdWQSZ0PUFBQUFBR0hiT05V

Graham, Emma-Jayne. 'Making Votives; Pain and Practice'. The Votive Project (Blog). Accessed 26 September, 2022. https://thevotivesproject.org/2020/09/15/making-votives/

Graham, Emma-Jayne. 'Mobility impairment in the sanctuaries of early Roman Italy'. In *Disability in Antiquity*, edited by Christian Laes et. al., 264-282. London and New York: Routledge, 2016.

Harvey, Graham. *Animism: Respecting the Living World*. New York: Columbia University Press, 2005.

Houlbrook, Ceri. 'The Lock-Love Charm: Folklore and Fashion'. *Tradition Today* 1, no. 9: 23-32.

Husain, Nazim, and Mohd Khalid. 'Aesthetic Significance of Solah Shringar (Sixteen Ornaments) in Unani Medicine'. *J. Complement. Altern. Med. Res* (2021): 69-81.

Johnson, Mark. *Embodied Mind, Meaning, and Reason*. London: University of Chicago Press, 2021.

Johnstone, Fiona and Kirstie Imber. 'Introducing the Anti-Portrait'. In *Anti-Portraiture: Beyond Likeness and Identity*, edited by Fiona Johnstone and Kirstie Imber, 1-24. London and New York: Bloomsbury, 2020.

Karma and Luck. Accessed January 8, 2022. https://www.karmaandluck.com/collections/womens-anklets-collection.

Kaur, Prabhjot, and Ruby Joseph. 'Women And Jewelry-The Traditional and Religious Dimensions of Ornamentation'. *Coherence* 3 (2012): 39-49.

Khalsa, Sahib S., and Rachel C. Lapidus. 'Can interoception improve the pragmatic search for biomarkers in psychiatry?' *Frontiers in Psychiatry* 7, no. 121 (2016): n.p.

Kirchhoff, Michael, Thomas Parr, Ensor Palacios, Karl Friston, and Julian Kiverstein. 'The Markov blankets of life: autonomy, active inference and the free energy principle'. *Journal of The Royal Society Interface* 15, no. 138 (2018): 20170792.

Latour, Bruno. *Reassembling the Social: An introduction to actor-network-theory*. Oxford: Oxford University Press, 2007.

Malchiodi, Cathy A. (ed.). *Handbook of Art Therapy*. New York: Guilford Press, 2011.

Morton, Timothy. *All Art is Ecological*. London: Penguin, 2021

Nestle, Frank O., Paola Di Meglio, Jian-Zhong Qin, and Brian J. Nickoloff. 'Skin immune sentinels in health and disease'. *Nature Reviews Immunology* 9, no. 10 (2009): 679-691.

Paine, Sheila. *Amulets: a world of secret powers, charms and magic*. London and New York: Thames & Hudson, 2004.

Pasqualini, Isabella, Maria Laura Blefari, Tej Tadi, Andrea Serino, and Olaf Blanke. 'The architectonic experience of body and space in augmented interiors'. *Frontiers in Psychology* 9, no. 375 (2018), n.p.

Qurashi, Jahanzeeb. 'Commodification of Islamic religious tourism: from spiritual to touristic experience'. *International Journal of Religious Tourism and Pilgrimage* 5, no. 1 (2017): 89-104.

Seth, Anil. *Being You: A New Science of Consciousness.* London: Penguin, 2021.

Shanafelt, Robert. 'Magic, miracle, and marvels in anthropology'. *Ethnos* 69, no. 3 (2004): 317-340.

Shusterman, Richard. *Body Consciousness: A Philosophy of Mindfulness and Somaesthetics.* New York: Cambridge University Press, 2008.

Thwaites, Annie. 'A history of amulets in ten objects'. *Science Museum Group Journal* 11, (2019): n.p.

Unschuld, Paul U., Hermann Tessenow, and Jinsheng Zheng. *Huang Di Nei Jing Su Wen: An annotated translation of Huang Di's inner classic–basic questions: 2 volumes.* Vol. 1. Univ of California Press, 2011.

Vaitl, Dieter. 'Interoception.' *Biological Psychology* 42, no. 1–2 (1996): 1-27.

Weinryb, Ittai (ed.). *Ex Voto: Votive Giving Across Cultures.* New York: Bard Graduate Center, 2016.

Wilburn, Andrew. *Materia Magica: the Archaeology of Magic in Roman Egypt, Cyprus, and Spain.* Ann Arbor: University of Michigan Press, 2012.

Wu, Jiayu. 'Research on the Application of Chinese Traditional Auspicious Elements in Modern Jewelry Design'. *Frontiers in Humanities and Social Sciences* 2, no. 3 (2022): 9-13.

CHAPTER 13

(Ad)dressing Wounds: A Trauma in Seven Act(or)s

Katharina Ludwig

Intro	*Into*
-duction –	*the hole*

It might prove helpful to provide a short introduction to the following text as it might sit—slightly uncomfortable or somewhat abstract—between contributions dealing with objects, thingliness and healing. This text does not involve a tangible object, nor a thing in the strict sense of the term, and rather than promoting notions of healing or cure it leans towards a concept of "un-healing" or keeping a wound open.

But let's start in the beginning. A recurring problem I encounter in my research on holes, and especially holes in text and language that I am specifically concerned with, is the lack of an object. It appears to me that it would seem much easier to describe something, to talk, or write about something that is ***there****—an object, a body—than addressing something*

K. Ludwig (✉)
Goldsmiths, University of London, London, UK
e-mail: info@katharinaludwig.com

D. Woolley et al. (eds.), *Wearable Objects and Curative Things*, Palgrave Studies in Fashion and the Body,
https://doi.org/10.1007/978-3-031-40017-9_13

that ***is not****—something that is unsayable, something that is commonly considered as a lack or an absence. Descriptions of the negative space of a hole are often nothing more than descriptions of the space around it. A troubling aspect however is that I believe the hole is an entity in its own rights and hence not a lack. However evasive it should appear, it should not only be defined through its peripheries.*

So, how to meet the challenge to speak or write of/from/with/through this absence, of unknowability and listen to unsayability? How to deal practically, theoretically and artistically with the unavailability and elusion of something?

As part of my research I experiment with a number of methods to make the problem of the non-object somewhat more accessible, addressable to me, to gain more insight inside (into?) the dark entrails of the hole. Two of them, that are connected to the topic of this publication and the following creative contribution and that I briefly introduce here, are rooted in a metaphorical realm of language and fictional narrative:

I situate the object of inquiry of my research and address in language and text. Language is the primary object I'm concerned with. It is an abstract body, yet a body it is. Text certainly has a body which lends it a certain physicality. A hole in the context of the body (of text) could be read as a metaphorical extrapolation into a lesion, cut—or wound, which also forms the etymological root of the term "trauma". The hole (the broken, disrupted, unsayable, unaddressable, unthinkable) could be considered as inscribed as a wound in the body of text. However the textual hole is not necessarily a lack, or empty, or even missing, even though it might resist direct address. Much rather holes can be regarded as portals connecting space and temporalities, as subsurface hiding spaces to gain momentum for subversive action or act as mouth-pieces for other unheard voices to pass through, echo and eclipse in polyvocality. Perhaps there exist other approaches than sealing, filling and closing a wound-hole? Langauge/textual holes inscribe themselves in a body of language as a possible symptom of woundedness (traumatisation) and it is this metaphor I employ speaking of wounds as a specific kind of hole and of the wounded text. In addition language generally operates as an object or body at different intersections between disciplines concerned with healing, and is object for a variety of explorations into ailment, illness, health, and cure.

From this linguistic, metaphorical consideration of the hole or wound I arrive in the practice part of my research at inventing or conjuring up fictionalised characters that assist me in addressing, interacting with, exploring, understanding, and approaching wounded language, wounds, lesions and their various histories, temporalities, affects, and implications. These characters predominantly feature as language characters (character might also refer to a typographical character such as a letter for example) that embody as texts, performative readings, videos, poems and at times costumes and installations accompanied by language and text-based elements. This is the sentiment from which the ongoing work cycle and the universe of the Woundlickers, which I introduced at the "Curative Things: Medicine/Fashion/Art Symposium", derived. It comprises different formations and embodiments of the character of the Woundlickers (see below for a more in-depth introduction of them) such as text, poem, reading, video, installation, printed publication and costumes, all circling around concepts of wounds and woundedness, temporalities and oral histories, contagion, infect and affect. The address of the wound, which is in the context of the Woundlickers a rather physical one, acts as one form of engagement or approach of the unsayable and the hole. It is a defence of brokenness and an opposition against flawed ideas of wholeness.

The following contribution I imagine to be regarded as an incoherent continuation of the world of the Woundlickers. It is a performance script of a play without a play, consisting of stage description and stage direction introducing, in addition to the Woundlickers, a further cast of characters. All of these characters embody different angles of how to approach holes/wounds/traumata—in words, deeds, disciplines and otherwise. They advocate or struggle with different strategies of care (medical, historical, psychoanalytical, sociological, theological, political, artistic).

The sole performance (on stage—a book could be considered as a sort of stage, too) will be the reading of the script, which exercises a choreography of language (on the page and by its reading), but also is a performance of a/the body of text. As a performance without performers in flesh and blood, it leaves the text and the voice suspended in an ongoing approach towards hole-ness.

Perhaps later, at a further stage, some performers could improvise on the information given by character description.

Stage Description

The Set

A hole has opened in the ground.

Dimmed lights, with one single bright spot pointing directly in/on–to the site of the hole.
The abyss is invisible from the point of view of the audience.

Existential considerations,
if this opening were ancient or new;
if it just opened or if it were fixed, gaping in exactly the same place for all times known;

if it was forcefully and violently opened
    —cut, dug, bored—
or opened by itself
    —ruptured, cracked, ripped—
or if it were a hole at all
or might not be a wound festering
or a mouth ajar in the ground;
belong to the same speculative realm as questions regarding its material conditions, and practical concerns relating to its appearance such as its depth or shallowness.

From what can be understood it remains unresolved
  if the hole is permanent
or only opens for a certain time;
  if it could be a tunnel
or portal,
  a way into
or out;
  if it could be a ceremonial site of ritualistic practice,
  the lesion of an ecological emergency
or a trace of any other kind of accident
or disaster.

A sombre atmosphere around the hole discloses however that the opening and impact of the cavernous, negative space constitutes an unusual, interrupting, cataclysmic event.

Nevertheless, the precise nature of this hole, as well as a definite conclusion on the classification of the body it bears/pierces, remains unclear. This is to say this hole embodies an unknowable, unsayable, ungraspable body. And yet it is physically there, in all its void, and therefore not devoid of substance—It's not an absence or a lack.

A number of characters have gathered around an abyssal opening in the ground.

The reason for the characters' gathering appears rather uncertain as to why the characters are where they are, what they are doing next to the open hole (they at times appear equally unknowing themselves), and where they came from. Their mysterious presence/dwelling, arranged circular around the hole, invites conjectures on if they were called or summoned, if they emerged from or through the opening of the hole. All surmises however remain inconclusive and fruitless. It is unclear/obscure what exactly drew them in the proximity of the hole and very little can be gathered on the characters gathering around the incision for now, beyond the fact that it can be assumed that all of them—one way or another—are involved in practices concerned with (w)hole-ness.

List of Characters

the SUTURESS *(a seamstress, an editor, a figure of the imaginary)*

The SUTURESS is specialised in anything woven together. She is proficient in whole making. A prodigy in close/thing: text, textures, textualities, textiles, tissue.

> TEXT—from Latin 'textus', tissue; from past participle stem of texere: 'to weave, to join, fit together, braid, interweave, construct, fabricate, build'

What is the difference between a sentence and a sewn? asks Susan Howe [1]
What is the difference between an editor, a reader or a seamstress?

[1] Susan Howe, *Spontaneous Particulars: The Telepathy Of Archives*, New York: New Directions, 2014, 19.

What the SUTURESS was taught (skills, techniques):

> To make a cut, to fabricate patterns,
> to fix, to fit,
> to sew, to stitch, to combine.
> To mend, to darn, to patch over and underneath holes.
> To wrap, to weft.
> To knot and to suture.
> To bast, to fold. To pleat, to lay and gather.
> To run threads and catch loose ends.
> To hem open seams. To finish, to not leave open/to close.
> To make wear/bear able.
> To seam (to make appear as)
> whole.

The SUTURESS has made whole a great number of broken, damaged, disrupted, hole-y text/iles. She has mended and darned the ➡ BODY WRITER's manuscripts, disconnected ramblings and staggering meanderings. She has sutured over textual holes, has closed them, and has connected disjoint limbs of the textual body. Her seams leave scars, scarcely noticeable to the reader or listener.

However with the number of holes multiplying in the ➡ BODY WRITER's text, with her words falling apart more and more in the face of her truncated sentences, her stumbling and rambling prose, the SUTURESS—due to being overworked and underpaid—begins to question the efforts of her labour.

Strewn around in her workshop the SUTURESS sees a torso linen-lined, several strewn pairs of legs and single arms, a hand, a wooden head, differently sized lasts for feet. A battleground of wounded bodies, detached limbs. The SUTURESS is struck by the un-whole-ness and fragmentation of the body, of her work. She, similar to the ➡ BODY WRITER, is surrounded by dismembered body parts.

Thoughts the SUTURESS tries to piece together:

The SUTURESS reflects on if the hole, the cut always comes first? Without the cut, the wound, without the hole no garment. And every garment is made from parts leaving holes open for parts of the body that is dressed. Each piece of text/ile, woven or knitted, spoken, sung or written, is constructed around holes.

And doesn't it mean to suture over a hole, to puncture tiny holes with the needle around it? To inflict additional wounds, open more holes in the procedure of repair? Of healing and mending? To her surprise her whole profession is not about the whole as she was taught—a deceptive illusion not more not less in retrospect—but about holes instead. And don't clothes, fashion also inscribe or mark a body, as Colette Soler says? [2] Don't they change one's form as comparable to a wound or cut in the flesh? Making the unbearable wearable.

The SUTURESS becomes increasingly alienated from what she was taught her work was about. Her disinterest in attempts of fixing, of repairing, in making whole something that never was whole but always hole grows immeasurably together with a previously undisclosed desire to resist filling and mending. She claims that she looks at her work differently now, that she gazed into the holes, into the cuts, the wounds in text/ile. They are not empty, they are not missing, they are not void or lack. According to the SUTURESS, to run needle and thread through the fringes of the hole, to forcefully draw the sides of a cut together, to achieve closure, to suture over a wound or hole, means to close the lips, the mouth of a cut, a wound—it silences, violently. The SUTURESS will vow to sew holes instead of making whole.

> *I fall, I fall.*
> *My scars today are beautiful,*
> *they all have the shape of an ellipsis[...]* [3]

* * *

the WOUND DRESSER *(a doctor, surgeon or medical worker)*

As a long-time practicing medical practitioner the WOUND DRESSER is deeply knowledgeable of different ways of curing wounds. He knows that the term *cure* derives from the Latin *curare—to care*, and that to cure therefore doesn't necessarily denote to heal. Rather it means to *mind*, to *treat*, to *attend* to wounds and comprises many acts of care. He doesn't consider himself a healer but much rather a specialist of wound care. A curator of wound(ed) objects in an operating theatre.

[2] Colette Soler, 'The Body in the Teaching of Jacques Lacan', *Quatro*, May, 1984, 1–19.
[3] Violette Leduc, *Die Bastardin*, Reinbek: Rowohlt, 1978. 27 (own translation).

Through his long and extensive studies, he became well acquainted with both historical and contemporary approaches and addresses towards wounds. *Wound* derives etymologically from the Greek term *trauma*, he has internalised.

The WOUND DRESSER knows about inner and outer wounds. He knows about mediaeval medical humoural theory as much as about the impact of humour on recovery.

The WOUND DRESSER knows about washing, cleaning, sucking and biting out wounds. He respects ➡ WOUNDLICKERS and mystics for their oral contribution towards wound care.

He knows about the disinfectant properties of saliva as much as he knows about the purifying qualities of fire, cauterising, purging and blood letting.

He knows about the use of contemporary disinfectants, too.

He knows about the balance of fluids such as blood, phlegm, bile and black bile.

He knows about needlework, surgical methods of suturing, of scarring and closing a wound.

The WOUND DRESSER knows equally a lot about making whole as about making holes: about amputation, -ostomies, wounding, cutting to rid the body of festering, inflammatory flesh.

The WOUND DRESSER knows of the importance of considerations of continuous wholeness of the body and the negative reputation of fragmentation. A hole-y, broken, wounded body was considered formless.

Regardless, he knows that the body was generally thought of as porous and permeable, full of holes, and that it could maintain this state even in the face of the hegemonic preferred ideal of wholeness, which turns out to be somewhat of a paradox, as do a lot of conceptions of the body—back then and today.

From his work as a first responder however, and this is also what brings him here, the WOUND DRESSER is well-versed on wet and dry wound dressings. Methods applied in that area haven't significantly changed over centuries, he never stops telling. To dress a wound, to anoint, to cover the lesion with textile, bandage or cloth, to soak up liquid, pus, blood, emerging from the hole. Wound fashion. A form of patching the ➡ SUTURESS is familiar with, too. A supposedly protective covering, a hiding of the hideous hole, which however runs the danger of festering underneath the dressing. A regular hygienic change of dressings proofs vital, the WOUND

DRESSER insists as much as he insists on curative measures with the goal of closing the wound. For the WOUND DRESSER to dress a wound is a form of address.

* * *

the WOUND ADDRESSER *(an analyst, presumably a Lacanian)*

For many years, WOUND ADDRESSERS have explored and mined the gloomy and murky wound tunnels, caves and wound-like portals leading to the underwor(l)ds of the subconscious, which—as an informed audience would immediately object—should be properly called the unconscious.

As archaeologists of the symptomatic sites of wounds the WOUND ADDRESSERS claim that the unconscious is structured like a language and that we in general only exist in language. Any/body can be represented in language, yet there is always something missing, the body (of text) is preconditionally incomplete, holey. WOUND ADDRESSERS therefore are experts in missing pieces and lack, and consequently unsatisfied desires of wholeness. This desire has to be articulated by verbally exploring the hole/wound, which actually is symptomatic of something else, the WOUND ADDRESSERS believe. The WOUND ADDRESSERS are looking for ways to address an unspeaking, unsaying wound. To speak through the wound, to the wound, to speak the wound. To achieve closure by disclosure. WOUND ADDRESSERS have seen that wounds are piercing through bodies, bodies of times, through linear temporalities, bodies of memory, bodies of language. They inscribe themselves on multiple levels of being. Hence, WOUND ADDRESSERS are highly interested in various holey businesses such as in cuts, traces, sutures and marks. Amputation, too, is central in the image of a chopped-off penis. Castration. A first cut. Bodily fragmentation generally plays a vital role in their practice and theories as a way to challenge an imaginary sense of completeness, which they regard as erroneous. The theories they stage mirror the workshop of the → SUTURESS.

The WOUND ADDRESSERS have developed different systems that should help in approaching the unsayable and even the unthinkable. They speak of different interconnected, knotted orders—really, symbolically and imaginarly. Similar to sailors and textile workers they have busied themselves with different kinds of knots to prevent things from undoing themselves, from shattering to pieces. They stand at the limits of knowing and saying, staring into an abyss, trying to interpret what is emitted. They know the circular movements the ➞ BODY WRITER encounters, too, of the impulse of moving around a symptomatic (textual) wound-hole, encircling, without reaching into, without filling, without accessing the hole—an almost ritualistic dance of ecstasy and suffering to the rhythm of a stuttering, incomplete, language—lalangue.

It is rather a heterogenous, corporeal and verbal ordeal of fundamental incompleteness: a gaping.[4]

* * *

the WOUNDLICKERS *(mystic-o-logical translators and transmitters of pain and trauma, highly infectious)*

> Licking wounds:
>
> expression metaphorically used to denote the time of recovery, recuperation and retraction after a defeat. In a medical sense: instinctive response to promote the healing process of an injury in oneself or others.

The WOUNDLICKERS' paramount tool is their tongues

Tongue tastes
Tongue tells
Tongue touches
Oral, organ/ic trinity: lick, lubricate, language

We have three tongues says Michel Serres.

Sprung/escaped from mythological tales and rhapsodic verse the WOUNDLICKERS wander the wor(l)d's woundscapes. Age-old mythological creatures, deities perhaps, the WOUNDLICKERS are drawn to wounds, to cuts, to openings. As wound dwellers they commonly can be found at sites of traumatic ruptures and wounds in different kinds of bodies. The WOUNDLICKERS' attraction to wounds results from a primary instinct: they feed from wounds by submerging their tongues deep into the pulsing flesh of the lesion. The WOUNDLICKERS press their mouths onto the flesh of the wound.

(Wide open mouth-wound.)

[4] Julia Kristeva, *Powers of Horror; an Essay on Abjection*, New York: European Perspectives: A Series of the Columbia University Press, 1982. 27.

They merge their mouths with the red pulsing tissue.

Tongues push
  deep,
    down,
      below. They detach parts of skin, calluses, scabs—their food.

Touching, kissing, licking wounds, taking filth by mouth, a mediaeval mythic affair: 'Never in my life have I tasted any food or drink sweeter or more exquisite',[5] mystic St Catherine of Siena has been reported to exclaim after drinking pus from a woman's festering, cancerous breast. She adds: 'Thou shalt swallow what inspires you with such horror'[6]

Desisting this detour, back to the WOUNDLICKERS: as one side effect, their licking cleans the wounds from dirt and debris. Saliva has wound-healing properties. It keeps the wounds moist, it accelerates blood clotting, and it acts as defence against infection. Another side effect, much rather for the WOUNDLICKERS themselves, has been reported: they become witness of the wounds' afflictions through licking. Their tongues become the wound's tongues. The WOUNDLICKERS share their tongues with deemed language-less, tongue-less wounds. With feeding they lend the wounds their tongues to speak. Consumption and digestion turn into translation. The WOUNDLICKERS tell of different tastes: tastes of loneliness, of doubt, of fear, of poverty, of illness, of oppression, of despair. Driving their tongues deep into wounds, emotions and memories of traumatic events become part of the WOUNDLICKERS' bodies. WOUNDLICKERS, as well as religious mystics, experience emotional raptures, delusions, sensory intoxication and somatisation of pain.

The WOUNDLICKERS become a living archive of traumata by absorption. Embodied practitioner of oral histories, from the lips of one wound into the mouth of the WOUNDLICKERS, into the gorge agape of another wound. A matter of collecting, filing and storing. Of translating, transmitting. Every information gained from wounds they licked, the knowledge of every disaster they witnessed is stored only temporarily,

[5] Caroline Bynum Walker, *Holy Feast and Holy Fast, The Religious Sigificance of Food to Medieval Women*, Berkeley, Los Angeles, London: University of California Press, 1988, 172.

[6] Raymond of Capua, *The Life of St. Catherine of Siena*, Dublin: James Duffy and Co. Limited, 2007, 93.

briefly, in the WOUNDLICKERS' system. But mind you, dear audience, they are contagious, infectious. Illness and cure. They spread remnants of emotive reactions, memories, histories broken down to minuscule particles—invisible but affective. Licked wounds become infected with knowledge and feeling of lesions of other times, places, people and histories. Along with their own trauma they contract and experience emotive memories of past inflictions. The WOUNDLICKERS demonstrate that wounds speak and tell, aren't silent, aren't empty, aren't mute. Many unheard voices speak from and through wounds. The WOUNDLICKERS would agree with the ➞ SUTURESS' observation: healing the wound would mean silencing here, closing the wound-mouth. Therefore the WOUNDLICKERS continue their labour, their work, their efforts, their gluttonous feasts: their licking of what is commonly thought of as lacking.

Emerging from the Abyss,
and re-entering it
that is life, is it not, Dear?[7]

* * *

the BODY WRITER *(an author, a poet, perhaps, some/any-body bearing a wound, a woman?, a figure of the symbolic)*

Women's writing is to write the body. [8] The BODY WRITER tries to write a body (of text). In vain. In pain. She struggles.

A visible ordeal. Beyond the common act and difficulty of writing. This very body, the body she wrestles to write, doesn't want to be written.
Doesn't want to become words.
Doesn't want to come into language.
Doesn't embody.

It resists and refuses. All that alludes to this body, which struggles to come into something that can just barely be called existence, to be a text at all, is the BODY WRITER's occupation and denomination as a writer. Over and over, as soon as the body begins to form, it, slippery, withdraws

[7] Emily Dickinson as quoted in Susan Howe, *Spontaneous Particulars: The Telepathy Of Archives*, New York: New Directions, 18.

[8] Hélène Cixous, Keith Cohen, and Paula Cohen, 'The Laugh of the Medusa', *Signs*, 1(4), 1976, 875–893.

itself. The paper violently rejects the trace of the pen, rises up against the touch and weight of words. The BODY WRITER seems to swallow her words, just barely formed, and choke on them. Her body paralyses in presence of the unwritten—unwritable—body of text. Language fails, often, and repeatedly, it fails in front of this body of text, too.

However it is not entirely true, dear audience, that the BODY WRITER cannot write at all. It is only certain parts, nevertheless important parts, that just seem to be impossible to put into words, to put into coherent thought even—to put onto paper.

The body the BODY WRITER attempts to write, this (whole) body eludes representation. It eludes inscription, of itself, in itself. Symbolically. Holey intractability of the unspeakable, one is inclined to think. But no, we have to answer, esteemed audience, the unwritten parts, abysses
ripped open
gaping
in the text,
voids devoid of words,

are in themselves, traces and marks. They are visible inscriptions cutting and wounding the text's texture. The BODY WRITER labours as wound-scribe inscribing the unbearable, insufferable as wound-holes.

Unwritable fractions dismember the body the BODY WRITER attempts to write. They open wounds in the surface of the flesh of the text. In her desperate attempt to word the unwordable the BODY WRITER writes body parts. Parts of a body of text. Words, symbols, and characters that surround the wound-hole. Fragmented fragments, detached, truncated. Woundscapes manifest between amputated body parts. Blood drips from cut faces. The body as a whole—continuous—remains unwritable, laments the BODY WRITER, while the informed audience, of course, is aware that these ideas of wholeness should today only be decaying relics of bygone times.

The fragments the BODY WRITER writes, however, are of a lesser importance. We have to draw our attention towards that which is situated in between them. Gaping open!

The BODY WRITER's writing has become a performance of a circular gesture, a swirling but stumbling, stammering staccato, a choreography of arranging words around an ungraspable event, of drawing the outline of holes with unrelated words, cutting sharp edges, the inside of the circle falls through, out into a beyond. Words gather around the fringes of an abyss, which becomes a representation of the unsayable, the unthinkable. A textual hole, outside language inside writing—un/b/reach/able.

And just like this the BODY WRITER is not writing fragments at all, but holes instead. Holes, wound-like openings in between/in the midst of words. This body of text will never be whole but hole, eternally broken, corrupt, disrupted. A writing struggling with and against wholeness simultaneously.

All literature is scarry. It celebrates the wound and repeats the lesion.[9]

* * *

the WOUNDED TEXT *(a body hole-y of language, a symptom of the real)*

( ) opens gaping wound-mouth
[ ] screams,
in silence
...breaks off
shatters
fractured fragments.
It shrivels and withers, it stutters, stumbles, it hiccups and gargles.
Sentence-rags, language-t-a-t-t-e-r-s stuttering spewed out. Incoherent, non-linear,—
the WOUNDED TEXT won't transport the reader.
It devours and swallows the reader.
It mauls and guzzles the writer, too.

The body of the text is fragile, soft, caves in, hangs and sags. It collapses without a skeleton, devoid of a narrative scaffold of linearity, of coherence to prop it up. It limps.

( ) Unfilled parenthesis( )
....................................never-ending ....
ellipses.. that continue beyond three dots, ...
punctuation marks puncture; mark the body!
truncated sentences, flayed grammar.

[9] Hélène Cixous, *Stigmata*, London and New York: Routledge, 2005, xi

It murmurs inside. It murmurs. Inside is the pain of speech the pain to say. Larger still. Greater than is the pain not to say. To not say. Says nothing against the pain to speak. It festers inside. The wound, liquid dust. Must break. Must void. [10]

* * *

the WORD-LASS *(a girl)*

The WORD-LASS doesn't speak words
The WORD-LASS listens
The WORD-LASS remembers
The WORD-LASS witnesses
The WORD-LASS collects
The WORD-LASS registers
The WORD-LASS records

The WORD-LASS occupies the role of a jester. She is silent, doesn't speak, as is commonly expected of the girl in a Roussaultian fashion.[11] "Putting a door in the female mouth has been an important project of patriarchal culture from antiquity to the present day,"[12] explains Anne Carson. But the WORD-LASS is also a working-lass. She gathers and records occurrences, she disrupts the plot, irritates the other characters, by her actions of archiving stories and hole-y remains. The role of the collector of tales is, as you certainly know, dear audience, often a work assigned to the realm of women. The WORD-LASS therefore embodies, with a nod to Hannah Ahrendt,[13] and Audre Lorde[14] a transformation of language into action.

* * *

the NARRATOR *(a voice)*

reading

[10] Theresa Hak Kyung Cha, *Dictee*, Berkeley, Calif.: University of California Press, 2009, 3.

[11] Jean-Jacques Rousseau, *Emile, or On Education*, 1763.

[12] Anne Carson, 'The Gender of Sound: Description, Definition and Mistrust of the Female Voice in Western Culture', *Resources of Feminist Research*, 23 (3): 1994, 24–31.

[13] Hannah Arendt, *Vita activa*, Munich: Piper, 2011.

[14] Audre Lorde, 'The transformation of silence into language and action', *Lesbian and Literature Panel.* Modern Language Association. Chicago, 1977.

SCENE 1, ACT 1

A number of characters have gathered around an abyssal opening in the ground.

A lot of theoretical knowledge which is not directly referenced but embedded in this piece of practice writing is discussed in greater detail and more appropriately credited in my forthcoming PhD thesis "The Hole: Notes Toward an Insurrectionary Poetics of the Wounded Text", Goldsmiths, University of London

CHAPTER 14

Crazy Jane Hats and Maria Medallions: Consuming, Collecting and Containing Love's Madness

Anna Jamieson

In late eighteenth- and early nineteenth-century England, female insanity became visible as never before. People heard stories, sang songs, collected mementoes, read poems and carried chapbooks which represented madwomen, and, in particular, women who were driven mad following a lover's death, disappearance or deceit. Now known as 'love's madness', this cultural craze saw novelists, dramatists, musicians, painters and printmakers celebrate a roster of deranged and delusional female characters, including Laurence Sterne's Maria of Moulines, William Shakespeare's Ophelia, William Cowper's Crazy Kate and Matthew Lewis's Crazy Jane. Across page, stage and canvas, these heroines were bestowed with features that codified their heartbroken pathology. Typically presented as young, tearful, beautiful and submissive, they roamed natural, nondescript settings,

A. Jamieson (✉)
University of Birmingham, Birmingham, UK
e-mail: a.jamieson@bham.ac.uk

D. Woolley et al. (eds.), *Wearable Objects and Curative Things*, Palgrave Studies in Fashion and the Body,
https://doi.org/10.1007/978-3-031-40017-9_14

adorned with downcast eyes, tear-stained cheeks, dishevelled clothing and a seemingly unthreatening disposition.

Alongside these cultural representations, a multitude of fashionable accessories, domestic goods and ephemeral items depicting the love-mad woman became available for contemporary consumers. With women enthusiastically assimilating love-mad objects into their personal assemblages, it became fashionable to allude to, and be associated with, the emotional states and elite ideals that these milder forms of madness came to evoke. As such, these years saw the condition of love's madness become commercialised, commodified, and, as this chapter explores, contained and controlled through cultural representations and consumer goods.

Not just a popular cultural archetype, love's madness was also understood as a real pathological condition, powered by the belief that heartbreak could genuinely drive a person mad. Though men were sometimes included in this diagnosis, the majority of discussion focused on lovelorn *women.*[1] Often described as 'erotomania', eighteenth- and nineteenth-century psychiatric medical texts claimed love was a prominent cause of insanity. Joseph Mason Cox's *Practical Observations on Insanity* (1806) included a chapter titled 'On Love, Its Modifications and Effects' and argued that 'Disappointment, Jealousy and particularly Seduction, as consequences of the passion, [are] too often causes of insanity'.[2] In 1811, Dr. William Black wrote that '"Love" was the fifth most common cause for admission at Bethlem, London's infamous asylum, after 'Misfortunes, Religion, Fever, Family & Hereditary'.[3] This belief was mirrored across cultural publications. Titled 'On Love', James Boswell's 1778 column in the *London Magazine* explained that 'Disappointed Love is one of the most frequent causes of madness, as every body may be convinced'.[4] In 1804, artist Joseph Farington reported in his diary that the greatest number of people confined to Bethlem were 'women in love'.[5]

[1] Roy Porter, 'Love, Sex and Madness in Eighteenth Century England', *Social Research* 53: 1986. 211–242 (219).

[2] Joseph Mason Cox, *Practical Observations on Insanity*, 2nd edn. London: C. & R. Baldwin, J. Murray, 1806. 25, 297, 306; Alexander Morison, *Outlines of Lectures on the Nature, Causes and Treatment of Insanity*, 4th edn. London.

[3] William Black, *A Dissertation on Insanity*. London: D. Ridgway, 1811.

[4] James Boswell, *Boswell's Column*, ed. Margery Bailey. London: William Kimber, 1951, 82.

[5] Joseph Farington, *The Diary of Joseph Farington*, ed. Kenneth Garlick, Angus Macintyre and Kathryn Cave, London; New Haven, CT; London: Yale University Press, 1978–83, vol. 6, 2288.

Despite this cultural and medical phenomenon, and the issues it raises about the relationship between health, illness and the body, scholarship in this area has proved relatively limited, particularly when compared with the extensive scholarship 'lavished', as Roy Porter described, on the Victorian madwoman.[6] Research on that era has been extremely fertile, with histories of late nineteenth-century hysteria and cultural figures such as Ophelia assuming a starring scholarly role.[7] The few scholars who have trained their focus on the cultural figure of the late eighteenth-century madwoman have tended to overlook the significance of the melancholic love-mad woman.[8] Homogenised within a line-up of more docile and pathetic love-mad figures, she is frequently conceived as a sentimental step en route to more transgressive, and noteworthy, modes of female insanity.[9]

Critically, different iterations of love-mad women related to the different classes, as suggested by her sartorial choices. Despite her humble origins, Sterne's Maria was often viewed as a more refined icon, donned in elegant, neo-classical dress. Ophelia's high birth meant that she too was aligned with the upper classes, depicted in white with a flower-crown adorning her head. In contrast, Crazy Kate was a young servant girl, impoverished and in tatty rags. Crazy Jane straddled these camps, sometimes portrayed in elegant garb, other times, as a scruffy country girl. These distinctions—some subtle, some not so subtle—impacted the way that each love-mad iteration was understood by contemporaries. Yet scholarship has tended to flatten these differences, characterising these love-mad women as straightforwardly saccharine, sentimental and harmless. More manic, ambiguous, sexualised or transgressive accounts of love's madness, both living and imaginary, certainly were available during this period. An opportunity has therefore been missed to reassess the ways

[6] Roy Porter, *Mind-Forg'd Manacles: A History of Madness in England from the Restoration to the Regency*. London: Athlone Press, 1987, ix.

[7] Elaine Showalter, 'Victorian Women and Insanity', *Victorian Studies* 23: 1980. 157–181; Gilman, Sander L. 1993. 'The Image of the Hysteric', in *Hysteria Beyond Freud*. eds. Sander L. Gilman, H. King, Roy Porter, G. S. Rousseau and Elaine Showalter, 345–436. Berkeley, CA: University of California Press.

[8] Jane Kromm, 'The Feminization of Madness in Visual Representation', *Feminist Studies* 20: 1994. 507–535.

[9] Elaine Showalter, *The Female Malady: Women, Madness and English Culture, 1830–1980*. London: Virago, 1987, 10–14; Helen Small, *Love's Madness: Medicine, the Novel and Female Insanity, 1800–1865*. Oxford: Clarendon Press, 1996, 12–14; Kromm, 'Feminization'.

that contemporaries interacted with this trope, alongside the varied emotional effects of this cultural encounter.

That said, the recent efforts of several scholars suggest a renewed attention towards the emotional function and transgressive possibilities of the love-mad archetype. Sterne's Maria has received increased critical attention, with William B. Gerard and Susan Lamb making important contributions on her role as a psychosocial empathetic prompt.[10] Sally Holloway's *The Game of Love* (2019) dedicated a chapter to cultural codes of romantic suffering, and the ways in which archetypal heroines helped eighteenth-century women conceptualise their own emotional turmoil.[11] Holloway offers a strong sense of the relationship between cultural heroines and lived experience, arguing that various love-mad examples 'shaped popular understandings of how a disappointed lover should (and should not) behave and wider perceptions of the consequences of failed relationships for courting women'.[12] Though she considers early modern experiences of lovesickness, Lesel Dawson's call for a reconceptualisation of the frail, weak and irrational lovesick woman resonates with these ideas. Dawson explores the *uses* of female lovesickness, brilliantly capturing the ways that the language of love's madness allowed female self-expression and self-fashioning to take place. Examining the potentially pleasurable or indulgent aspects of this trope, Dawson argues that elite women were well aware of the cultural codes that melancholy or lovesickness represented—including learning, loneliness and interiority.[13]

This chapter powers these reassessments via a material, object-based approach. Historians have long conceptualised the final decades of the eighteenth century as witnessing a consumer revolution, whereby goods

[10] William B. Gerard, 'Laurence Sterne's "Poor Maria" as Model of Empathic Response', in *The Palgrave Handbook of Affect Studies and Textual Criticism*, eds. Donald R. Wehrs and Thomas Blake, 2017. 481–512. Basingstoke; Hampshire: Palgrave Macmillan; Gerard, William B. '"All that the heart wishes": Changing Views toward Sentimentality Reflected in Visualizations of Sterne's Maria, 1773–1888'. *Studies in Eighteenth-Century Culture* 2005, 34: 197–269; Susan Lamb, *Bringing Travel Home to England: Tourism, Gender and Imaginative Literature in the Eighteenth Century*. Newark, DE: University of Delaware Press, 2009.

[11] Sally Holloway, *The Game of Love in Georgian England: Courtship, Emotions and Material Culture*. Oxford: Oxford University Press, 2019, 123.

[12] Holloway, *Game of Love*, 128.

[13] Lesel Dawson, *Lovesickness and gender in early modern English literature*. Oxford: Oxford University Press, 2008, 93–94.

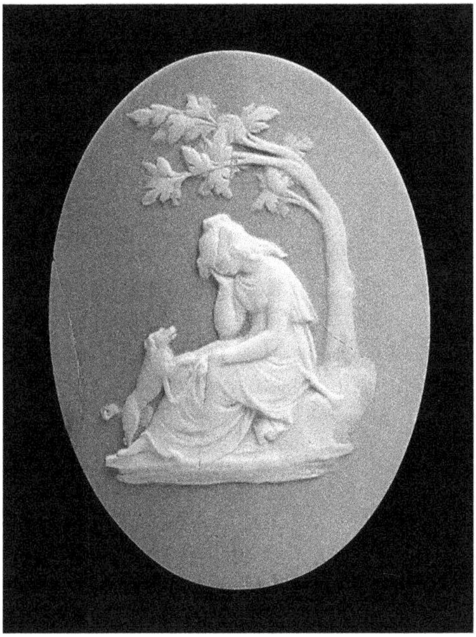

Fig. 14.1 Jasperware Buckle Ornament, after a design by Lady Elizabeth Templetown, made by Josiah Wedgwood and Sons, about 1785, England. Museum no. 464-1890. ©Victoria & Albert Museum, London

were increasingly designed for *pleasure* rather than *need*.[14] With the eighteenth century constituting a transitional moment in the commercialisation of romantic customs, numerous fashionable articles which commercialised love's madness became available for consumption.[15] This chapter explores this material phenomenon via various wearable objects that connect health, fashion and art: including belt buckles and pieces of jewellery that depicted Laurence Sterne's melancholic archetype, Maria of Moulines (Fig. 14.1), and the 'Crazy Jane Hat', a headpiece allegedly worn at fashionable parties throughout the 1790s.

The ubiquity and popularity of objects relating to Maria means that they still feature prominently in fashion and stoneware collections, easy to find via a quick Google search. The Crazy Jane Hat, on the other hand,

[14] Neil McKendrick, John Brewer and J. H Plumb, eds. *The Birth of a Consumer Society: The Commercialization of Eighteenth-Century England*. London: Europa Publications Limited, 1982.

[15] Holloway, *Game of Love*, 18; Small, *Love's Madness*, 13; Catherine M. Gordon, *British Paintings of Subjects from the English Novel, 1740–1870*. New York, NY; London: Garland, 1988, 73–6, 79, 87–9.

proves far more elusive. Only fleetingly mentioned in a biography of the creator of Crazy Jane in the 1850s, the hat is a beguiling source for the historian of material culture. Like Jane herself—who, despite her cultural profusion, proves the least visible of the love-mad heroines across scholarship—the hat has not been the focus of any sustained critical analysis. It thus functions as a mysterious sartorial item, made even more so as details of what it looked like do not survive. Nor does it appear to exist in any physical collection.

In line with historians who present a compelling model of the nexus of eighteenth-century experience, emotion and objects, this chapter excavates the layers of meaning attached to these wearable love-mad objects, questioning what it meant to incorporate them into the fashioned body, and to remove them once at home. It connects arguments about the role of fictionalised late eighteenth- and early nineteenth-century madwomen to the wider historiography of material culture, consumerism and emotions. In doing so, it characterises love-mad items as containers for an array of feelings and fears connected to mental illness and health, functioning as protective emotional artefacts. By linking the consumption of love-mad objects to more complex psychic processes linked to containment, control and even comfort, the chapter demonstrates that the putatively harmless condition of love's madness had more powerful psychological effects than scholars have previously acknowledged.

14.1 Visualising Love's Madness

Love's madness was part of a wider cultural phenomenon which saw the exhibition of a mild form of nerves function as a signifier of one's virtue. Within the broader dynamics of eighteenth-century sensibility, whereby being emotionally expressive and sensitive to one's external surroundings was a marker of genteel behaviour, a nervous episode or disposition could demonstrate an individual's genteel and refined character even further. Contemporary physicians George Cheyne and James Adair argued that the elite classes were disproportionately affected by an array of 'sinking, suffocating and strangling Nervous Disorders', their 'extraordinary refinement and sensibility' meaning that they were particularly sensitive to their exterior surroundings. As a result, such nervous diseases became aspirational.[16]

Nevertheless, some forms of madness were of course understood as extremely serious and plenty of commentators warned of the dangers of emotional outbursts toppling into full-blown derangement, particularly for the 'weaker' sex.[17] With the new taxonomy of eighteenth-century nervous disorders linked to frail bodies, the weaker physicality of women was commonly viewed as intensifying the likelihood of genuine mental disorder. Despite this, exhibiting a milder form of madness—of which love's madness was an important strand—was still seen as in keeping with refined, fashionable and sentimental expectations of gentility, so long as it was carefully managed.[18]

A mild form of madness was not just accepted—at times, it was celebrated. Dawson has shown that during the Renaissance, the 'dress, language, and posture associated with melancholy were available to women both as a form of expression and a means of self-fashioning', a method used to exhibit elevated social status and intellectual disposition.[19] The same was true of women in the late eighteenth century. Several portraits of aristocratic women from this period explicitly reference melancholy, utilising familiar signs to indicate the sitter's sensibility and elite status. John Raphael Smith's engraving after a painting by George Carter, titled *Miss Carter in the Character of Maria* from 1774, was the first visual representation of Sterne's Maria. 'Maria of Moulines' first appears in the

[16] George Cheyne, *The English malady or, A treatise of nervous diseases of all kinds, as spleen, vapours, lowness of spirits, hypochondriacal, and hysterical distempers, etc.* London: Strahan, 1733, 3; Carolyn Day and Amelia Rauser, 'Thomas Lawrence's Consumptive Chic: Reinterpreting Lady Manners's Hectic Flush in 1794', *Eighteenth-Century Studies* 49: 2016. 455–474 (457).

[17] G. L. Barker-Benfield, *The Culture of Sensibility: Sex and Society in Eighteenth-century Britain*. Chicago, IL: University of Chicago Press, 1992, 2–3.

[18] The high-profile illness of King George III in the late 1780s undoubtedly contributed to a more positive conceptualisation of nervousness within contemporary popular culture, along with its affiliation with the elite classes. Framed as a mild and fleeting pathology, George III and the royal court employed the language of nerves to underplay the severe implications of a mentally ill sovereign, with the King himself reassuring his court that: 'I'm nervous, I'm not ill, but I'm nervous'. See Frances Burney, *Diary and Letters of Madam D'Arbly*, ed. C.F. Barrett. London: Coburn, Hurst and Blackett, 1854. vol. 4, 239; Ida Macalpine and Richard Hunter. *George III and the Mad-Business*. Allen Lane: The Penguin Press, 1969.

[19] Dawson, *Lovesickness and gender*, 96.

ninth volume of Sterne's *Tristam Shandy* (1767), and again in *A Sentimental Journey* (1768). Once a 'quick witted and amicable maid', Maria is now melancholic, grief-stricken and haunted by the death of her lover. Sometimes depicted alone, at other times with her male companion, the 1770s saw Smith's representation joined by others from Joseph Wright of Derby and Angelica Kauffman, which were widely exhibited. Across these depictions, Maria is set in a bucolic landscape, dressed in white, with loose flowing hair and a sorrowful expression.[20]

The mood captured in Carter's painting—which depicts his daughter, Miss Carter—is one of isolated melancholy, a mood that this young woman was happy to emulate.[21] Gerard's analysis of this portrait/subject painting notes that Miss Carter's straining dog (a representation of Maria's sole companion, Sylvio) here becomes a neatly groomed French poodle, rather than a breed more in keeping with Sterne's initial portrayal of Maria as a local country girl. Testifying to Porter's comments that sensibility 'afforded a mode of melancholy in which ladies *par excellence* could participate',[22] this substitute 'hints at the character's popularity among the middle and upper-classes, who might possess a similar pet'.[23] Similarly, George Romney's *Mrs Crouch* (1787) shows a woman fully embracing the iconography of lovesick pensiveness. The esteemed actress and opera singer wears a plain white dress and is seated beside a substantial tree trunk, beyond which a ship carrying her husband sails towards the horizon. Toying with the chain of a portrait miniature that shows her spouse, Mrs. Crouch is depicted as a devoted wife, complete with a natural backdrop and pretty features.[24] The love-mad woman's dedication to her absent lover reinforces the unrelenting loyalty of the sitter: alongside refinement and emotional expressivity, channelling love's madness bestowed virtues of fidelity and steadfastness to a woman's character. The rural setting and tree, along with Mrs. Crouch's good looks and expression of pensive contemplation, positions Romney's portrait within a wider visual schema surrounding this acceptable mode of love's madness. These portraits suggest a fluid visual vocabulary within both subject painting and

[20] For more on Maria's melancholic iconography, see W.B. Gerard, 'All that the heart wishes', 238–240.

[21] Gerard, *Visual Imagination,* 142.

[22] Porter, *Mind-Forg'd Manacles*, 244.

[23] Gerard, *Visual Imagination*, 142.

[24] Julius Bryant, *Kenwood, Paintings in the Iveagh Bequest.* New Haven, CT; London: Yale University Press, 2003, 388.

portraits, as features including the loose white dress, downcast expression and coastal surroundings were repeated across works of both celebrated women and love-mad archetypes. Yet a woman's affinity with melancholic or love-mad characteristics was not only displayed through gesture, countenance or behaviour. As we see with the repeated motif of the loose white dress, it was also demonstrated through fashionable articles.

14.2 The Case of the Crazy Jane Hat

In 1796, a poem by Matthew Lewis captured the public imagination. Following the success of his Gothic novel *The Monk,* the poem described an alleged episode which occurred during Lewis's evening walk in the grounds of Inveraray Castle, when staying at the Duke of Argyll's estate in Scotland. The story went that Lewis and a female companion had stumbled across 'a poor mad Woman [...] at whose appearance the Lady was much alarmed'.[25] The four-stanza poem tells of the meeting between this woman, the broken-hearted 'Crazy Jane', and the female passer-by—presumably Lewis's companion. Abandoned by her lover Henry, Crazy Jane expounds her plight to this obliging female spectator.

Functioning as an instructive tale of immoral behaviour, Jane's story of ill-fated attachment was, according to Lewis's biographer, infused with such romance, suspense and adventure as to gain 'a degree of popularity scarcely yet abated'.[26] By 1799, the lyrics had been put to music by leading female composer Harriet Abrams.[27] This publicity saw the poem published across the day's leading periodicals and newspapers, with Abram's rendition becoming a mainstay of Britain's performance circuit. Bound in ballad books or sold as single sheet scores, the ballad was heard by a wide cross-section of society, from music halls, streets and alehouses to elite performance spaces. By the early nineteenth century, Jane was the subject of a popular chapbook, *The Tragical History of Miss Jane Arnold, Commonly called Crazy Jane [...] Founded on Facts*, written by Sarah Wilkinson.[28] Periodicals and newspapers advertised a popular Crazy Jane opera and

[25] *Courier*, 27 March 1799; *Star and Evening Advertiser*, 27 March 1799.

[26] Margaret Baron-Wilson, *The Life and Correspondence: With Many Pieces in Prose and Verse Never Before Published*. London: Henry Colburn, vol. 1, 1839, 188.

[27] Leslie Ritchie, *Women writing music in late eighteenth-century England: social harmony in literature and performance*. London; New York, NY: Routledge, 2016, 110.

[28] Sarah Wilkinson, *The tragical history of Miss Jane Arnold, commonly called Crazy Jane and Mr. H. Percival... Founded on Facts*. Stirling, 1820.

ballet.[29] A print, several woodcut illustrations and a watercolour joined this cultural medley, and by the 1830s, it was reported that a 'Crazy Jane Hat' had been all the rage in the century's final decades.[30]

The Life and Correspondence of M. G. Lewis, written by Margaret Baron-Wilson and published in 1839, is the only publication that documents this mysterious item. Baron-Wilson described how the hat was 'worth mention, because it shows the extraordinary popularity which one of the merest trifles from Lewis's pen was then capable of obtaining'. Speaking of the ballad, she explained:

> After the usual complimentary tributes from barrel-organs, and wandering damsels of every degree of vocal ability, it crowned not only the author's brow with laurels, but also that of many a youthful beauty, in the shape of a fashionable hat, called the 'Crazy Jane hat'.[31]

No longer surviving in any collections, other contemporary recollections from the period frustratingly fail to mention this item. Its existence as a 'missing object' aligns it with arguments put forward by curator and historian, Glenn Adamson. Accounting for the phenomenon of loss within the study of material culture, Adamson charts his fruitless search to find a single British domestic footstool dated before 1800, despite seeing representations of such an item in the second plate of William Hogarth's *Marriage a la Mode* (1745).[32] Yet the footstool, he maintains, 'was no less important to eighteenth-century Britain for being absent'.[33] Rather than proving fruitless or problematic, Adamson insists that asking questions about lost objects is a productive enterprise, their absence becoming a matter of historical interest in its own right.[34]

This advice chimes with others working across the medical humanities and the discipline of material culture more broadly. In *Manifesto for a Visual Medical Humanities*, Fiona Johnstone stresses that 'visual artefacts can facilitate the suspension of certainty and function as sites for

[29] *Morning Chronicle*, 23 March 1805; *Monthly Mirror*, 19 June 1805.

[30] Baron-Wilson. *Life and Correspondence*, 189.

[31] Baron-Wilson. *Life and Correspondence*, 189.

[32] Glenn Adamson, 'The Case of the Missing Footstool: Reading the Absent Object', in *History and Material Culture: A Student's Guide to Approaching Alternative Sources*, ed. Karen Harvey, 192–207. New York, NY; London: Routledge, 2007.

[33] Adamson, 'Missing Footstool', 194.

[34] Adamson, 'Missing Footstool', 192–193.

productive doubt'.[35] Johnstone's advice to embrace ambiguity speaks to the work of Jules David Prown and Karen Harvey who, when faced with an absence of personal responses and inventories when researching specific objects, have encouraged approaches which use creative imagining 'to understand why an object is the way it is, or provokes the way it provokes'.[36] In the absence of contemporary discussions of the hat, alongside the issue that I do not have access to the object itself to analyse, my approach towards this missing object mobilises similar methods, relying upon its reported existence and popularity, along with a sprinkling of speculation, to excavate its meaning to late eighteenth-century society.

Through these speculations, various hypotheses come to the fore. Perhaps the Crazy Jane hat was a mere flash in the pan? Or such a unique piece that only a few were ever made—although Baron-Wilson's comment that 'many a youthful beauty' wore the hat suggests otherwise. A more likely explanation is that it was more of a generic item than first assumed. Rather than bearing an obvious, literal reference to Crazy Jane, identifiable for the modern researcher, the hat may have been recognisable to contemporaries in a different way. It may have borne a particular style, having been worn by a specific performer of the ballad or as part of a costume in a theatrical production. Gill Perry's discussion of the fashionable 'Abington cap', worn by celebrity actress Frances Abington, illuminates this idea. Perry tells of this cap becoming popular in the 1750s and 1760s, recounting how one theatre manager described that 'Abington's cap was so much the taste with ladies of fashion, that there was not a milliners shop window, great or small, that was not adorned with it, and in large letters ABINGTON appeared to attract the passer by'.[37] The hat was similar to a small pointed cap adorned with feathers and red flowers worn by Abington

[35] Fiona Johnstone, 'Manifesto for a Visual Medical Humanities', *Medical Humanities*, 2018, https://blogs.bmj.com/medical-humanities/2018/07/31/manifesto-for-a-visual-medical-humanities/. Accessed 1 April 2022.

[36] Jules David Prown, 'Mind in Matter: An Introduction to Material Culture Theory and Method', *Winterthur Portfolio* 17: 1982, 1–19 (7–10); Karen Harvey, 'Introduction: Historians, Material Culture and Materiality', in *History and Material Culture: A Student's Guide to Approaching Alternative Sources*. New York, NY; London: Routledge, 2009, 2. I have used this methodology in additional research on the lived experience of women's mental illness and material culture during this period; see Anna Jamieson, "Comforts in her Calamity': Shopping and Consumption in the Late Eighteenth-Century Madhouse', *Eighteenth-Century Studies* 55: 2021, 82–102.

[37] Gill Perry, *Spectacular Flirtations: Viewing the Actress in British Art and Theatre, 1768–1820*. New Haven; CT; London: Yale University Press, 2007, 218, f.n. 64.

in a later portrait, Thomas Hickey's *Frances Abington as Lady Baby Lardoon in 'The Maid of Oaks' by John Burgoyne* (1775). Yet without this visual reference and association with Abington, the cap's meaning would probably be lost.[38] While today we might miss the sartorial cues which connect the Crazy Jane hat to its love-mad heroine, the contemporary viewer may have immediately recognised its style or decorative features, helping to explain the apparent invisibility of this supposedly popular item.

Raising issues around fashion and celebrity, sensibility and mental illness, this accessory prompts the question: what did it mean for a woman to purchase, own, wear or gift a hat associated with Crazy Jane and love's madness? If we take the craze surrounding Abington's hat as an example, we can understand Jane's popularity as operating within the dynamics of *fashion*, rather than madness. To wear the hat was not to pay homage to Jane and her love-mad pathology; rather, it referenced a popular actress, singer or performance associated with Crazy Jane, aligning the wearer with fashionable society and its genteel entertainments. The identity of the 'fair maid' that Crazy Jane originally directs her advice to supports this idea. On the night of this alleged meeting, Lewis was enjoying an evening stroll with the daughter of his host: Lady Charlotte Campbell, later Bury, a woman described by the *Belle Assemblee* as 'the most distinguished ornament of the fashionable circle'.[39] With the beautiful and stylish Campbell being the first woman to be associated with Jane, wearing such an item was a way to connect with, or at least aspire to, the beauty, elegance and refinement of Campbell and her clique.

A more exaggerated iteration of this ritual can be found in early nineteenth-century Paris. Following a performance of Hamlet, the straw worn in the hair of the female actress playing Ophelia—a reference to the use of straw as asylum bedding—became 'all the rage of Parisian high fashion'.[40] The fact that elegant, elite women were walking around Paris with straw in their hair is not to suggest that women were literally attempting to look like they had escaped from La Salpêtrière, Paris's infamous

[38] Perry, *Spectacular Flirtations,* 121.

[39] *Belle Assemblee,* London, 1809. For more on Campbell, see Amelia Rauser, *Art in the Age of Undress: Art, Fashion and the Classical Ideal in the 1790s.* New Haven, CT; London: Yale University Press, 2020, 21–23.

[40] Susan Lamb, 'Applauding Shakespeare's Ophelia in the Eighteenth Century: Sexual Desire, Politics, and the Good Woman', in *Women as Sites of Culture: Women's Roles in Cultural Formation from the Renaissance to the Twentieth Century,* ed. Susan Shifrin, 105–123. Hampshire: Ashgate Publishing, 2002.

asylum. Rather, the incorporation of these features into one's fashioned body and public assemblage was linked to their connotations with high society and the celebrated status of a prestigious performer. In 1800, the *Monthly Magazine* reviewed the latest musical Crazy Jane spin-off—a ballad titled *Henry's Return; the Sequel to Crazy Jane*—favourably, stressing how it was well received by the 'fashionable clientele for whom the pieces were written'.[41] Donning the hat or wearing a sprig of straw allowed eighteenth-century women to situate themselves alongside celebrated individuals, becoming part of this 'fashionable clientele'. Via this reading, women such as Mrs. Crouch were not necessarily concerned about referencing love-mad melancholy *specifically* in their portraits. Rather, it was about aligning themselves with a fashionable trope and those 'youthful beauties' who were at its heart.

That said, there was more at stake here than the desire to emulate a glamorous clique. In one of the only mentions of the hat within secondary literature, literary critic Helen Small states that 'with Crazy Jane millinery, female insanity reached its nadir, becoming a fashion accessory: madness quite literally à la mode'.[42] The hat's popularity suggests that it *was* fashionable to allude to, and be associated with, certain emotional states and characteristics that milder forms of madness evoked: of emotional expressivity, fine feeling and an innately sensitive disposition. The enthusiastic assimilation of love-mad objects into women's personal assemblages demonstrates this point. Clearly, material objects were used as self-fashioning props through which love-mad characters such as Maria and Jane, and their positive associational qualities, could be referenced.

Extremely popular in the 1770s and 1780s, an amazing array of Wedgwood stoneware and jewellery depicted Maria of Moulines. Alongside stoneware, Sterne's melancholic heroine appeared as an isolated motif on a range of jewellery, including earrings, medallions, buckles and bracelets, all marketed with the female consumer in mind.[43] As with Harriet Abrams's ballad, it was a woman, Lady Templetown, who created Maria's popular Wedgwood motif. Gerard has argued that 'it was important for Wedgwood to credit a contemporary English woman [...] with the image to complete its appeal to its target audience', reinforcing the

[41] *Monthly Magazine*, August 1800, vol. 61, 67.

[42] Small, *Love's Madness*, 13–14.

[43] William B. Gerard, *Laurence Sterne and the Visual Imagination*. London; New York, NY: Routledge, 2016, 147.

triangulation between Jane, her female creator and her female audience.[44] Following Templetown's basic composition of a solitary woman, dog and tree, this motif appears in a portrait of the Duchesse d'Orléans by Élisabeth Louise Vigée from 1789. 'Not only is the noblewoman depicted dressed in a loose, unstructured peasant costume like Maria's', Gerard writes, 'but she is also wearing a Wedgwood belt buckle medallion of the character, probably set in cut steel'. The Duchess's sombre gaze, pensive attitude and explicit reference to Maria reveals how this archetype was 'far more than a character in a book, but rather a regular and prominent resident in the popular imagination'.[45] This popularity was not just about cultural interest, but a desire to be associated with Maria and her mild pathology, demonstrating the illness's emotional ramifications, and its connections with the fashionable trend of sensibility.

Melancholy was not the only 'fashionable' illness during this period. Historian Carolyn Day's 2017 book *Consumptive Chic* (2017) explored how consumption related to contemporary ideals of beauty and class within eighteenth-century fashionable society.[46] In an earlier article co-authored with Amelia Rauser, Day analysed the aesthetic dimensions of this relationship within Thomas Lawrence's *Portrait of Catherine Grey, Lady Manners, as Juno* from 1794. The article convincingly argues that Lawrence's portrait used 'the tubercular as a visual shorthand for beauty, genius, and sensibility', employing a language of blushing, stooping posture and exaggerated thinness as indicators of the sitter's sensibility.[47] Here, women do not merely don accessories linked to tuberculosis. Rather they *assimilate* these visual markers into their physical body and complexion.

Day and Rauser have stressed that it was a tubercular *mode* of beauty, rather than the literal development of the disease, that Lawrence sought to highlight in his painting of Lady Manners.[48] Even so, they still suggest that some women were willing to make various physical sacrifices, even if just on the canvas, to evoke this fashionable aesthetic. The visualisation of the physical thinness of one's body or the curvature of one's spine serves as a

[44] Gerard argues that Wedgwood's stoneware 'appealed predominantly to female taste'. See Gerard, *Visual Imagination*, 147.

[45] Gerard, *Visual Imagination*, 147–9.

[46] Carolyn Day, *Consumptive Chic: A history of beauty, fashion and disease*. London; New York, NY: Bloomsbury, 2017.

[47] Day and Rauser, 'Hectic Flush', 467.

[48] Day and Rauser, 'Hectic Flush', 458.

far more embodied marker of illness than the poses displayed, and the airs adopted, within portraits and paintings of love-mad women. In contrast, expressions of melancholy as part of the fashioned body functioned rather differently. These were part of a *temporary* sartorial assemblage, of the evocation of a melancholic *mood*, rather than symbolising full-blown assimilation of an illness into the physical body.

Be it a sprig of straw in one's hair, a piece of jewellery for Maria, or a hat for Jane, these arguments characterise love-mad articles as associative symbols that linked their wearers or owners to the sought-after emotional qualities that the convention evoked. Thinking about wearing these objects in public, their removable nature in private feels important too. The fact that material expressions of love's madness could be removed, put away, even discarded once worn, meant that women were in control of their potent emotional references: they were handled on their own terms. At the same time, this act of ownership speaks to an additional layer of control: that of the unruly threat of love's madness itself. As these objects embarked on a lifecycle of their own, undergoing various consumptive processes across a variety of scenarios, their meaning adjusted accordingly. Collective signifiers of cultural currency and fashionability at some moments, at others they served as more complex embodiments of private emotional meaning, as the final section of this chapter will explore.

14.3 Bringing Madness Home

What happened to the love-mad object when brought into the home? Susan Stewart's analysis of the role of miniature objects as souvenirs, and their place as identity definers for the people who bought, collected and carried them, is useful when answering this question. 'The souvenir', Stewart says, 'reduces the public, the monumental, and the three-dimensional into the miniature, that which can be enveloped by the body'.[49] Collapsing distance into proximity, Stewart characterises souvenirs as objects which facilitate private reflections and thought processes; a material container through which public cultural encounters can be digested in private.[50]

[49] Susan Stewart, *On Longing: Narratives of the Miniature, the Gigantic, the Souvenir, the Collection*. Durham, NC; London: Duke University Press, 1993, 137–138.

[50] Stewart, *On Longing*, 135.

A love-mad accessory tied to a cultural encounter functions similarly. On the one hand, for those who encountered Crazy Jane as part of a genteel performance or had viewed a painting of Maria at the Royal Academy, bringing an item associated with her back home was another way to engage with this fashionable trope, thus enacting one's material participation in the love-mad craze and a person's membership in this emotional, expressive and genteel community. But these objects clearly carried additional meaning. Calling to mind Sara Ahmed's arguments on the 'stickiness' of 'things', and Daniel Miller's on the ways in which objects 'breathe out emotions with which they have been associated', [51] they might harbour auspicious associations, not necessarily linked to love's madness but serving as a memento of happier times at plays, galleries or performances with loved ones. In this sense, they become tokens of positive memories, perhaps gaining the same kind of emotional value experienced when thumbing through a dogeared theatre programme found forgotten in a drawer, reusing a tote bag from a favourite museum, or pinning a ticket from a music concert to the fridge.

Arguing for the 'significant material-history component to the history of emotions', Rob Boddice maintains that 'we can think of objects as elicitors of emotions, only insofar as we remember that an object does not elicit the same emotions in all people'.[52] Likewise, an object's meaning could change depending on its placement. Markers of sociability and one's emotionally expressive character when worn in public, this meaning might shift in a new setting: when taken off, stowed in a cupboard, hung on a hook or concealed in the intimate space of a woman's pocket. Across these spaces, a more complex set of feelings might unravel.

As discussed, love's madness was not merely a positive paradigm of illness that advertised one's pensive interiority and emotional depth. Despite being a disorder sometimes associated with more positive expressions of feeling, this expression could also be dangerous. The aforementioned chorus of medical men who included love on their lists of primary causes of insanity helped crystallise the difference between a mild bout of disappointed love and a severe case of full-blown love's madness, arguing that

[51] Sara Ahmed, 'Happy Objects', in *The Affect Theory Reader*, eds. Melissa Gregg and Gregory J. Seigworth, 29–51. Durham, N.C: Duke University Press, 2008; Daniel Miller, *The Comfort of Things*, Cambridge: Polity Press, 2008.

[52] Rob Boddice, *The History of Emotions*. Manchester: Manchester University Press, 2018, 38.

the latter could be fatal. Another issue was the love-mad woman's sexuality. Crazy Jane's story in particular welcomed a more sensualised and erotic reading, through its assertion that sexual impropriety and the loss of her virtue caused Jane's descent into madness. Certain lines and lyrics from the poem and ballad, such as 'he was false, and I undone', surely piqued the interest of the singer, listener or reader. With Jane's insanity taking hold *after* the act of sexual intercourse, the poem functioned as a morality tale, warning its female readers about the consequences of losing one's virginity.[53] Susan Lamb has similarly argued that Sterne's *A Sentimental Journey* 'was not universally read as sexually innocent'. In fact, it could be interpreted as 'downright bawdy', alerting us to the degree to which sexuality was at issue in the text.[54]

Some women expressed explicit disdain for the trope. Feeling patronised by Samuel Richardson after reading descriptions of the love-mad behaviour of Lady Clementina della Porretta in *Sir Charles Grandison* (1753), Lady Mary Wortley Montagu wrote that the author 'should be better skilled in physic than to think fits and madness any ornament to the character of his heroines'.[55] We cannot presume that all women would have enjoyed the love-mad craze; thinking about the more ambiguous, unpopular or deviant aspects of the love-mad story disrupts the notion that the lovesick woman functioned purely as an unthreatening emblem of a mild pathology, or as vehicles of straightforward sentimentality.

For some, feelings of erotic desire, anger, shame, fear or intoxicating love felt or remembered when encountering a performance taking place in a theatre, or a song heard in a rowdy tavern, might transfer to the souvenir and be experienced, virtually, at home. No longer a mere symbol of an emotional trend, the object itself becomes a repository for a woman's feelings surrounding sexual transgression or immoral behaviour,

[53] Relatively little has been written on the subject of virginity and eighteenth-century love's madness. Though Porter asked 'how did people see the relations between sex and insanity? Within the traditional models of madness, could the lusts of the flesh by responsible for the overthrow of the mind?', he gave few definitive answers. Sexual frustration has previously been interpreted as prompting insanity, with Lamb arguing that during this period, 'experts and the public alike believed that lack of gratification rather than the desire itself' could cause madness. See Porter, 'Love, Sex and Madness', 220; Lamb, 'Applauding Shakespeare's Ophelia', 107.

[54] Lamb, *Bringing Travel Home*, 159. See also Gordon, *British Paintings*, 79.

[55] Brimley Johnson, ed. 1925. *Letters from Lady Mary Wortley Montagu*, London: Everyman's Editions, 465.

inviting associated emotions of guilt, shame or fear. Stewart has noted how miniature objects embody imagined experiences within the realms of fantasy, suggesting that their associative function stretched to sexual and seductive imaginings.[56] Serving as alluring proxies through which individuals might navigate typically frowned-upon thoughts, some women may have enjoyed the unsavoury and titillating elements of the madwoman's sexual misbehaviour that the love-mad object conjured. Others may have utilised the trope to express feelings of anger, passion, even revenge. Dawson has stressed that the language surrounding lovesickness provided a vital means of expressing negative emotion, allowing 'individuals to criticize those who have mistreated them whilst still appearing as passive victims'.[57] Contained within these fashionable accessories, these feelings might intensify when they were handled at home.

On the other hand, with the love-mad story serving as an important moral lesson, its associations with immorality and ensuing poverty might have bolstered the object's moralistic power. Through this lens, it functioned as a corrective tool, a material memento of a fall from grace which ensured good behaviour in the future. Pieces of jewellery were surely passed down through family lines, from woman to woman, linked to family histories of broken hearts, lost loves and the dangerous effects of sex outside of marriage. They might also have functioned as markers of a woman's superiority, either when worn in public or perused in private, symbolising the owner's own avoidance of falling into the naive trap which caught the love-mad heroine.

Finally, the purchasing and possession of these items could also stand in for the metaphorical ownership of the concept of love's madness itself. The financial transaction of acquiring a brooch, buckle or hat, of paying for a product linked to a love-mad pathology, may have alleviated or downplayed the disarming threat of the disorder—subject to one's own mental health and personal situation. A woman familiar with the experience of mental collapse after the death of a husband may have felt distressed when engaging with certain renditions of the love-mad trope. Someone dealing with an adulterous marriage might well have found some of Jane's lines ('think him false / I found him so') painful to recount. With the period's cultural commentators peddling the alarming consequences of disappointed love, collapsing these fears into wearable,

[56] Stewart, *On Longing*, 139.
[57] Dawson, *Lovesickness*, 8.

familiar and easy-to-handle objects could circumvent the ideological and social dangers they represented. Reducing these fears into a small hand-held form made them tangible, controllable, even comforting. An illness often characterised through boundless, excessive and unrestrictive imagery, love's madness is rendered to something recognisable, contained and curbed within the material and the three-dimensional. For anyone who had struggled with their health, suffered from a broken heart or had taken care of a mentally ill family member or friend, these processes linked to consumption and ownership may have assisted their fears and feelings about mental illness, even endowing the love-mad object with protective and talismanic properties.

This reading is best conceptualised within the spatial parameters of the pocket. Characterising tie-on pockets as 'thresholds' which articulated relationships between 'interior and exterior, secrecy and disclosure, self and other', the work of Barbara Burman and Arianne Fennetaux on eighteenth-century women and their pockets has broadened understanding on how women interacted with certain pocketable items.[58] Worn between inner and outer wear, the physical positioning of the pocket between skin and garment meant that these were spaces 'where intimate scenarios were projected and explored'.[59] These projections and explorations might, in turn, transfer onto objects placed inside. Within these mobile vessels of intimacy, sexuality and emotional life, a pocketable love-mad item like a Maria medallion takes on further ideological import concerning a woman's identity and her innermost, private thoughts. Be they sexual, protective or talismanic, keeping these items so close to the body could intensify their meaning.[60] For some woman, pocketing a love-mad medallion might speak to private desires, the madwoman standing in for a

[58] Barbara Burman and Ariane Fennetaux, *The Pocket: A hidden history of women's lives, 1600–1900*. New Haven, CT: Yale University Press, 2020; Barbara Burman, 'Pocketing the Difference: Gender and Pockets in Nineteenth-Century Britain', *Gender and History* 14: 2002. 447–69 (447–8); Ariane Fennetaux, 'Pockets, Consumption and Female Sociability in Eighteenth-century London', 2017, https://www-cc.gakushuin.ac.jp/~20070019/Abstract2017/Fennetaux.pdf. Accessed 15 January 2022. Fennetaux explains how from the end of the seventeenth century, 'every woman, regardless of her rank or status, had one or several pairs of tie-on pockets, which were detachable items of clothing rather like bags worn under a woman's skirt and accessed through slits in her overdress'. See Ariane Fennetaux, 2008, 'Women's Pockets and the Construction of Privacy in the Long Eighteenth Century', *Eighteenth-Century Fiction* 20: 307–334 (308).

[59] Fennetaux, 'Women's Pockets', 333.

[60] Fennetaux, 'Women's Pockets', 319, 330, 333.

sexually expressive surrogate. Perhaps the eighteenth-century woman, unhappy in love, found herself fiddling with the piece of jewellery hidden away in her pocket when nervous, and seeking comfort. We can therefore read the pocketed love-mad item as guarding the beholder from the threat of mental deterioration or functioning as a lucky charm against a broken heart. While their precise meanings are manifold, the act of purchasing, wearing, pocketing or putting away these items could assist the owner's own fears surrounding mental deterioration or the threat of the unruly, dangerous madwoman herself.

14.4 Conclusion

This chapter has characterised love-mad objects as miniature vehicles through which historical actors could explore a range of issues relating to identity: love, sexuality, morality and health. In her text, *The Self and It: Novel Objects,* Julie Park argues that 'the eighteenth-century self reached its most lively articulation through the material objects we traditionally consider as trivial imitations or supplements of the human: dolls, machines, puppets, wigs, muffs, hats, pens, letters, bound books, and fictional narratives'.[61] Identity, Park maintains, is embodied through these inanimate objects, which become media through which individuals can not only acquire knowledge about others, but also the self.[62] Park's arguments resonate with those made throughout this chapter about objects that depicted Maria and Jane, positioning them as important conduits through which eighteenth-century individuals could explore both the era's ideological complexities, and themselves. Wistfully thinking about a husband, lover or admirer, pondering the more sexualised aspects of the love-mad woman's tale, thinking about one's own brush with mental illness or rolling one's eyes at a male writer's overly sentimental prose: all these processes were bound to and embodied by the love-mad object.

Despite the absence of a paper trail documenting the responses the love-mad object provoked, their very existence and dissemination reveal interest and engagement with them. These objects existed, people owned them, and many of them have survived. In the same way that we as researchers remain wary of retrospectively diagnosing historical actors

[61] Julie Park, *The Self and It: Novel Objects.* Stanford, CA: Stanford University Press, 2010, 95.

[62] Park, *Self and It*, xviii, xv.

with modern illnesses, I do not wish to retrospectively endow eighteenth- and nineteenth-century actors with a pluralistic understanding of twenty-first-century mental illness. Yet a material approach clearly provides greater texture to these attitudes, in line with Porter's assertion that eighteenth-century madness was 'unbound'; that it 'wore many faces', and could be 'cosmic, comic, clinical or casual'.[63] Expanding our conceptualisation of love's madness, these sartorial and material interventions reveal that the condition was frequently celebrated and embraced. Love-mad souvenirs had the power to function as symbols of one's involvement in an emotional community and a souvenir of happy times. They also served as conduits of correction and moralistic storytelling, or as protective containers, alluring yet provocative psychological souvenirs associative of a complex cocktail of feelings including shame, guilt, fear or betrayal. Holding, containing and keeping at bay all manner of fears surrounding madness, ultimately these objects offered a reassuring barrier or talisman against the pathology itself, in ways that proved protective and comforting, and reminded the owner to be wary of excessive feeling, and to take care.

References

Adamson, Glenn. 'The Case of the Missing Footstool: Reading the Absent Object'. In *History and Material Culture: A Student's Guide to Approaching Alternative Sources*, ed. Karen Harvey, 192–207. New York, NY; London: Routledge. 2007.

Ahmed, Sara. 'Happy Objects'. In *The Affect Theory Reader*, eds. Melissa Gregg and Gregory J. Seigworth, 29-51. Durham, N.C: Duke University Press. 2008.

Barker-Benfield, G. L. *The Culture of Sensibility: Sex and Society in Eighteenth-century Britain*. Chicago, IL: University of Chicago Press. 1992.

Baron-Wilson, Margaret. *The Life and Correspondence: With Many Pieces in Prose and Verse Never Before Published*. London: Henry Colburn, vol. 1. 1839.

Black, William. *A Dissertation on Insanity*. London: D. Ridgway. 1811.

Boddice, Rob. *The History of Emotions*. Manchester: Manchester University Press. 2018.

Boswell, James. *Boswell's Column*, ed. Margery Bailey. London: William Kimber. 1951.

Brimley Johnson, ed., *Letters from Lady Mary Wortley Montagu*. London: Everyman's Editions. 1925.

Bryant, Julius. *Kenwood, Paintings in the Iveagh Bequest*. New Haven, CT; London: Yale University Press. 2003.

[63] Porter, *Mind-Forg'd Manacles*, 18.

Burman, Barbara. 'Pocketing the Difference: Gender and Pockets in Nineteenth-Century Britain'. *Gender and History* 14: 2002. 447–69.

Burman, Barbara and Ariane Fennetaux. *The Pocket: A hidden history of women's lives, 1600–1900*. New Haven, CT: Yale University Press. 2020.

Burney, Frances. *Diary and Letters of Madam D'Arbly*, ed. C.F. Barrett. London: Coburn, Hurst and Blackett, vol. 4. 1854.

Cheyne, George. *The English malady or, A treatise of nervous diseases of all kinds, as spleen, vapours, lowness of spirits, hypochondriacal, and hysterical distempers, etc.* London: Strahan. 1733.

Dawson, Lesel. *Lovesickness and gender in early modern English literature*. Oxford: Oxford University Press. 2008.

Day, Carolyn. *Consumptive Chic: A history of beauty, fashion and disease*. London; New York, NY: Bloomsbury. 2017.

Day, Carolyn and Amelia Rauser. 'Thomas Lawrence's Consumptive Chic: Reinterpreting Lady Manners's Hectic Flush in 1794'. *Eighteenth-Century Studies* 49: 2016. 455–474.

David Prown, Jules. 'Mind in Matter: An Introduction to Material Culture Theory and Method'. *Winterthur Portfolio* 17: 1982. 1–19.

Farington, Joseph. *The Diary of Joseph Farington*, ed. Kenneth Garlick, Angus Macintyre and Kathryn Cave. London; New Haven, CT: Yale University Press, 1978–1983. vol. 6.

Fennetaux, Ariane. 'Women's Pockets and the Construction of Privacy in the Long Eighteenth Century'. *Eighteenth-Century Fiction*. 20: 2008. 307–334.

Fennetaux, Ariane. 'Pockets, Consumption and Female Sociability in Eighteenth-century London'. 2017. https://www-cc.gakushuin.ac.jp/~20070019/Abstract2017/Fennetaux.pdf. Accessed 15 January 2022.

Gerard, William B. '"All that the heart wishes": Changing Views toward Sentimentality Reflected in Visualizations of Sterne's Maria, 1773-1888'. *Studies in Eighteenth-Century Culture* 34: 2005. 197–269.

Gerard, William B. 'Laurence Sterne's "Poor Maria" as Model of Empathic Response'. In *The Palgrave Handbook of Affect Studies and Textual Criticism*, eds. Donald R. Wehrs and Thomas Blake, 481–512. Basingstoke; Hampshire: Palgrave Macmillan, 2017.

Gerard, William B. *Laurence Sterne and the Visual Imagination*. London; New York, NY: Routledge. 2016.

Gilman, Sander L. 'The Image of the Hysteric'. In *Hysteria Beyond Freud*. eds. Sander L. Gilman, H. King, Roy Porter, G. S. Rousseau and Elaine Showalter, 345–436. Berkeley, CA: University of California Press. 1993.

Gordon, Catherine M. *British Paintings of Subjects from the English Novel, 1740–1870*. New York, NY; London: Garland. 1988.

Harvey, Karen. 'Introduction: Historians, Material Culture and Materiality'. In *History and Material Culture: A Student's Guide to Approaching Alternative Sources*. New York, NY; London: Routledge. 2009.

Holloway, Sally. *The Game of Love in Georgian England: Courtship, Emotions and Material Culture*. Oxford: Oxford University Press. 2019.

Jamieson, Anna. '"Comforts in her Calamity": Shopping and Consumption in the Late Eighteenth-Century Madhouse.' *Eighteenth-Century Studies* 55: 2021. 82–102.

Johnstone, Fiona. 'Manifesto for a Visual Medical Humanities'. *Medical Humanities*. 2018. https://blogs.bmj.com/medical-humanities/2018/07/31/manifesto-for-a-visual-medical-humanities/. Accessed 1 April 2022.

Kromm, Jane. 'The Feminization of Madness in Visual Representation'. *Feminist Studies* 20: 1994. 507–535.

Lamb, Susan. 'Applauding Shakespeare's Ophelia in the Eighteenth Century: Sexual Desire, Politics, and the Good Woman'. In *Women as Sites of Culture: Women's Roles in Cultural Formation from the Renaissance to the Twentieth Century*, ed. Susan Shifrin, 105–123. Hampshire: Ashgate Publishing. 2002.

Lamb, Susan. *Bringing Travel Home to England: Tourism, Gender and Imaginative Literature in the Eighteenth Century*. Newark, DE: University of Delaware Press. 2009.

Macalpine, Ida and Richard Hunter. *George III and the Mad-Business*. Allen Lane: The Penguin Press. 1969.

Mason Cox, Joseph. *Practical Observations on Insanity*, 2nd edn. London: C. & R. Baldwin, J. Murray. 1806.

McKendrick, Neil, John Brewer and J. H Plumb, eds. *The Birth of a Consumer Society: The Commercialization of Eighteenth-Century England*. London: Europa Publications Limited. 1982.

Miller, Daniel. *The Comfort of Things*. Cambridge: Polity Press. 2008.

Morison, Alexander. *Outlines of Lectures on the Nature, Causes and Treatment of Insanity*, 4th edn. London. 1848.

Park, Julie. 'The Self and It: Novel Objects'. Stanford, CA: Stanford University Press. 2010.

Perry, Gill. *Spectacular Flirtations: Viewing the Actress in British Art and Theatre, 1768–1820*. New Haven; CT; London: Yale University Press. 2007.

Porter, Roy. 'Love, Sex and Madness in Eighteenth Century England'. *Social Research* 53: 1986. 211–242.

Porter, Roy. *Mind-Forg'd Manacles: A History of Madness in England from the Restoration to the Regency*. London: Athlone Press. 1987.

Rauser, Amelia. *Art in the Age of Undress: Art, Fashion and the Classical Ideal in the 1790s*. New Haven, CT; London: Yale University Press. 2020.

Ritchie, Leslie. *Women writing music in late eighteenth-century England: social harmony in literature and performance.* London; New York, NY: Routledge. 2016.

Showalter, Elaine. 'Victorian Women and Insanity'. *Victorian Studies* 23: 1980. 157–181.

Showalter, Elaine. *The Female Malady: Women, Madness and English Culture, 1830–1980.* London: Virago. 1987.

Small, Helen. *Love's Madness: Medicine, the Novel and Female Insanity, 1800–1865.* Oxford: Clarendon Press. 1996.

Stewart, Susan. *On Longing: Narratives of the Miniature, the Gigantic, the Souvenir, the Collection*. Durham, NC; London: Duke University Press, 1993.

Wilkinson, Sarah. *The tragical history of Miss Jane Arnold, commonly called Crazy Jane and Mr. H. Percival … Founded on Facts.* Stirling. 1820.

Periodicals

Courier
Belle Assemble
Star and Evening Advertiser
Monthly Magazine
Monthly Mirror
Morning Chronicle

Index[1]

[1] Note: Page numbers followed by 'n' refer to notes.

D. Woolley et al. (eds.), *Wearable Objects and Curative Things*, Palgrave Studies in Fashion and the Body,
https://doi.org/10.1007/978-3-031-40017-9